The Drug Expert

A Practical Guide to the Impact of Drug Use in Legal Proceedings

The Drug Expert
A Practical Guide to the Impact of Drug Use in Legal Proceedings

Craig W. Stevens, Ph.D.
Professor of Pharmacology
OSU-Center for Health Sciences
Tulsa, OK, United States

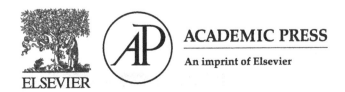

ACADEMIC PRESS

An imprint of Elsevier

Academic Press is an imprint of Elsevier
125 London Wall, London EC2Y 5AS, United Kingdom
525 B Street, Suite 1650, San Diego, CA 92101, United States
50 Hampshire Street, 5th Floor, Cambridge, MA 02139, United States
The Boulevard, Langford Lane, Kidlington, Oxford OX5 1GB, United Kingdom

Notices
Knowledge and best practice in this field are constantly changing. As new research and experience broaden our understanding, changes in research methods, professional practices, or medical treatment may become necessary.

Practitioners and researchers must always rely on their own experience and knowledge in evaluating and using any information, methods, compounds, or experiments described herein. In using such information or methods they should be mindful of their own safety and the safety of others, including parties for whom they have a professional responsibility.

To the fullest extent of the law, neither the Publisher nor the authors, contributors, or editors, assume any liability for any injury and/or damage to persons or property as a matter of products liability, negligence or otherwise, or from any use or operation of any methods, products, instructions, or ideas contained in the material herein.

Library of Congress Cataloging-in-Publication Data
A catalog record for this book is available from the Library of Congress

British Library Cataloguing-in-Publication Data
A catalogue record for this book is available from the British Library

ISBN 978-0-12-800048-9

For information on all Academic Press publications
visit our website at https://www.elsevier.com/books-and-journals

Publisher: Andre Gerharc Wolff
Acquisition Editor: Erin Hill-Parks
Editorial Project Manager: Sam W. Young
Production Project Manager: Joy Christel Neumarin Honest Thangiah
Cover Designer: Christian J. Bilbow

Typeset by SPi Global, India

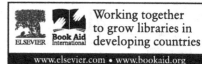
Working together
to grow libraries in
developing countries

www.elsevier.com • www.bookaid.org

Table of Contents

About the Author

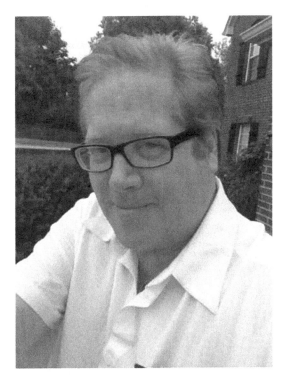

Craig W. Stevens, Ph.D., is a Professor of Pharmacology at OSU-Center for Health Sciences in Tulsa, Oklahoma. Over the past twenty years, he moonlighted as a Drug Expert in more than 85 legal cases. Working for both the defense and the prosecution, and the plaintiff or the defendant, Dr. Stevens provided expert pharmacology consulting in both criminal and civil proceedings. He has testified on drug issues ranging from sedative-hypnotic drug effects in the elderly, the cognitive impact of anticancer agents, and the impact of antiepileptic drugs on criminal behavior, to alcohol abuse and homicide in Native Americans, vehicular manslaughter under the influence of prescription medications, and lethal injection drugs used to carry out the death penalty. For further information on Dr. Stevens and drug issues in the courts see www.drugexpert.org

Preface

Each year I urge the first-year medical students to repeat the mantra "we love drugs" during the intro lecture of the Medical Pharmacology course. Repeating this mantra helps overcome the negative images that the word "drug" or "drugs" conjures up in our brains. The learning process occurs best in a mind unclouded by negative bias, and I want the med students (read "future physicians") to learn as much about drugs, and to remember as many drugs as they can. I admit that students repeating the "we love drugs" mantra is a pedagogic device with unproven efficacy. But most people hear the word "drug" and think of illegal drug use. They imagine someone snorting cocaine, shooting up heroin, or smoking marijuana. Some people may conjure up the image of bars and alcohol, and some fewer yet may think of cigarettes and nicotine. Very few people hear the word "drug" and think of aspirin or Lipitor®. But all medicines are also drugs. Medicines are just drugs with a business plan.

The word "drug" is used by pharmacologists to mean any substance which alters something or some process in a living thing, with humans the living thing for purposes of this book. Drugs are chemicals found in nature or made in a lab. The term "drug" applies to all legal and illegal substances, prescription and nonprescription medicines, and controlled or freely available substances. Drugs may be medicines, herbal remedies, or any form of tobacco or alcohol. Alcohol is a very special drug in society, sometimes listed alongside drugs as if in a different category. Nothing irritates a pharmacologist more than the phrase "drugs and alcohol," as if alcohol is not a drug. Alcohol is an easily abused, widespread used, and extremely dangerous drug. It is a credit to the persuasive powers of the alcohol industry and media that alcohol abuse and obvious intoxication is nefariously embedded in our common culture as a laughable social media event, rather than a serious problem for individuals and society. (Think of the movie *Arthur*, starring Dudley Moore, as the epitome of this "funny" drunk character.) With consistency in drug policy, there would be FDA regulation (after all, it is called the Food *and Drug* Administration) of alcohol, as any other dangerous drug. If that were to happen, then beer and other alcohol drugs might be displayed and sold in the Health & Pharmacy area of major retailers, like all other over-the-counter (OTC) drugs. Perhaps there would even be prescription and nonprescription beer!

The bottom line is that there is a world of drugs that affects our bodies and brain. The drugs that affect the brain cause changes in thought and behavior. Chronic use of drugs causes physical changes in brain structure. These drug-induced changes in thought and behavior often coincide with civil actions and legal offences, which may then be brought to the court by one party or the prosecution. Whether drug use is at the heart of the legal proceedings or is a contributing factor, the impact of the specific drugs in each case needs to be examined by a drug expert.

This book is not a polemic on whether there is too much drug use in our society (there is) but rather an examination of drug use by individuals during actions that lead to legal proceedings. In moonlighting as a consultant with defense law firms and prosecuting attorneys as a "drug expert" (a role more officially known as a Pharmacology Litigation Consultant or Pharmacology Expert Witness) I've had the opportunity to work with a number of attorneys, do drug research, write litigation reports, give depositions, and testify in court. This book was written to convey the crucial pharmacolegal issues that arose from my involvement in over eighty cases, and to provide a guide to other pharmacologists and attorneys in their jobs as expert witnesses or hiring attorneys. Following an introductory chapter examining drug use in our society, real-life cases will be used to provide an initial narrative for each chapter.

Early chapters relay simpler cases and introduce the reader to basic concepts in pharmacology and the legal system. At the same time, practical advice on working as a drug expert and working with a drug expert is incorporated in each chapter. Later chapters highlight more complex issues in pharmacolegal cases, which move the book beyond merely a how-to guide for drug experts and the attorneys who hire them, to a discussion of current drug issues in a legal context. A second thread running through the book is to provide background on common drugs encountered in the court system, which will be useful to law students, attorneys, and pharmacologists, as well as the interested general public. The book ends with a chapter on the drugs used for lethal injection in the prison system. Perhaps in no other arena is the presence of a pharmacologist drug expert so sorely needed.

Each chapter is listed in the table of contents with subheadings to assist with finding a particular drug or pharmacolegal issue. An extensive index is included for searching of specific drugs or legal terms. Appendices provide a list of contact information for pharmacology departments at medical schools across the United States (a sourcebook for hiring attorneys), and numerous samples of documents used and produced by drug experts and the attorneys who hire them.

Finally, a bit of a legal stipulation here. First, just like they say in the old detective movies, the names have been changed to protect the innocent. The narrative section that starts each chapter is a fictionalized account of a real-life case that led to an attorney picking up the phone and engaging a drug expert. Second, no part of this treatise should be taken as legal or medical advice, and any use of the research examples or pharmacolegal strategies presented herein is done solely as an independent act of the reader.

And remember, *we love drugs*.

Craig W. Stevens, Ph.D.

Professor of Pharmacology, OSU-Center for Health Sciences, Tulsa, OK, United States

Acknowledgments

Many thanks to the fine people at Elsevier who helped and encouraged this project from the long-awaited proposal stage to the final production of the book you now hold. I especially appreciate the assistance of Erin Hill-Parks, who encouraged me to develop this project, Sam Young, who managed the project, and Joy Honest Thangiah who brought us to the finish line. A special thanks to Christian Bilbow for the cover design. I thank the editors at Elsevier for their proof-reading and editing of the manuscript, but of course, any errors remaining are all *mea culpa*.

I also recognize the important role that the following attorneys and legal scholars played in the development of my second career as a drug expert: Kurt Arras, Erin Barnhart, David Bean, Eric Berger, Michael Blue, Brian Boeheim, Allen Bohnert, Mark Bonner, Johnny Bruce, Stuart Campbell, David Carpenter, Michael Carr, Seth Caywood, Mark Cooper, Terrill Corley, Jim Craig, Jeff Dasovich, Deborah Denno, Matt Devlin, Roy Dickinson, Jay Dunham, Travis Dunn, Benjamin Faulkner, Robin Feeney, Judith Finn, Ciera Freeman, Marion Fry, Tom Ganem, Patti Ghezzi, Kurt Glassco, Daniel Graves, Matthew Haire, Catherine Hammarsten, Martin Hart, Steve Horton, Derek Ingle, Jim Jennings, Mike Jones, Linda Kaufmann, Marty Keach, Courtney Kelly, Paul Kolker, Robin Konrad, Montgomery Lair, Tony Laizure, Karen Langdon, Josh Lee, Randy Long, Linda Lye, Randy Lynn, Shannon McMurray, Andrea Medley, Jason Messenger, James Milton, Mark Mitchell, Steve Modovsky, Stan Monroe, Pansy Moore-Shrier, Jan Moreno, Thomas Mortensen, Robert Murdock, Mark Myles, Kevin Nedwick, Margaret Nicholson, Rob Nigh, Elizabeth Oglesby, Matthew Ottoway, Kirsten Palfreyman, Dustin Phillips, Larry Pinkerton, Katie Polonksy, Trevor Reynolds, Larry Roberson, Gene Robinson, Robert Rode, Adam Rusnak, Jay Self, Richard Shallcross, Allen Smallwood, Jeff Smith, Daryl Sohn, Derrick Teague, Richard Tennent, Curtis Thomas, Haylie Treas, Scott Troy, Jerry Truster, David Van Meter, Jason Waddell, Emily Washington, Bradley West, Aarin Williams, John Williams, Justin Williams, Rene Williams, Rob Williams, Brian Wood, Nadia Wood, Carol Wright, and John Zelbst. A special acknowledgment goes to Rabon Martin, one of the most interesting lawyers I've had the pleasure to work with, who passed away from this world all too soon. His dedication to providing legal services to the underserved and indigent population was admirable.

Much appreciation goes to the past and present Deans, Associate Deans, and Department Chairs at Oklahoma State University, Center for Health Sciences and the College of Osteopathic Medicine in Tulsa, Oklahoma. I enjoy a successful career as a Professor of Pharmacology and an exciting second career as a Drug Expert due to their unfettered encouragement and support.

Finally, I thank my parents, for their early instilment of books and a love of knowledge, and my five children and their mates for their constant source of laughter and joy. I want to especially acknowledge the unending devotion of my wife, the *real doctor*, which makes it all worth it. Her love is the ultimate drug. This book is dedicated to her.

Craig W. Stevens, Ph.D.

Professor of Pharmacology, OSU-Center for Health Sciences, Tulsa, OK, United States

Chapter 1

What a Long Strange Trip It's Been: Our drugged society

Drug Use by Americans—Drugs and Mental Illness—Drugs and Crimes

Drug Effects on Brain and Behavior—Drug Use and the Legal System

We live in a drugged society. There are drugs all around us and inside us. In the last 40 years we've witnessed the meteoric rise of the medical-pharmaceutical complex. Drug companies made more drugs. Physicians prescribed more drugs. Patients took more drugs.[1] Witness the emergence of "celebrity" drugs; those drugs marketed so well and used by so many that they achieve widespread name recognition, like Lipitor®, Ambien®, and Viagra®.

The growth in the mass media marketing of prescription drugs began when the Food and Drug Administration (FDA) clarified its rules on drug advertising in 1997.[2] This government action gave the green light for Big Pharma to launch highly successful direct-to-consumer TV commercials and magazine ad campaigns. It is now commonplace for Viagra® or Cialis® commercials appear when families are gathered around the TV, giving rise to the unique juxtaposition of erectile dysfunction and grandma in the room. There is the veterinary drug market with numerous canine and feline versions of human-approved drugs.[3] This includes many canine psychotherapeutic drugs, like antidepressants and antianxiety drugs, commonly called "doggie downers." The picture comes to mind of an overmedicated American man walking an overmedicated dog, stopping a little too long at each fire hydrant.

This introductory chapter will present recent data on overall drug use in America, drugs and mental illness, the linkage between drugs and crime, and the effects of drugs on brain and behavior. The chapter ends with an overview of the pharmacolegal issues of drug use and an introduction to the increasing role of the drug expert in legal matters. Chapters following this introductory text provide guidance to pharmacologists and attorneys working to incorporate testimony by drug experts into the court record and highlight actual pharmacolegal issues from real-life, drug expert cases. The final chapter of the book outlines the pharmacology of lethal injection, a sordid tale of clinical drugs misused for the lethal injection of condemned inmates. The involvement of the author in lethal injection litigation on behalf of the State and the inmates is the foundation for this closing chapter.

Drug Use by Americans

Americans love drugs. It is probable that the reader has at least one drug in his or her body at this very moment. Most likely it is caffeine, a brain stimulant, delivered in a convenient dosing form such as a cup of coffee, or tea, or an energy drink or soda pop. Eighty percent of the America's population voluntarily use caffeine daily, many others unknowingly ingest caffeine in their diets.[4] Or perhaps you have the stimulant nicotine in your blood, efficiently delivered by numerous devices ranging from a hand-rolled cigarette to a rechargeable electronic cigarette (e-cig), or chewing tobacco, or chewing gum (Nicorette®). Maybe you have a medical condition, like chronic pain, or diabetes, or hypertension, or all three, and take drugs as prescribed by your physician. Most of the drugs used to treat these chronic conditions remain in your bloodstream around the clock, 24-7. Or you have a headache and recently took ibuprofen (Advil®) or acetaminophen (Tylenol®) which remains in your system for the rest of the day. Some of you may have gone to a bar last night, leaving remnants of ethanol in your blood from having one,

---

[1] Kantor ED et al. (2015). Trends in prescription drug use among adults in the United States from 1999–2012. JAMA 314: 1818–1830.

[2] Weinmeyer R (2013) Direct-to-consumer advertising of drugs. AMA J. Ethics 15:954–959.

[3] Beyene B, Tesega B (2014) Rational veterinary drug use: Its significance in public health. J. Vet. Med. Anim. Health 6:302–8.

[4] Hodge JG, Scanlon M (2010) The consumable vice: caffeine, public health, and the law. J. Contemp. Health Law Policy 27:76–119. This article is a real eye-opener in describing the number of food and beverages gratuitously supplemented with caffeine and the insidious nature of caffeine in our daily lives.

The Drug Expert. https://doi.org/10.1016/B978-0-12-800048-9.00001-8

or two, or three drinks too many. Readers in Colorado, Washington state, or practically everywhere, may have smoked marijuana earlier today or in the last day or two.[5] Your pothead bodies contain the active ingredient of marijuana, tetrahydrocannabinol (THC), sequestered in fat cells and being slowly released back into the bloodstream, metabolized by the liver, and excreted out in the urine. A few of you are chipping away on illegal drugs like cocaine or methamphetamine, leaving long-lasting metabolites detectable in your bloodstream and urine. A larger number of you are abusing prescription drugs, not taken under any doctor's orders, and obtained illegally from a "friend" or relative or a dealer or someone else's medicine cabinet. These legal drugs used illegally leave the tell-tale signs of the parent drug molecules or drug metabolites in your bloodstream as well.

The following first section presents the results of new research studies, and industry and government reports that detail the use of drugs in America. The overall thrust of this section is to show that all kinds of different drugs are used at inordinately high frequencies and among an unusually large number of people in America. The focus in this section is on four sectors of societal drug use, namely, prescription drugs, nonprescription drugs, alcohol, and illegal drugs.

Prescription drug use

No other country in the world comes close to the United States in the volume of drug consumption. Americans are the number one among all peoples, cultures, and countries in drug use per capita, measured as drug consumption per person, for both legal and illegal drug substances.[6] The Kaiser Family Foundation reports that for the year 2018, the total number of prescriptions filled at retail pharmacies across the United States was 3,787,398,033.[7] Divide this number into the estimated U.S. population in 2018[8] (327,167,434) and you get 11.6 prescriptions per capita. That is enough prescriptions written for each newborn, child, and adult in the United States to get a prescription drug filled each month for about a year.

In the United States, retail sales of prescription drugs in the year 2018 brought in a total of $378 billion and some change.[9] With about 3.78 billion prescriptions filled, we get an average prescription price of about $100, which seems a little high, but may represent the skewing of the price curve by newer, higher-priced medications.[10] Additionally, with health insurance or Medicare paying for some or all of the cost of our medicine, and various levels of co-pays contributed by the consumer, we really have no idea of the true price of each prescription filled. Retail prescription drugs are subsidized products, made cheaper to the consumer by third-party health insurance or government subsidies. The profits from the $378 billion in sales of prescription drugs are divvied up between the retailer/wholesaler, like Walgreens[11] or CVS Health, and drug companies, like Pfizer. Headquartered in New York City, Pfizer is one of the world's most profitable pharmaceuticals firm with revenues of $53.6 billion dollars in 2018.[12]

While the numbers of prescription drugs filled in the United States is enough for everyone to get one prescription filled each month, a recent study by the Mayo Clinic gives us an idea of who is getting all these prescriptions filled, and what types of prescription drugs are taken.[13] Using nearly all men, women, and children residing in a single county in Minnesota, the Mayo researchers were able to examine the electronic prescription records of 142,377 people. This is such a large sample size that, to a first approximation, the conclusions of the study have general validity for the whole nation. Nearly 7 out of 10 people were prescribed at least one drug in the year 2009. It is no wonder that the pharmaceutical industry is called "Big Pharma" with 70% of Americans buying and using their products. Even more telling, about half of these drug users were prescribed two or more drugs, and another fifth are taking as many as five or more prescription drugs. Overall, women and the elderly received more prescriptions than males and other age groups.

As expected, the most commonly prescribed class of drugs was antibiotics, with 17% of the population written a script for a Z-Pak® or another antibiotic. The second-most common type of drugs were antidepressants, like Prozac® and Zooloft®,

---

5 Marijuana, also spelled marihuana in legal contexts, has an extremely long elimination time from the body. See Cary PL (2005) The marijuana detection window: determining the length of time cannabinoids will remain detectable in urine following smoking. National Drug Court Institute, Drug Court Rev. 5:23–58.

6 United Nations Office of Drug Control, World Drug Report 2010 at *www.unodc.org/unodc/data-and-analysis/WDR-2010.html*.

7 Kaiser Family Foundation report (2015) Total number of retail prescription drugs filled at pharmacies. IMS Health Incorporated Special Data Request at *kff.org/other/state-indicator/total-retail-rx-drugs*.

8 USA Census population on December 31, 2017 from *www.census.gov*.

9 Kaiser Family Foundation report (2015) Total retail sales for prescription drugs filled at pharmacies. IMS Health Incorporated Special Data Request (*kff.org/other/state-indicator/total-sales-for-retail-rx-drugs*).

10 The average price of a filled prescriptions increased $65 in 2014 to $100 per prescription in 2018.

11 Walgreens is the number one drugstore chain in the USA, and with the recent acquisition of the UK's Boots chain, is the largest drugstore chain in the world. In accord with its number one status, Walgreens paid the largest fine to date of $80 million to the United States Drug Enforcement Agency (DEA) for improper distribution and dispensing of the opioid controlled substances hydrocodone and oxycodone. From "Walgreens Agrees to Pay a Record Settlement of $80 Million for Civil Penalties under the Controlled Substances" DEA Press Release Number 954-660-4602, June 11, 2013.

12 Pfizer 2018 annual statement at: *https://s21.q4cdn.com/317678438/files/doc_financials/Quarterly/2018/q4/Q4-2018-PFE-Earnings-Release.pdf*.

13 Zhong W et al. (2013) Age and sex patterns of drug prescribing in a defined American population. Mayo Clinic Proceed. 88:697–707.

prescribed to 13% of the population. The third most common drug class prescribed to 12% of the population was opioid analgesics (painkillers), with the well-known examples being hydrocodone (in Lortab® and Vicodin®) and oxycodone (OxyContin®).

Americans love all drugs but they really, truly love opioid drugs. This love has gotten totally out of hand, with Americans consuming 80% of the global opioid drug supply while making up only about 5% of the world's population.[14] Focusing on the opioid analgesic drug, hydrocodone, we use and abuse hydrocodone to such an extent that 99% of the global hydrocodone supply is consumed by Americans (5% of the world population). That is enough hydrocodone so that every adult in America could be medicated with the standard dose of hydrocodone every 4h for 1 month.[15]

Prescription opioids are analgesic drugs, used to treat moderate to severe pain.[16] Opioids are abused for their euphoric effects, targeting the same brain receptors as heroin. Unfortunately, opioid analgesics are extremely dangerous drugs that can easily lead to addiction and death from respiratory depression. Unintentional death from prescription opioids is at epidemic levels, far outnumbering the combined death toll from heroin and cocaine overdose deaths.[17] The deaths of celebrities Heath Ledger, Philip Seymour Hoffman, Prince, and Whitney Houston are just four of the overdose deaths attributed to prescription opioid abuse in recent years. In spite of all the public information and media coverage of prescription opioid abuse and overdose death, some physicians prescribe opioids to their patients without full realization of the dangers of opioid addiction and overdose. We will see a civil case later in the book where death from prescription opioid overdose led to a physician charged with improper prescribing practices and medical negligence. Other types of drugs that are prescribed to millions of Americans include sleep medications, like Ambien®, and antianxiety agents, like Xanax®. In the chapters ahead, the use of legal prescription drugs, including antidepressants, opioid analgesics, sleep medications, antianxiety drugs, antiseizure agents, and others, will be examined in the context of civil and criminal proceedings.

Nonprescription drug use

There are two types of pharmaceutical drugs available in the United States and most countries: prescription drugs and nonprescription or over-the-counter (OTC) drugs. Prescription drugs require a physician's written, FAXed, or computer-transmitted prescription (e-script) written for a particular individual. Nonprescription or OTC drugs don't require a doctor's prescription and are widely available to all individuals in drugstores, grocery stores, mass merchandizers (like Walmart or Target), gas stations, and convenience stores. In the United States, both prescription and nonprescription drugs are approved and regulated by the FDA.

Some OTC drugs, like celebrity or blockbuster prescription drugs, are household names. Most people are familiar with the trade names of Advil®, Nyquil®, Robitussin DM®, Mucinex®, and Tylenol®.[18] Nonprescription or OTC drugs are sold in numerous formulations and products that present the buyer with a dizzying array of choices, much like going down the breakfast cereal aisle in the supermarket. In the popular OTC pain reliever category, the neighborhood Walgreens store carries 70 aspirin-containing products and 198 nonaspirin drug products.[19] There are 204 OTC drug products in the adult cold and cough medicine category. Many of these cold and flu products contain mixtures of various drugs including nonopioid pain relievers, cough suppressants, decongestants, and antihistamines. OTC combination medicines increase total drug exposure compared with prescription drugs, which are mostly single drug products. For example, the combination OTC product, Nyquil® Severe Cold & Flu Nighttime Relief®, contains four active ingredients: acetaminophen, for pain and fever; dextromethorphan, for cough suppression; doxylamine, an antihistamine; and phenylephrine, a decongestant.

Many nonprescription or OTC drugs started off as prescription drugs. When a drug is available as an OTC medicine, it was usually approved and marketed as a prescription medicine first.[20] After years or decades on the prescription drug market, prescription drugs with a good safety profile may be switched to OTC status by the drug company working with the FDA to gain approval. Even though the OTC drug market as a whole is <10% of the prescription drug markets, an "Rx-to-OTC switch" can mitigate declining sales due to a generic competitor and extend the life cycle of a drug.[21] The FDA

[14] Manchikanti L, Singh A (2008) Therapeutic opioids: a ten-year perspective on the complexities and complications of the escalating use, abuse, and nonmedical use of opioids. Pain Physician 11:S63–S88.

[15] Centers for Disease Control (2011) Vital signs: overdoses of prescription opioid pain relievers-United States, 1999–2008. MMWR 60:1487–92.

[16] Brenner GM, Stevens CW (2013) Pharmacology, 4th Ed. Saunders/Elsevier, Philadelphia/London.

[17] Volkow ND et al. (2014) Medication-assisted therapies-tackling the opioid-overdose epidemic. New Engl. J. Med. 370:2063–66.

[18] In September, 1982, seven people took cyanide-laced Tylenol® in Chicago and died. This triggered a national scare resulting in stores nationwide to pull Tylenol® from their shelves. The person who tampered with the Tylenol® bottles and laced pills with cyanide was never apprehended. As it was this crime that led to tamper-proof packaging and tamper-proof laws, we can all thank the unknown perpetrator for the difficulty we have now opening almost anything, like medicine bottles, food packages, and drinks. See Bartz S (2012) The Tylenol Mafia: Marketing, Murder, and Johnson & Johnson. CreateSpace Amazon Publishers.

[19] From an online search of the closest Walgreens to my office, filtered by products actually in stock at the store.

[20] Cohen J et al. (2013) Assessing the economic impact of Rx-to-OTC switches: systematic review and guidelines for future development. Med. Econ. 16:835–44.

[21] Mahecha LA (2006) Rx-to-OTC switches: trends and factors underlying success. Nat. Rev. Drug Discov. 5:380–5.

reviews the safety data and proposed OTC drug labeling and if all goes well, there quickly appears a new, heavily advertised box or bottle in the pharmacy section. Some drugs remain marketed as both prescription drugs and nonprescription drugs, with the OTC version of the drug available in a different formulation or with a lowered dosage strength. The movement of drugs from prescription-only to nonprescription OTC drugs is a continual process, with monthly announcements by the FDA of the drugs making this switch on the FDA website.

Americans love taking drugs that they can buy without a prescription more than drugs that need a prescription. Whereas the Mayo study before showed that 70% of the population had at least one prescription filled in a year, a 2012 report from the Consumer Healthcare Products Association found that 81% of the American population bought at least one OTC drug product in a year.[22] Retail sales of OTC drug products reached about $34 billion in 2017.[23] Although the OTC drug market is more fragmented than the prescription drug market, many of the OTC branded products are from drug companies which are owned by a Big Pharma company. Case in point, NyQuil® is branded as a Vicks® product, from the original Vick Chemical Company established in 1809, and later acquired by Proctor and Gamble in 1985.[24]

Like prescription drugs, many nonprescription OTC drugs are abused and taken for nonmedical purposes, that is, to get high. OTC drug abuse is easier, and easier on the wallet, than abusing prescription drugs. Additionally, it is not a crime to possess Benadryl® tablets or Robitussin DM® cough syrup or any OTC drug. There is no need to go to the doctor and get a prescription for an OTC drug. Anyone, including teenagers and children, can buy OTC drugs which are widely available in almost any type of store or gas station. As a result, there is a great deal of OTC drug abuse in America, especially among the youth and adolescent.[25] The next chapter introduces our first drug expert case, which centers on abuse of an OTC drug product containing an antihistamine. Excessive doses of this antihistamine-containing product were taken by a teenager who survived the drug doses, but because of the psychotic effect of the OTC medication did not make it through the night.

Alcohol use

Alcohol remains the true "over-the-counter" drug. In some cases, especially when purchasing the pocket-sized half-pints kept behind the cashier, alcohol is literally passed *over the counter* to the customer. Most OTC drugs today are not actually passed "over-the-counter" but thrown into a shopping basket by the consumer directly off the shelf in the supermarket or drugstore. The "over-the-counter" term for nonprescription drugs is from the early days when there were no prescription-only medications and all drugs were passed over the pharmacist's counter.

The active ingredient in all alcoholic beverages is ethanol. Ethanol is a simple molecule, with only two carbon backbone atoms. It is the excretion product of yeast, which is actually a type of microorganism in the fungus Kingdom. Ethanol is produced by fermentation. Fermentation is the biological process in yeast and other microorganisms whereby sugars are converted into energy for the yeast cell. The yeast cells then release ethanol and carbon dioxide as metabolic waste product. Essentially, ethanol is yeast piss.[26]

"Alcohol and drugs" is a common phrase that makes a drug expert cringe. Alcohol is a drug; there is no way around it. But historically, alcohol got mixed up with prohibition and *La Cosa Nostra*, and ended up being regulated by a federal agency called the Bureau of Alcohol, Tobacco, Firearms and Explosives, known commonly as the ATF, housed in the Department of Justice. The ATF's mission with regard to alcohol is to reduce smuggling and trafficking activity, decreasing funds derived from illegal alcohol trafficking available to criminal and terrorist organizations, and significantly reduce alcohol tax revenue losses to the States.[27] Since January 1, 2003, the Alcohol and Tobacco Tax and Trade Bureau in the Department of the Treasury became responsible for regulating the alcohol and tobacco industries, removing the tax and industry regulation burden from the ATF. Now, alcohol production, importation, wholesale distribution, advertising, and labeling is regulated by the Alcohol and Tobacco Tax and Trade Bureau.

Alcohol remains the only legal and most commonly used drug in the United States that is not regulated as a drug. Perhaps following the path of tobacco regulation, alcohol will become a drug by new laws, and included under FDA

---

[22] Consumer Healthcare Products Association (2015) The Value of OTC Medicine to the United States. 2014 White Paper, CHPA. Available at *www.chpa.org*.

[23] Consumer Healthcare Products Association (2015) Retail sales of OTC medicines at *www.chpa.org*.

[24] The Vick Chemical Company was established in 1809 and its most famous product, Vick's VapoRub®, saw sales increase from $900 million to $3 billion in 1918, the year of the deadly Spanish flu epidemic in America. University of North Carolina, Louis Round Wilson Special Collect. Library, Richardson-Vicks, Inc., 1885–1995.

[25] Conca AJ, Worthen DR (2012) Nonprescription drug abuse. J. Pharm. Pract. 25:13–21.

[26] We will skip the obvious scatological analogy of the release of the carbon dioxide gas in yeast cells.

[27] ATF website at *www.atf.gov/content/alcohol-and-tobacco*.

regulation.[28] Or maybe there will be a legal recognition of alcohol as a food, or more specifically a beverage. After all, alcoholic beverages are nothing but fermented forms of foodstuffs that can be taken in their original forms; it is grape juice that becomes wine, grain slurries that transform into beer, and molasses that turns to rum. But alcohol is not a food, although some people seem to live on beer. If alcohol was a food it would already be regulated by the Food and Drug Administration, the FDA. Neither is alcohol an illegal drug like heroin, but alcohol has exceedingly more detrimental effects on society than all illegal drugs combined.[29] So because alcohol is not regulated like legal drugs by the FDA, and alcohol is not an illegal drug like heroin and hounded by the DEA, there is some credence to using the phrase "drugs and alcohol." Alcohol is a different "drug" than any other drug in our society. This does not mean that our repugnant view of the phrase "drugs and alcohol" is relaxing, just that alcohol is a very *special* nondrug drug.

The contribution of alcohol to our drugged society cannot be overstated. As a single agent, ethanol is the number one legal drug used and abused by Americans. Slightly more than half (52.2%) of Americans age 12 or older report regular use of alcohol, with about half of those reporting "binge" drinking in the last month.[30] In comparison, the number one illegal drug, marijuana, is used regularly by about 7.5% of the American population that are 12 or older. More people using alcohol does not mean that alcohol is more addicting than marijuana, although it may be. It's just that alcohol products are so widely available, heavily advertised, and socially acceptable. If the trend continues toward state and perhaps federal legalization of marijuana, it is possible that the number of marijuana users would increase and approach the level of alcohol users.

The volume of beer, wine, and liquor sold in 2016 was enough for every man, woman, and child in America to consume 2.35 gallons of pure ethanol (200 proof alcohol).[31] The alcoholic beverage industry in the United States drank in about $234 billion in retail sales in 2017.[32] In comparison, prescription drugs bring in retail sales of $378 billion a year, and nonprescription or OTC drugs ring up $34 billion in sales.

Tobacco use delivers nicotine to the brain. Nicotine is a stimulant drug that acts on the brain and is addictive, but may be more addictive when delivered in the form of tobacco than by itself.[33] However, nicotine effects on brain and behavior are mild and not associated with major changes in behavior or psychomotor effects. Nicotine, for example, does not affect one's ability to drive a motor vehicle. No legal cases are found where being under the influence of nicotine is linked to criminal or civil proceedings. Yet nicotine in tobacco products is a common legal drug that in 2012 was currently used by 27.3% of all Americans aged 18 or older.[34] The U.S. tobacco industry had sales of nearly $96 billion in 2010.[35] So while tobacco drug use is the leading cause of preventable death in the United States, killing more than 480,000 people annually,[36] tobacco use per se does not impact the legal system directly as do other drugs. In contrast, alcohol use has a tremendous impact on criminal and civil proceedings. There are three examples in this book where different aspects of alcohol use were factors in civil or criminal cases.

Illegal drug use

The use of illegal drugs by individuals occurs in every society that has illegal drugs. The legality of a drug, whether as a medicine or socially used drug, is entirely dependent on where the drug user is located. For example, a marijuana user that takes one step in any direction from the iconic Four Corners Memorial at the southwestern corner of Colorado changes the legal status of the marijuana joint in the user's pocket. One step northwest, into Utah, or one

---

[28] After more than a decade of wrangling in Congress, including the infamous denial by the heads of the tobacco industry before the Senate that nicotine was not an addictive drug, the Family Smoking Prevention and Tobacco Control Act was signed into law by President Obama in 2009 and gave the FDA authority to regulate the manufacture, distribution, and marketing of tobacco products to protect public health. However, enactment of some sections is still being fought by the tobacco industry. For example, graphic warnings on cigarette packs were found unconstitutional by the DC Circuit Court. See Husten CG, Deyton LR (2013) Understanding the tobacco control act. Lancet 381:1570–1580.

[29] Rehm J et al. (2011) Global burden of disease and injury and economic cost attributable to alcohol use and alcohol-use disorders. Lancet 373:2223–33.

[30] Substance Abuse and Mental Health Services Administration (2015) Results from the 2013 National Survey on Drug Use and Health: summary of national findings. Rockville, MD, at *www.samhsa.gov*.

[31] Haughwout SP et al. (2018) Apparent per capita alcohol consumption: national, state, and regional trends, 1977–2016. National Institute on Alcohol Abuse and Alcoholism Division of Epidemiology and Prevention Research Alcohol Epidemiologic Data System.

[32] *https://www.statista.com/topics/1709/alcoholic-beverages/*.

[33] There are numerous other chemicals in burning tobacco that appear to modulate the addictiveness of nicotine, at least in rats. This may be an argument in favor of e-cigarettes which only deliver nicotine vapor and not the vast array of other tobacco chemicals. See Hall BJ et al. (2014) Differential effects of non-nicotine tobacco constituent compounds on nicotine self-administration in rats. Pharmacol. Biochem. Behav. 120:103–108.

[34] Surgeon General's Report (2014) The Health Consequences of Smoking-Fifty Years of Progress, U.S. Department of Health and Human Services. Figure represents total tobacco use including cigarettes, smokeless tobacco (i.e., chewing tobacco or snuff), cigars, or pipe tobacco. Missing from this data is the large and growing number of e-cig, or "vape" users.

[35] Reportlinker (2014) Tobacco industry market research and statistics. *reportlinker.com/ci02053/Tobacco.html*.

[36] Surgeon General's Report (2014) *op. cit.*

step southwest into Arizona, or southeast into New Mexico, and the user is committing a state crime in possessing that particular plant product. One step back to the "Rocky Mountain High" state and the marijuana joint is legal again, at least according to state law. The feds, in the form of DEA agents, could arrest anyone in the United States, in any state, for marijuana possession as it remains a Schedule I Controlled Substance under Federal Law. Federal Drug Law trumps state drug law.[37] Taking a broader worldview, federal and state laws in the United States allow the unabated use of alcohol. Hop a flight to Saudi Arabia and one arrives in a country where alcohol is illegal, with draconian punishment for its sale and use. The punishment for getting caught for alcohol offenses in Saudi Arabia is a public whipping.[38] Like in the real estate business, when it comes to drug use and drug laws, it's all about location, location, location.

When the location is America, bring your party hat. Recent studies by the World Health Organization (WHO) show that Americans have the highest incidence of lifetime use of cocaine and marijuana, compared to seventeen countries around the world.[39] Americans were also among the top users of tobacco. The 17 countries in the study were Colombia, Mexico, United States, Belgium, France, Germany, Italy, Netherlands, Spain, Ukraine, Israel, Lebanon, Nigeria, South Africa, Japan, People's Republic of China, and New Zealand. According to the Office of National Drug Control Policy, Americans spend more than any other country on illicit drugs, buying more than 100 billion dollars' worth of cocaine, marijuana, heroin, and methamphetamine annually.[40] The biggest illegal drug marketplace in the world is on the streets of America.

The illegal use of drugs in America over the last five decades followed the availability and development of specific drugs and formulations. As shown in Table 1.1, each decade is noted for a particular illicit drug in vogue during that decade. The first wave of baby-boomers in the 1960s that rocked the boat were the hippies, fueled by an illegal drug diet of marijuana and LSD. The 1970s saw the return of opioid-addicted Vietnam vets who first tasted the rich heroin produced in

TABLE 1.1 Trends in illegal drug use in the United States over last five decades.

Decade	Trending illegal drugs	Cultural characterizations
1960s	Marijuana, LSD	The hippie movement, the psychedelic age
1970s	Heroin	The Golden Triangle, the veteran addict
1980s	Powder cocaine	The disco culture, the rise of the cocaine cartels
1990s	Crack cocaine	The crack epidemic, the inner-city crisis
2000s	Methamphetamine	The home-cooker, the scourge of rural America
2010s	Emerging drugs of abuse,[a] K2, "Spice," other synthetic cannabinoids, "bath salts" "flakka"	Emerging drugs of abuse, the rise of the synthetic drugs

[a] *K2, or "Spice" contain mixtures of cannabinoid substances that are synthetic analogs of the natural cannabinoid and active ingredient of marijuana, THC. These synthetic cannabinoids are more dangerous and lead to greater ER admissions than natural marijuana use. Other emerging drugs of abuse include "bath salts," a family of drugs containing one or more synthetic chemicals related to cathinone, an amphetamine-like stimulant found naturally in the Khat plant; "Krokodil," a synthetic form of a heroin-like drug called desomorphine, made by combining codeine tablets with various toxic chemicals including lighter fluid, gasoline, and industrial solvents; "N-bomb," refers to synthetic hallucinogens that are being sold as legal substitutes for LSD or mescaline; "Syrup," prescription-strength cough syrup containing codeine and promethazine mixed with soda, and "Flakka," a synthetic stimulant alpha-pyrrolidinopentiophenone (α-PVP).*

---

[37] There are 23 states where medical marijuana is legal (Arizona, Arkansas, Connecticut, Delaware, Florida, Hawaii, Illinois, Louisiana, Maryland, Minnesota, Missouri, Montana, New Hampshire, New Jersey, New Mexico, New York, North Dakota, Ohio, Oklahoma, Pennsylvania, Rhode Island, Utah, West Virginia) and 9 states and a district with legalized recreational marijuana (Alaska, California, Colorado, Maine, Massachusetts, Michigan, Nevada, Oregon, Vermont, and Washington DC). The Supreme Court decision in *Gonzales v. Raich,* used the Commerce Clause of the United States Constitution to determine that the feds may criminally prosecute the production and use of home-grown marijuana even in states with approved medical marijuana use. *Gonzales v. Raich (previously Ashcroft v. Raich), 545 U.S. 1 (2005).*

[38] Public whipping or *flogging,* done by lashes with a stiff cane against the buttocks, causes severe injury. See Iakobishvili E (2011) Inflicting Harm: Judicial corporal punishment for drug and alcohol offences in selected countries. Report from the International Harm Reduction Association.

[39] Degenhardt L et al. (2008) Toward a global view of alcohol, tobacco, cannabis, and cocaine use: findings from the WHO World Mental Health Surveys. PLoS Med. 5:e141.

[40] Office of National Drug Control Policy (2014) What America's Users Spend on Illegal Drugs: 2000–2010.

the Golden Triangle.[41] In the 1980s there was the disco craze, powered by powder cocaine. The 1990s saw the full bloom of the crack cocaine epidemic, a cheaper, smokable form of cocaine. The new millennium and following decade swelled with the internet-enabled manufacture of methamphetamine. The decade of the 2010s, so far, looks like the decade of the synthetic and designer drugs.

Overall illegal drug use in America increased between 2008 and 2014 according to the national survey conducted by the Substance Abuse and Mental Health Services Administration, SAMHSA.[42] Their *National Survey on Drug Use and Health* reported that 24.6 million Americans 12 or older were current illicit drug users (past month use), equal to 9.4% of the total population, or about 1 person in 10.[43]

Marijuana is the number one illicit drug. Of the 9.4% of the population currently using illicit drugs, marijuana use makes up about 80% of illicit drug use. The number two class of illicit drugs is prescription drugs that are used for non-medical reasons or diverted from the intended recipient. These nonmedical prescription drugs are mostly opioid analgesics that are fueling the current opioid overdose epidemic. People abusing prescription drugs make up about 30% of illicit drug use. About 7% of illicit drug use is due to cocaine, and 5% due to the use of hallucinogens, like LSD or MDMA ("X" or "Ecstasy"). About 2% of drug abusers use methamphetamine and only about 1% of current illicit drug use is due to heroin use. The percentages add up to more than 100% due to multiple illicit drug use by the same person. As mentioned before, illicit drug users in the United States spend about $100 billion annually on cocaine, heroin, marijuana, and methamphetamine.

One remedy to the large illicit drug problem is to legalize illegal drugs and therefore make them legal drugs. Countries, states, or localities which do this will see a tremendous drop of illegal drug use. For example, we can be sure that the states of Colorado and Washington saw a tremendous drop in the illegal use of marijuana since January 1, 2014, when recreational use of marijuana was made legal in those two states. This is not simply a facetious attempt at wordplay, but to stress that legalization remains a debatable option for drug laws in this country. Many European countries decriminalized "soft" drugs like cannabis (marijuana) while "hard" drugs like cocaine and heroin are fully prosecuted. The Netherlands and the infamous "coffee shops" of Amsterdam come to mind. In Portugal, illegal drug use with simple possession brings an offender directly into a treatment system, bypassing any criminal proceeding altogether.[44]

Drugs and Mental Illness

It is clear that many Americans take drugs illegally to self-treat their own brand of mental illness. A whopping 70% of drug abusers have comorbidity of mental illness, specifically anxiety and mood disorders.[45] Conversely, 63% of people diagnosed with general anxiety disorder and 54% of those diagnosed with major depression abuse drugs.[46] This means that many people abusing drugs may not do so if properly treated for mental disorders. One of the factors of the "Perfect Drug-Storm" that gives us an astronomical level of drug use in America is the lack of a decent mental health care system. For many years, treatment of mental illness was not covered adequately or at all by insurers, although improved mental health coverage is mandated under the Affordable Care Act of 2010, known either affectionately or derisively depending on your political party as *Obamacare*. Ideally, mentally ill individuals in our society would be diagnosed and treated with behavioral or cognitive therapy and one or more of the commonly used psychotropic drugs, and go on their merry way. Unfortunately, due to many factors beyond the scope of this book, this is not the case. But one reason for the suboptimal treatment of the mentally ill is the social stigma attached to mental illness. Because mental illness is a dysfunction of the brain, the traditional seat of the "soul" and the misunderstood organ of "free will," illnesses of the brain carry with them all

---

[41] The Golden Triangle is one of Asia's two main opium-producing and heroin-processing areas. It is an area that includes the mountain fields of Myanmar, Laos and Thailand in Southeast Asia. The Golden Triangle has been one of the most extensive poppy cultivation areas of the world since the middle of the last century. In the early 21st century, Afghanistan became the world's largest poppy cultivator. This area is called the Golden Crescent. See Talpur A, George TP (2014) A review of drug policy in the Golden Crescent: towards the development of more effective solutions. Asian J Psychiatry 12:31–35.

[42] This is the latest data available: Substance Abuse and Mental Health Services Administration (2014) Results from the 2013 National Survey on Drug Use and Health: Summary of National Findings, U.S. Department of Health and Human Services. At: *www.samhsa.gov/atod*.

[43] To bring these numbers home, I often think of my medical school class which has about 100 students per year. As I look upon this group, I can imagine 10 of them currently using illicit drugs. If one thinks of heavily peopled places, like Grand Central Station in New York, it is easy to imagine hundreds of illicit drug users swirling around in a seething morass of humanity.

[44] Gonçalves R et al. (2015) A social cost perspective in the wake of the Portuguese strategy for the fight against drugs. Int J Drug Policy 26:199–209.

[45] Hartwell KJ et al. (2009) Biologic commonalities between mental illness and addiction. Prim. Psychiatry 16:33–39.

[46] Blanco C et al. (2014) The latent structure and comorbidity patterns of generalized anxiety disorder and major depressive disorder: a national study. Depress. Anxiety 31:214–222.

sorts of cultural baggage. From the crazy caveman cast out from the tribe, to the homeless schizophrenic babbling in Times Square, people with diseases of the brain that effect outward behavior are given a leprous distance.[47] Only about 10% of the people in this country that need treatment for drug abuse receive any treatment[48] and less than half of Americans with mental illness receive any treatment.[49] Americans are also the number one country in the world for mental illness. In a WHO Mental Health Report, the prevalence of any psychiatric disorder in the past year was the highest in the United States, at 26.4% of the adult population.[50]

Self-medication for anxiety

Anxiety disorders have the highest prevalence of all mental disorders in America, with a lifetime prevalence of 31% of U.S. adult population reporting an anxiety disorder. In any one year, 18% of the adult population is suffering from an anxiety disorder.[51] As we will see in a following section explaining the actions of drugs on the brain, the neurons in the brain at baseline are revved up and ready to go. This general tonus of an excitatory state is kept in check by a large cadre of smaller inhibitory neurons. In anxiety disorders, one of the problems is a lack of inhibitory neuron activity or a genetic deficiency in these neurons so that the excitatory neurons run unopposed. In this case, central nervous system (CNS) depressant drugs are helpful. The classic drugs for treating anxiety are benzodiazepines, like alprazolam (Xanax®) and diazepam (Valium®). Because the benzodiazepines are addictive, antidepressants like fluoxetine (Prozac®) and sertraline (Zoloft®) are now the first-line drugs used to treat anxiety. But for the untreated anxious among us, a major drug problem is the abuse of benzodiazepines, like Xanax®, to self-treat anxiety. The mellow smoke of burning marijuana is also often used to self-treat anxiety disorders; there is a strong positive correlation between anxiety disorders and cannabis use.[52]

Self-medication for mood disorders

Mood disorders include bipolar disorder (manic-depressive disease) and major depressive disorder. Annually, about 10% of the U.S. adult population is diagnosed with a mood disorder.[53] The classic drugs to treat depression are the antidepressants, like Prozac® and Zoloft®. These agents are not addictive, and produce no pleasurable or rewarding effects on the brain. Antidepressants work by increasing levels of serotonin and/or norepinephrine brain neurotransmitters, and this action alleviates depression in most patients.[54] However, as mentioned before, less than half of the people that have mood disorders receive treatment for their disease and many resort to self-medication. The comorbidity of substance abuse and mental illness is highest for persons diagnosed with bipolar disorder, reaching 60% in this patient population.[55] For people with major depression, substance abuse rates are about 40% for alcohol abuse and 17% for other types of drug abuse. Postpartum depression, a subtype of major depression, affects 14% of women in the first 3 months after birth. These women abuse drugs at a higher rate than nonpregnant or pregnant women, with postpartum alcohol abuse ranging from 30% to 49% and other drug abuse ranging from 5% to 9%.[56]

Self-medication for schizophrenia

Schizophrenia is a serious mental disease that afflicts about 1% of the population.[57] To a first approximation, schizophrenia is a simple disease noted by the overabundance of the neurotransmitter dopamine released in the frontal cortex, the

[47] While women with mental illness are no longer burned at the stake for being witches, overuse of new antidepressants and antipsychotics aimed at women may produce a generation of *Stepford Wives*. Indeed, daytime drama TV shows aimed at women viewers should be called "dope operas" not "soap operas" given the pervasive drug ads now playing during commercial breaks.

[48] Substance Abuse and Mental Health Services Administration (2013) Results from the 2012 National Survey on Drug Use and Health: summary of national findings. Rockville, MD.

[49] Wang PS et al. (2005) Twelve-month use of mental health services in the United States: results from the National Comorbidity Survey Replication. Arch. Gen. Psychiatry 62:629–640.

[50] Uwakwe R, Otakpor A (2014) Public mental health – using the mental health gap action program to put all hands to the pumps. Front. Public Health 2:33.

[51] Kessler RC, Chiu WT (2005) Prevalence, severity, and comorbidity of twelve-month DSM-IV disorders in the National Comorbidity Survey Replication (NCSR). Arch. Gen. Psych. 62: 617–627.

[52] Kedzior KK, Laeber LT (2014) A positive association between anxiety disorders and cannabis use or cannabis use disorders in the general population—a meta-analysis of 31 studies. BMC Psychiatry 14:136.

[53] Kessler RC, Chiu WT (2005) *op. cit.*

[54] Brenner GM, Stevens CW (2013) *op. cit.*

[55] Pettinati HM et al. (2013) Current status of co-occurring mood and substance use disorders: a new therapeutic target. Am J Psychiatry 170:23–30.

[56] Chapman SL, Wu LT (2013) Postpartum substance use and depressive symptoms: a review. Women Health 53:479–503.

[57] Power RA et al. (2014) Genetic predisposition to schizophrenia associated with increased use of cannabis. Mol Psychiatry 19:1201–1204.

area of the brain that controls thought and behavior. Typical antipsychotic drugs used to treat schizophrenia are dopamine antagonists, which block the action of the overabundant dopamine release causing schizophrenia. Twelve percent of schizophrenics have comorbid drug abuse or drug dependence disorders in any given year and about 25% of schizophrenics self-medicate with marijuana.[58]

There are unending reports of untreated mental illness leading to crimes and incidents that make the national news. Besides the high school, college, and movie theater mass shootings, recent newspaper headlines include "Mother Talked about Demons before Driving Child-Filled Minivan into Ocean," "Florida Executes Schizophrenic Man Who Believed He Was Prince of God," "Gunman Storms Way into Western Psychiatric Institute, Kills One," and the almost humorous[59] "Mandela Interpreter Claims Schizophrenic Episode." In these unfortunate cases and many others, the person exhibiting the bizarre behavior was found to be an untreated schizophrenic. All the psychiatrists and pharmacologists in the nation know that there are sound treatment options with numerous antipsychotic drugs that have a good chance of controlling the aberrant and psychotic behaviors produced by schizophrenia. Ironically, the lack of drug use is also a major area of pharmacology-related litigation. In a case forthcoming, the author has testified on the lack of pharmacotherapy for a schizophrenic released from prison without continuing health care. Without antipsychotic medications, the psychosis of schizophrenia returned and a heinous criminal act ensued. The requirement for transitional care of released felons is in the correctional guidelines of states, yet one that is often overlooked by underfunded state correctional agencies.

Drugs and Crimes

Drugs and crime go hand in hand. Probably the first cavemen to discover mead, an alcoholic drink from fermented honey, drank too much and started fighting. This led to the first drug-induced homicide, or *Cro-Magnocide* if you will. In this manner, drugs and crime have a direct link, with crime being facilitated or outright caused by drug intoxication. Direct drug crime is due to a pharmacological effect of the drug that alters the brain and behavior in a fashion so that the individual is more likely to commit the crime. This is the first of three types of drug impact on crime: a direct pharmacological effect of the specific drug that is a contributing or sole factor in the commission of a crime. Data to support this assertion are presented next. The second impact of drugs on crime is when drug users undertake criminal activity to support their drug addiction. Third, drugs impact the legal system by their imposed illegality. Some drug laws and sentencing guidelines cry out for the testimony of a drug expert due to their decidedly un-pharmacological nature and unjust statutes.[60]

There is good evidence that many crimes are committed under the influence of one or more drugs. The National Institute of Justice, which is the research, development, and evaluation agency of the U.S. Department of Justice, began a new research program called the Arrestee Drug Abuse Monitoring (ADAM) program in 2000.[61] ADAM was designed to determine the prevalence of illegal drug use in male arrestees, with surveys and urine testing of up to ten different types of drugs. Although the ADAM program provided important drug use data in this crucial population, congressional budget cuts forced its termination in 2004. The Office of National Drug Control Policy, in the Executive Office of the President, renewed the program in 2007 calling it ADAM II. The ADAM II program is the only federal survey that uses a bioassay, namely, urinalysis, to verify the validity of self-reported drug use. However, again stating budget cuts, the program was discontinued after 2013 and is not likely to return. A final report on ADAM II results was issued by the Office of National Drug Control Policy in January, 2014, and its findings are reviewed next.[62]

Survey data on illegal drug use and urine drug tests were obtained from male arrestees within 24 h of booking. The four most common illegal drugs detected were marijuana, methamphetamine, opioids,[63] and cocaine. Averaged among all the sites of the ADAM II program, 82.9% of male arrestees in 2013 were positive in urine tests and the self-reported use of marijuana. Methamphetamine use was self-reported and detected in 62.9% of arrestees and opioids in 50% of arrestees.

---

[58] Asher CJ, Gask L (2010) Reasons for illicit drug use in people with schizophrenia: Qualitative study. BMC Psychiatry 10:94.

[59] This tragicomedy occurred during the speeches at Nelson Mandela's eulogy. Apparently, the deaf-language interpreter, Thamsanqa Jantjie was a schizophrenic with inadequate training in English to sign-language translation. His hand gestures were the equivalent of nonsense babbling. Kulish N, NY Times, Dec. 12, 2013.

[60] One example, the amount of cocaine in a seized crack cocaine sample translated to a much longer prison sentence than the same amount of cocaine in seized powder cocaine. See Chapter 11 *I Want a New Drug*.

[61] Hunt D, Rhodes W (2001) Methodology Guide for ADAM. National Institute of Justice, U.S. Department of Justice, Washington, DC.

[62] Hunt D, Chapman M (2014) 2013 Annual Report, Arrestee Drug Abuse Monitoring Program II. Washington, DC: Office of National Drug Control Policy, Executive Office of the President.

[63] Opioids is the preferred terms for all endogenous (endorphins) and the various types of exogenous (morphine, oxycodone, heroin, etc.) chemicals that act on opioid receptors. Opiates is an older term used for alkaloid opiate drugs before the discovery in the 1970s of the endogenous opioid peptides (endorphins) that act like the brain's own morphine. The clinically used drug class of opioids are called opioid analgesics.

Opioids included both prescription opioid analgesics, like hydrocodone and oxycodone used illegally, as well as the more minor use of heroin. Cocaine and its metabolites were self-reported and detected in 38.2% of arrestees. Of course, these detection rates for marijuana, methamphetamine, opioids, and cocaine sum up to be <100% due to some arrestees using multiple drugs. Multiple drug use was detected in an average of 26.1% of arrestees among the sample sites.

Overall, it is clear that people who are arrested for crimes use illegal drugs at a much greater rate than the general population. Despite the fact that a large proportion of ADAM II arrestees tested positive for illegal drugs in 2013, only about 25% of all arrestees had ever been enrolled in an outpatient drug or alcohol treatment program; <30% had ever participated in any inpatient drug or alcohol treatment program. Given the comorbidity of substance abuse and mental illness, it is telling that only 3.7% of arrestees were ever admitted for inpatient mental health or psychiatric treatment.

The direct effect of drugs on crimes is also seen in the annual crime statistics provided by the Federal Bureau of Investigation (FBI).[64] The FBI groups all crimes into three main categories: Crimes against Persons, Crimes against Property, and Crimes against Society. Using the rough metric of law enforcement assessment of drug and alcohol intoxication, a finer association between drug use and specific types of crimes is found. For example, Crimes against Persons includes assault, homicide, kidnapping, and sexual offenses. The latest dataset from 2012 shows that the greatest prevalence of alcohol use is associated with assault offenses. The greatest prevalence of illegal drug use is associated with homicide offenses. Unfortunately this dataset does not record specific drugs but lumps all abused drugs except alcohol into the category of illegal drugs. For Crimes against Property, alcohol use was most prevalent in bribery cases and illegal drugs most strongly associated with stolen property offences. Crimes against Society include drug offenses, gambling, prostitution, pornography, and weapons law violations. Alcohol was associated most strongly with weapons law violations and drug use with drug offenses. Indeed, in 52.2% of all drug or narcotic offenses, the offender was under the influence of illegal drugs. It seems that many drug dealers forgot the golden rule about not sampling their own merchandize.

Secondly, crimes are also committed to maintain the income to support a substance abuse disorder by the purchase of illegal drugs. In a survey published from the Bureau of Prison Statistics of the U.S. Department of Justice (DOJ), 17% of State and 18% of Federal prisoners committed their crime to obtain money for drugs.[65] Additionally, 32% of State offenders and 26% of Federal inmates were under the influence of illegal drugs at the time of their crime. Like the ADAM II program, this drug research program of the DOJ was lost to other federal budget priorities, and the last report available is from 2004.

Thirdly, illegal drugs promote crime simply by possessing them or selling them. On December 31, 2016, the United States held an estimated 1.51 million persons in state and federal prisons.[66] In federal prisons, nearly half (47%) of the prison population were incarcerated for drug offenses. In state prisons, most offenders were there due to violent felonies, with 16% convicted on drug offenses. There were another 731,200 incarcerated persons in local jails and, considering offenders on probation (3,673,100) and parole (874,800), there was a total of 6,613,500 persons under adult correctional system control in 2016.[67] These numbers give rise to the shocking statistic that 1 in 38 adults are under correctional system control.

It is clear by this point in the chapter that Americans heavily use all kinds of drugs, from the "safe" nonprescription cold remedies to the nastiest, dangerous drugs that are today's emerging drugs of abuse, like the opioid analog called *Krokodil*.[68] It is clear also that many Americans abuse drugs to self-treat underlying mental illness, reflecting a glaring deficit in the health care system for the treatment of mental illness. Finally, drugs and crime intersect in three important ways: Firstly, illegal drugs promote crime from the direct pharmacological action of the drug, like a paranoid *tweeker* after binging on methamphetamine who assaults a police officer. Secondly, persons with a substance abuse disorder often commit crimes to maintain an income for their addiction. Thirdly, illegal drugs promote crime due to their innate status as illegal drugs, with criminal acts ranging from simple possession of a wee bit of a minor drug to the high-level, multikilogram international narco-trafficking of cocaine tonnage. This last aspect of drugs and crime is pursued with a zealous intent for prosecution that leads to the United States having the highest percentage of its citizens incarcerated, and the droll iteration of

---

[64] National Incident-Based Reporting System (2012) Drugs/Narcotics and Alcohol Involvement by Offense Category Table, USA Department of Justice, Federal Bureau of Investigation, Criminal Justice Information Services Division.

[65] Mumola CJ, Karberg JC (2006) Drug Use and Dependence, State and Federal Prisoners, 2004. U.S. Department of Justice, Office of Justice Programs, Bureau of Justice Statistics, Washington, DC.

[66] Carson EA (2018) Prisoners in 2016, U.S. Department of Justice, Office of Justice Programs, Bureau of Justice Statistics, Washington, DC.

[67] Kaeble D, Cowhig M (2018) Correctional Populations in the United States, 2016, U.S. Department of Justice, Office of Justice Programs, Bureau of Justice Statistics, Washington, DC.

[68] *Krokodil* is a particularly nasty opioid drug full of toxic impurities that originated in the Eastern bloc countries and was recently found in the USA. See Katselou M et al. (2014) A "krokodil" emerges from the murky waters of addiction. Life Sci. 102:81–87. *Krokodil* is from the Russian "Крокодил" (crocodile), so-named as injections of *Krokodil* cause severe necrosis and gangrene of the surrounding area. For readers with a strong stomach, there are Google images available of the drug's necrotizing effect.

overcrowded prisons and the failed war on drugs in our society.[69] The drug expert has an important role in fighting irrational drug sentencing guidelines and the efforts of a drug expert in such a case is presented in an upcoming chapter.

We now sit in intermission, perhaps in awe of the amount and prevalence of drug use, and the insidious nature of drugs in our society. Legal or illegal, pill or powder, lozenge or lager, drugs are everywhere in our lives and are here to stay. The pharmaceutical industry saves countless lives every day with safe and effective products used by millions of Americans. However, some legal and illegal drugs destroy American cities and American families. They continue to do so every day. How is this possible?

Drug Effects on Brain and Behavior

Not all drugs have an effect on brain and behavior. Taking an aspirin will not get you high, although relief of headache pain itself can be somewhat rewarding. Antibiotics are not sold illegally on college campuses, and a street market for antihypertensive drugs does not exist. There are no reports of a statin drug being abused, and diabetics are not known for abusing their injectable insulin. However, there are many drugs that affect the brain, either by direct pharmacological effects or neurotoxic effects, or both.

A primer on neuropharmacology

To understand drug effects on the brain we first need to come to a basic understanding of the brain. The brain is not as complex as it is hyped up to be. Sure it is loaded with billions of brain cells, called neurons, with each neuron linked to about 10,000 other neurons.[70] But to a first approximation, the brain and its neurons are a binary system; neuronal activity can only be excited or inhibited when acted on by drugs or neurotransmitters. Neurotransmitters are the brain's own set of drugs. Neurotransmitters and exogenous drugs (taken or administered) often share the same set of targets in the brain, called drug receptors.

Neurons project long extensions of their cell bodies in thin fibers out to one another. When two of these neural fibers meet, they form a junction with a small gap, called a synapse. At the synapse, neurons transmit a signal from one neuron to the next by release of neurotransmitters. A neuron on one side of the synapse releases the neurotransmitter and the neuron on the other side of the synapse has receptors for the neurotransmitter. Many drugs that affect the brain mimic neurotransmitters by acting on the same drug receptors as do neurotransmitters in the synapse. In this way, CNS[71] drugs lead to effects on the brain by altering the function of the brain's own neurotransmitters and receptors. Depending on which groups of neurons in the brain are affected by drugs, there is a change in neuronal activity that results in altered thoughts, memories, and behaviors. Consciousness is thought to be an emergent property of neuronal ensembles in the brain.[72] How exactly the activity of brain neurons gives rise to conscious phenomena and their alteration by drugs is not known, but such a detailed understanding of consciousness will be worth a *Nobel Prize* or two.

A good example of a drug affecting brain and behavior is the action of morphine or other opioids on brain neurons. There are specialized nerve pathways and neurons that transmit pain information throughout the CNS. These pain neurons are abundant with opioid receptors, which are proteins that span across the cell membrane and signal when opioids bind to them. Opioid drugs fit into the opioid receptors like a lock and key.[73] Opioid receptors exist on pain neurons for the use of our own endogenous opioid painkillers, the endorphins. Morphine and other opioids are such good analgesics because humans long ago discovered that the juice from the unripe pod of the poppy plant contains a substance, later isolated to be morphine, which binds to the same opioid receptors as our own endorphins.[74] When opioid receptors on pain neurons are activated by an opioid molecule binding to them, either from endogenous endorphins or an exogenous opioid, the pain neuron undergoes a chain of molecular events that lead to the suppression of neuronal activity. Decreased pain neuron activity results in decreased pain neurotransmission, providing analgesia and perceived by the patient as pain relief. We will see in

---

[69] Alexander M (2010) The New Jim Crow: Mass Incarceration in the Age of Colorblindness. New York: The New Press.

[70] There are 10^{12} or about 1 trillion neurons in each of our brains. See Kandel ER, Schwartz JH (1985) Principles of Neural Sciences, 2nd Edition, Elsevier Scientific Publishing Company: New York, NY. A trillion neurons seemed like a really large number when I first learned it as a graduate student in the 1980s; it seems smaller now in light of the Mideast wars costing $4 trillion and the current U.S. national debt of $18 trillion.

[71] CNS stands for Central Nervous System, i.e., the brain and spinal cord.

[72] This is one view. According to neuroscientist Sam Harris, consciousness is an illusion. See Harris S (2014) *Waking Up: A Guide to Spirituality Without Religion*, Simon & Schuster: New York, NY.

[73] More realistically, considering the small size of the drug molecule and the large size of the drug receptor protein, the analogy of a drug binding to a drug receptor is more like a gnat on an elephant's arse.

[74] Stevens CW (2009) The evolution of vertebrate opioid receptors. Front Biosci (Landmark Ed.) 14:1247–1269.

one of the following chapters that the action of opioids at other brain areas, such as brainstem neurons that drive breathing, leads to the major opioid adverse effect of respiratory depression and death.

Other drugs that affect brain function have a more general effect and target more neurons than opioid drugs. The highly used and abused drugs classified as sedative-hypnotics affect large numbers of neurons throughout different functional areas of the brain. The brain is composed of excitatory neurons and inhibitory neurons. Like their name implies, excitatory neurons excite the nervous system and produce thought, speech, and behavior. Inhibitory neurons are outnumbered by the excitatory neurons by about ten to one,[75] and exist to keep the excitatory neurons in check. It is your excitatory neurons that are activated as you read and process this sentence and your inhibitory neurons that fire to keep you from reading the words out loud. The sedative-hypnotic agents, including barbiturates and benzodiazepines, cause increased inhibition of brain neurons. Use of sedative-hypnotic drugs is often seen in driving under the influence cases and other cases of aberrant behavior.

Drugs that alter brain function do so by direct pharmacological action or a direct neurotoxic effect. The drugs that are addictive and abused also activate reward pathways along with a direct pharmacological effect. Rewarding drugs all act by the same brain mechanism with the final common pathway producing increased dopamine release in a particular place in the brain. Drugs can also affect the brain by direct destruction of neurons, a neurotoxic effect. Some drugs activate rewarding pathways and also exert a neurotoxic effect, especially with long-term use. Alcohol, methamphetamine, and MDMA (Ecstasy, "X") are good examples of rewarding and neurotoxic drugs.

Rewarding drugs

There is a group of neurons in the brain that are devoted to reinforcing behaviors good for the survival of the species. The number one priority for any species, from virus and bacteria to rodents and humans, is to make more of that species. In humans, this is accomplished by the reward contingency of human copulation,[76] which provides a tremendous boost of reward in the brain if done correctly. Eating is also good for the survival of the species and with it comes activation of the reward system in the brain. The main neurotransmitter of the reward pathway is *dopamine*, released onto neurons in the *nucleus accumbens*. The frequency and amount of dopamine released onto the neurons of the nucleus accumbens is directly related to the intensity of the reward.[77] Rewarding drugs usurp this basic brain function to produce the same brain state as the natural reward, only a thousand times more potent. Rats will lever press until death to self-administer cocaine and other addictive drugs that cause the release of dopamine at the nucleus accumbens.[78] Intravenous heroin abusers describe the "rush" after heroin use as it quickly enters the brain and describe it as "orgasmic pleasure" and the euphoria of heroin use is correlated with the release of dopamine in the nucleus accumbens.[79]

Repeated drug use leads to changes in the brain's reward system. The drug-using brain enters a pathological or disease state characterized by physical changes in the brain. The director of the National Institute on Drug Abuse (NIDA), Nora Volkow, besides leading the largest drug abuse research program in the world, is also a premier neuroscientist working on detecting brain changes following chronic drug abuse.[80] Her research on humans using advanced brain imaging techniques shows that dopamine receptors are decreased in cocaine addicts. There is also a loss in gray matter volume, which is a measure of the loss of brain cells, with continued drug abuse. Most importantly with regard to crimes committed by individuals with a drug abuse problem, the function of the brain's frontal cortex is impaired in drug addicts. The frontal cortex is the part of the brain that controls impulsivity, decision-making, planning, and the ability to resist drug taking. These brain alterations, and many others, that occur with habitual drug use provide the physical evidence that substance abuse disorders are a behavioral manifestation of an underlying brain disease. Bottom line for people who seriously abuse drugs is that they are not in it for the kicks but are mentally sick.[81]

---

[75] Basua K et al. (2008) Novel strategy to selectively label excitatory and inhibitory neurons in the cerebral cortex of mice. J Neurosci Methods 170:212–219.

[76] Human orgasm produces an increase in the blood levels of endorphins, consistent with an increase in brain endorphins which is likely responsible for euphoria and other postcoital brain drug effects. Nicoli RM, Nicoli JM (1995) Biochimie de l'éros. *Contraception, fertilité, sexualité* 23:137–144. Due to the opioid reward of endorphins, some people become addicted to sex. Same for eating, gambling, running, and a myriad of other reinforcing behaviors.

[77] Koob GF, Bloom FE (1988) Cellular and molecular mechanisms of drug dependence. Science 242:715–723.

[78] Bozarth MA, Wise RA (1985) Toxicity associated with long-term intravenous heroin and cocaine self-administration in the rat. JAMA 254:81–83.

[79] Seecof R, Tennant FS (1986) Subjective perceptions to the intravenous "rush" of heroin and cocaine in opioid addicts. Am. J. Drug. Alcohol Abuse 12:79–87; Volkow ND et al. (2009) Imaging dopamine's role in drug abuse and addiction. Neuropharm. 56 (Suppl 1):3–8.

[80] Volkow ND et al. (2012) Addiction circuitry in the human brain. Annu. Rev. Pharmacol. Toxicol. 52:321–336.

[81] While poor decision-making may lead to individuals starting drug use, the continued abuse of drugs creates a state of mental disease. NIDA, the leading government institute for research on drug abuse, recognizes that treating drug-involved offenders decreases substance abuse and reduces associated criminal behavior. Chandler RK et al. (2009) Treating drug abuse and addiction in the criminal justice system. JAMA 301:183–190.

Neurotoxic drugs

There are some commonly used drugs that are neurotoxic to the brain. One of the most neurotoxic drugs used without much thought to ensuing brain damage is alcohol. The widespread availability and cultural acceptance of alcohol masks the fact that alcohol is a neurotoxic drug with devastating effects on brain function and behavior. Alcoholism, termed alcohol use disorder, is a type of substance abuse disorder and a chronic medical disease classified in diagnostic listings alongside other mental disorders such as schizophrenia and depression.[82] Alcohol use is associated with neurotoxicity and cognitive impairment which is manifest by difficulties in memory, attention (ability to concentrate), planning ahead, motor (movement) control, visuospatial performance (locating and reacting to objects), and obviously affects behavior such as driving a motor vehicle.[83] Chronic alcoholics often become so dependent on ethanol that they stop eating a healthy, balanced diet. The result can be general malnutrition and a specific deficiency in vitamin B_1 (thiamine). Lack of vitamin B_1 contributes to the neurotoxicity of alcohol and damages the central and peripheral nervous systems. This pathological state is known as *Wernicke's disease*. If not treated, Wernicke's disease develops into a more serious disorder called *Korsakoff's psychosis*, which is characterized by profound amnesia (memory loss) and other severe cognitive impairments. Although alcohol-induced Wernicke's disease can be treated and reversed if it is detected early, the brain toxicity linked with Korsakoff's psychosis is mostly irreversible.[84]

A second major class of drugs that aren't abused but becoming well known for their neurotoxic effects are the drugs used to treat cancer. Generally known as chemotherapeutic agents, these types of drugs are among the most dangerous drugs to use, that is, they have small therapeutic windows. Cancer chemotherapy often walks the fine line between killing the cancerous tumor cells and killing the patient. While the use of these chemotherapeutic agents is beneficial in a number of different types of cancers, adverse effects that are commonly seen include peripheral and central neurotoxicity, the latter leading to a decrease in cognitive (mental) function.[85] This neurotoxicity is noted in a large number of medical studies and there are numerous papers documenting cognitive decline in cancer patients.[86] Cognitive dysfunction that is manifest by severe memory, attention deficits, and other problems occurs in up to 70% of chemotherapy-treated cancer patients. The adverse cognitive effect of chemotherapy is so common that a term has circulated among cancer patients and their doctors naming it "chemobrain" or "chemofog." Although not generally appreciated by the oncology community or their cancer patients, cancer is now considered a strong risk factor for long-term cognitive deficits and dementia.[87]

Classes of drugs affecting brain and behavior

Table 1.2 lists the classes of the most commonly used drugs that have effects on brain and behavior. Three levels of classification are shown starting with overall drug type, then drug class, and for some agents, further classification into drug subclass. A short description of some CNS effects is summarized in the last column. Examples of behaviors affected are also given under this column heading.

Drug Use and the Legal System

We've seen that drug use in our society is rampant by examining prescription, nonprescription, alcohol and illegal drug use. We've explored drug use as self-treatment for mental disorders and the linkage between drugs and crime, as well as a more detailed look at drug action in the brain and the mechanisms of drug addiction. To set the stage for thinking about the impact of drugs on legal cases, consider a man involved in a motor vehicle accident that kills the driver of another car. The man is uninjured in the crash but a hospital blood draw is taken for a toxicology screen and comes back positive for benzodiazepines and opioids. The trier-of-fact, whether it be judge or jury, needs an expert opinion addressing a number of questions for fair adjudication of the defendant: What tests were used in the toxicology screen? Are they preliminary or confirmatory tests? What blood levels of drugs were detected? Can the blood levels of drugs predict drug impairment? What are the brain effects of the drugs? Did the man have a prescription for the drugs? Do blood levels of the prescription drug support proper use of drug? What is the effect of two types of drugs used together? This is a sampling of the many possible questions to

---

[82] Diagnostic and Statistical Manual of Mental Disorders, Fifth Edition: DSM-5™ (2013) American Psychiatric Association, Arlington, VA.

[83] Svanberg J, Evans JJ (2013) Neuropsychological rehabilitation in alcohol-related brain damage: a systematic review. Alcohol Alcohol. 48:704–711.

[84] Svanberg J, Evans JJ (2013) *op. cit.*

[85] Mandilaras V et al. (2013) The impact of cancer therapy on cognition in the elderly. Front Pharmacol. 4:48.

[86] Ahles TA et al. (2012) Cancer- and cancer treatment-associated cognitive change: an update on the state of the science. Clin Oncol. 30:3675–3686.

[87] Heflin LH et al. (2005) Cancer as a risk factor for long-term cognitive deficits and dementia. J Natl Cancer Inst. 97:854–856.

TABLE 1.2 Classes and examples of drugs affecting brain and behavior.

Drug type	Drug class	Drug subclass	Examples	Brain and behavioral effects
CNS depressants	Alcohol	–	Beer, liquor	As a general class, CNS depressants increase the activity of brain neurons. CNS depressants also activate reward pathways leading to drug dependence. Adverse effects include sedation, motor incoordination, and cognitive impairment. Paradoxical reactions leading to behavioral disinhibition can also occur. Agents such as the popular Z-drugs used for treating insomnia are also associated with complex behaviors and suicide.
	Antiepileptics	Barbiturates	Phenobarbital (Luminal®)	
	Antihistamines	First generation	Diphenhydramine (Benedryl®), Hydroxyzine (Atarax®)	
	Sedative-hypnotics	Barbiturates	Pentobarbital (Nembutal®), Sodium thiopental (Pentothal®)	
		Benzodiazepines	Diazepam (Valium®), Alprazolam (Xanax®)	
		Z-drugs	Zolpidem (Ambien®), Zaleplon (Sonata®).	
	Opioid analgesics	Prescription opioids	Morphine, Hydrocodone (Lortab®), Oxycodone (Oxycontin®)	
		Illegal opioids	Heroin	
CNS stimulants	Amphetamines	–	Amphetamines (Adderall®), Methylphenidate (Ritalin®), Methamphetamine	As a general class, CNS stimulants increase the activity of brain neurons. CNS stimulants also activate reward pathways leading to drug dependence. Adverse effects include brain and cardiac toxicity, and cognitive impairment with long-term use.
			MDMA (Ecstasy), synthetic stimulants (bath salts)	
	Cocaine	–	Crack cocaine, powder cocaine	
CNS hallucinogens	Strong hallucinogens		LSD, Peyote (cactus), Psilocybin (magic mushrooms)	Intense to mild visual distortions, and perceptual disturbances. Little to mild reward pathway activation. Toxicity associated with synthetic cannabinoids.
	Mild hallucinogens		Marijuana, synthetic cannabinoids ("K2", "Spice")	
Psychotherapeutic agents	Antidepressants	Tricyclic antidepressants	Amitriptyline (Elavil®)	Little abuse of psychotherapeutic agents, none or slight activation of reward pathways. Evidence of increase thoughts and behaviors leading to suicide with antidepressants.
	Antidepressants	SSRIs	Fluoxetine (Prozac®), Sertraline (Zooloft®)	
	Antipsychotics	Typical	Chlorpromazine (Thorazine®)	
		Atypical	Risperidone (Risperdal®)	
Neurotoxic drugs	Alcohol	–	Beer, liquor (spirits)	Direct neurotoxic effects observed especially with long-term use. Severe cognitive impairment can result.
	Antineoplastic[a] agents	Cytotoxic agents	5-Flourouracil (5-FU), Cisplatin (Platinol®)	

[a] Antineoplastic agents are drugs used to fight cancer; neoplasm means "new growth."

address for both the prosecution of this man and for his defense if indicted.[88] The drug expert, as a pharmacologist, is the best person to answer these questions.

In this final section, the impact of drug use in cases before the court, both civil and criminal, is explored and the role of the drug expert introduced. First, a brief overview of civil and criminal jurisdiction, types of lawsuits commonly encountered by a drug expert, and overview of drug tort cases.

Types of legal cases

There are two types of legal cases that bifurcate the majority of all grievances in society: criminal or civil.[89] In a criminal case, the state or federal government acts on behalf of the victim and files a lawsuit against an individual, the defendant. In a civil case, an individual, the plaintiff, brings suit against another individual, the defendant, to right a particular wrong. The laws covering this type of civil case are called tort law. *Tort* is a word derived from the Latin, *tortum* or "injury," the same root that gives us the word "torture." Tort law exists "to make the injured party whole again," usually by forcing the opposing party to pay reparations or damages. Toxic torts are injury lawsuits filed against an individual or corporation for damages due to the toxic effects of a chemical or drug. Most pharmaceutical tort cases are mass tort or class-action lawsuits, as drugs are consumed by thousands if not millions of people.[90] These are the types of class-action lawsuits often seeking additional litigants by law firms advertising on late-night, cable TV shows.[91] Some drug toxic tort cases may not be suitable as class-action mass torts as establishing the same injury in all litigants may not be possible. Often drug toxic torts are part of a multidistrict litigation (MDL) process which joins litigants claiming damage by the same drug in combined litigation in a single federal district court.[92] In this way, pretrial processes such as discovery and expert witness testimony can be uniform and shared among all cases.

The drug expert

A complete analysis of a legal case that involves a medication or other drug that may have affected the alleged illegal or civil action requires consideration of multiple factors involved in the drug use. These include the physical properties of the drug, the formulation of the drug, its pharmacological effects, and the pharmacokinetics of the drug.[93] Additionally, for prescription drugs, there is analysis of the clinical scenario that led to the prescribing of a particular drug to an individual, the doses administered, possible adverse effects, and the monitoring of drug effect and drug levels. A pharmacologist litigation consultant, simply called a drug expert, is needed for this analysis. A drug expert is also employed on pharmaceutical toxic tort cases, providing an expert opinion on the likelihood of adverse effects in a drug product liability case. A drug expert can also play a role in the application of drug sentencing guidelines, providing a rational interpretation to reflect the latest medical and scientific research on drugs, drug use, and drug effects.

There is a disjunction between the easy availability of powerful and dangerous prescription drugs promulgated by physicians to their patients and the ultimate responsibility for actions that occur when patients take the drugs. A good example of the current legal thinking about drug use is reflected in the FDA warnings found on many CNS depressant medications about brain effects, for example with the benzodiazepine, alprazolam (Xanax®) "Because of its CNS depressant effects, patients receiving Xanax® should be cautioned against engaging in hazardous occupations or activities requiring complete mental alertness such as operating machinery or driving a motor vehicle."[94] Note the FDA warnings do not say that driving is absolutely contraindicated; it is not written "Don't drive while taking Xanax® or you will crash and kill yourself or

---

[88] Although the drug expert will mostly work for the defense, the prosecution should also consult a drug expert to see if drug-related charges are warranted. The prosecution may rely less on drug experts as their own employees testify (which may present a conflict), and due to the lack of funds to hire an outside drug expert. My experience is that the prosecution does not always perform due diligence to see if a legitimate drug impact was present. However, there is a group of district attorneys in a rural jurisdiction that used my services on three occasions and showed admirable prosecutorial constraint based on my findings.

[89] Much of the following introductory material is from Baumgras A (2010) Basic Legal Structure and Organization. In Miller NS (Ed.) Principles of Addiction and the Law: Applications in Forensic, Mental Health, and Medical Practice. Academic Press: San Diego, CA.

[90] Schaffzin D (2013) Warning: Lawyer Advertising May Be Hazardous to Your Health! A Call to Fairly Balance Commercial Solicitation of Clients in Pharmaceutical Litigation. 8 Charleston L. Rev. 319; University of Memphis Legal Studies Research Paper No. 131.

[91] Some recent TV mass tort lawsuit ads include the antipsychotic drug risperidone (Risperdal®), for causing breast development in young boys (gynecomastia), and the anti-diabetes drug rosiglitazone (Avandia®), for causing cardiovascular injury and death.

[92] Pierce T (2014) It's Not Over 'Til It's Over: Mandating Federal Pretrial Jurisdiction and Oversight in Mass Torts. 79 Missouri Law Review 27.

[93] Pharmacokinetics literally means "drug movement" and is divided into four phases; *absorption* of the drug, *distribution* of the drug from the blood to the tissues, *metabolism* of the drug by the liver, and *elimination* of the drug usually by excretion by the kidneys and urine. These four phases are often referred to by the popular acronym, ADME.

[94] Xanax® Prescribing Information, available in the Physicians' Desk Reference (PDR).

somebody else." The FDA reflects the spirit of the law throughout the land that it is the responsibility of the individual taking the drug to know how the drug affects their brain. That is fine in a society *not* living under the influence of many powerful brain drugs readily prescribed by physicians, but leaving the decision to drive in the mind of a drug user is problematic as the pharmacological effects of drug use itself often cause impairment of the decision-making process. It is likely that existing drug laws place too much responsibility on the individual and not enough on the drug, pharmaceutical companies, and physicians. There is a much medical and pharmacological data on drug effects in humans that needs to be considered before the legal assignment of blame. The drug expert is the professional that can shed light on these and many other issues.

In spite of the large number of criminal and civil cases involving drugs, a report from the Judicial Center shows that expert witnesses are underutilized in criminal cases, both by the prosecution and the defense, and that most experts in civil ligation are physicians.[95] As further elaborated in the next chapter, physicians are not adequately trained in pharmacology to carry out the scientific analysis of drugs and their use. Additionally, the prosecution often uses a police lab employee, a laboratory forensic toxicologist without an advanced degree, to provide expert testimony which is inherently prejudicial and often goes unchallenged, especially in indigent cases represented by an appointed public defender. The drug expert is a neutral party and serves as a consultant to the prosecuting or defense attorney, an expert witness for the plaintiff or the defendant.

Americans are the world's biggest drug users. This is due to a unique set of multifactorial conditions impinging on American society, creating the "The Perfect Drug-Storm." Further exploration of the drug-crazed situation in the United States is beyond the scope of this book, but will be fully explored in a forthcoming treatise. What this chapter shows is that Americans use drugs at a volume and frequency higher than any other national grouping of people. There is a price to pay for high levels of drug use in America, whether it be increased motor vehicle accidents or epidemic levels of prescription opioid overdose deaths.[96] Drugs, in all of their various forms and formulations, are here to stay. The genie is not going back in the pill bottle. Given that we live in a society overrun with drug use, one of the key issues now is dealing with drug impact on the legal system. The testifying pharmacologist, or drug expert, determines whether a drug was more likely than not a factor in a person's behavior, illness, injury, or death.[97] The cases in the following chapters are based on the real-life experiences of a drug expert and illustrate the diverse drug issues that are present in our justice system.

---

[95] Krafka C et al. (2002) Judge and attorney experiences, practices, and concerns regarding expert testimony in federal civil trials. Psych. Public Pol. Law 8:309–332.

[96] Centers for Disease Control and Prevention (2102) CDC Grand Rounds: Prescription Drug Overdoses—a U.S. Epidemic. MMWR 61:10–13.

[97] Zedeck MS (2010) *Expert Witness in the Legal System: A Scientist's Search for Justice.* Lauriat Press: Pittsburgh, PA.

Chapter 2

A Parent's Worst Nightmare: Drug-Induced Psychosis and Deadly Police Force

Over-the-Counter Drug Abuse—Benadryl® and the Brain

Testing for Drug Use in the Recently Dead—Finding the Drug Expert

The Drug Expert's Initial Contact With an Attorney

[Narrative]
Nineteen year-old Jimmy was the last child living at home with Mr. and Mrs. Cattoni.[1] The Cattoni family lived in a small three bedroom house located in an aging development. Jimmy's parents found marijuana in his room recently, and most nights Jimmy stayed out late or in his room listening to heavy metal rock. Last Saturday night, Jimmy came out of his room and confronted his parents who were watching TV. He became violent and his father called the police. The police arrived nine minutes later and approached the front door. Sergeant Roberts was accompanied by his partner, Officer Ted Daniels. The police entered and Mrs. Cattoni gave a brief account of the incident and stated that their son was in his room down the hall. Roberts walked down the hall and knocked loudly yelling for Jimmy to come out and talk to them. Jimmy told them to go to hell. The police banged on the door with increasing urgency while Jimmy continued to swear at them. After Roberts yelled that they would break down his door and come get him, Jimmy finally threw open his door. He was waving a machete and in a highly agitated state. As he stepped towards Roberts, Daniels drew his service revolver and shot Jimmy once in the chest. Jimmy Cattoni died within minutes as the bullet pierced the apex of his heart causing massive internal hemorrhage. Afterwards, the police scene investigators cataloged the contents of Jimmy's room and found a half-empty bottle of Benadryl®. The medical examiner's report of the deceased included a toxicology report from postmortem blood samples. THC, the active ingredient of marijuana, and diphenhydramine, the active drug ingredient in Benadryl®, were detected and quantified in the decedent's blood samples. The parents of the deceased teen filed a wrongful death lawsuit against the Police Department and Officers Roberts and Daniels. The Police Department was represented by a large firm and the lead attorney on the case hired a drug expert, a local medical school pharmacologist, to determine the effects, if any, marijuana and Benadryl® had on the decedent's behavior at the time of the shooting.

Over-the-Counter Drug Abuse

As elaborated in Chapter 1, nonprescription or OTC drug abuse is rampant in our society. Nonprescription drug abuse is defined as the use of an OTC drug product in a manner not indicated on the label.[2] OTC drug abuse includes such actions as taking more drug than recommended, or in the present chapter case, taking high doses of an OTC drug for its mind-altering effects on the brain. Another aspect of OTC drug abuse is self-medicating for health problems not indicated on the label. For example, using popular cold and cough remedies every night to get to sleep is OTC drug abuse. National survey data indicate that about 3.1 million persons aged 12 years and older abuse OTC drugs at least once in their lifetime, with 3.7% prevalence of OTC drug abuse among adolescents younger than 18 years of age.[3] An alarming 26% of 9th graders reported abusing OTC cough medicines to get high, which was greater than the 25% of them using marijuana for the same reason.

---

[1] Although this narrative and others are based on actual cases, the names of individuals, attorneys, and law firms were changed, and in some cases, additional material was added to round-out the narrative and outcome.

[2] Conca AJ, Worthen DR (2012) Nonprescription drug abuse. J. Pharm. Pract. 25:13–21.

[3] Substance Abuse and Mental Health Services Administration (SAMHSA) Results from the 2008 National Survey on Drug Use and Health (NSDUH): National Findings, September 2009.

Of the 6841 Emergency Department admissions in California from 2006 to 2007, most adolescent admissions (ages 12–17) were for stimulant prescription abuse or OTC drug abuse, whereas ER admissions for abuse of opioid prescription drugs were most common for adults 18 years and older.[4] In the demographic group of 18–25 year olds, drug abuse using freely available OTC drugs is growing at a rate of nearly 5% per year.[5]

The two most abused OTC drugs are dextromethorphan (DM) and diphenhydramine. Many nonprescription cold and cough remedies contain both DM and diphenhydramine, however these two drugs will be considered individually.

Dextromethorphan (DM) is a drug that was developed from CIA and Navy-sponsored research in the 1950s.[6] The goal of this classified project was to identify a nonaddictive substitute for the use of codeine as a cough suppressant. Codeine is an opioid, and besides providing pain-relief, codeine also exerts a cough suppressant, or antitussive effect. Antitussives work by decreasing activity of neurons in the part of the brain that causes coughing. After trying many chemicals, DM was selected as it suppressed cough but was not addictive to experienced opioid users.[7] DM is an active ingredient in a large number of OTC cold and cough remedies including Mucinex-DM®, Vicks DayQuil Cough®, Pertussin ES®, Tylenol Cold and Cough Nighttime®, Robitussin DM®, and Children's Robitussin Cough Long-Acting®.

Dextromethorphan abuse

Almost as soon as dextromethorphan hit the market, reports of DM abuse appeared in the medical journals.[8] OTC remedies containing DM are legal, relatively cheap, and easily available. Many parents would not question the discovery of cough medicine in their kid's bedroom but would be seriously concerned if they found a bag of marijuana. But a drug-to-drug comparison reveals that cough medicines containing DM and other abused OTC drugs send more young adults to the ER than use of marijuana. In the last decade, there was an increased number of dextromethorphan abuse cases in the ER and this was largely due to increased admissions for adolescents.[9] The even younger fetal population is also affected by OTC drug and specifically DM abuse. DM use during pregnancy increases the prevalence of congenital malformations in the fetus.[10]

Dextromethorphan taken at normal doses suppresses cough by inhibiting the cough reflex neurons in the brain. DM does this by inhibiting the neurons that fire when irritants are present in the respiratory tract. DM blocks the receptors that excitatory neurotransmitters activate with respiratory irritation. Like the antihistamine drug diphenhydramine, DM is an antagonist drug.

An important concept applicable to most all drugs is the idea of *selectivity*. Drugs are selective for their targeted receptor within their normal dose range. At higher doses, drugs can lose their selectivity and interact with other drug receptors that are not part of their beneficial or therapeutic targets. At normal doses, DM acts as an antagonist (receptor blocker) at excitatory neurotransmitter receptors in the cough center of the brain. At high doses consistent with drug abuse, DM acts at other receptors and in other ways to produce the mind-altering effects sought by abusers.[11]

Normal therapeutic doses of dextromethorphan are 15–30 mg[12] taken three or four times a day. Mild intoxication, noted by tachycardia, hypertension, vomiting, euphoria, loss of motor coordination, and giggling or laughing is reported with a dose of 100–200 mg DM.[13] At higher doses, in the range of 1000–1500 mg DM is noted by confusion, agitation, hallucinations, seizures, and loss of consciousness. As a 12-oz bottle of Robitussin DM contains 710 mg of DM, therefore drinking

---

[4]   Gonzales R et al. (2011) Prescription and over-the-counter drug treatment admissions to the California public treatment system. J Subst. Abuse Treat. 40:224–229.

[5]   Lessenger JE, Feinberg SD (2008) Abuse of prescription and over-the counter medications. JABFM 21:45–54.

[6]   Classified papers obtained from the Department of Defense by a FOIA request at *www.dod.mil/pubs/foi/logistics_material_readiness/acq_bud_fin/02-A-0846RELEASE.pdf.*

[7]   The addictive potential of dextromethorphan and other drugs was tested on imprisoned heroin addicts held at a Kentucky penitentiary. From 1935 until 1975, the U.S. Public Health Service funded drug research using heroin addicts at this penal institution, called by inmates and staff "The Narcotic Farm." See Nancy D. Campbell, J.P. Olsen, Luke Walden (2008) The Narcotic Farm: The Rise and Fall of America's First Prison for Drug Addicts. Abrams: New York, NY.

[8]   Degkwitz R (1964) Dextromethorphan (Romilar®) as an intoxicating agent. Nervenarzt 35:412–414.

[9]   Bryner JK et al. (2006) Dextromethorphan abuse in adolescence. Arch. Pediatr. Adolesc. Med. 160:1217–1222.

[10]   Einarson A et al. (2001) The safety of dextromethorphan in pregnancy. Chest 119:466–469.

[11]   Chary M et al. (2014) Signs and symptoms of dextromethorphan exposure from YouTube. PLoS One 9:e82452.

[12]   The "mg" stands for "milligram," a common unit of the metric system. A milligram (mg) is 1/1000th of a gram. A gram, abbreviated with just a "g," is about the weight of a paperclip. A microgram (µg or mcg) is 1/1000th of a mg, and the nanogram (ng), you guessed it, is 1/1000th of a µg. Most prescription drug doses are in mg. For units heavier than a gram, we have the kilogram (kg) which is 1000 times the weight of a gram. Kilogram quantities are associated with large amounts of illegal drugs (e.g., a "kilo" of cocaine). The United States, along with Liberia and Myanmar (old Burma), remain the only countries in the world that have not adopted the metric system as their official system of measurement.

[13]   Mayhew M (2007) Dextromethorphan abuse. J. Nurse Pract. 3:650–651.

even half a bottle would produce strong intoxication. Drinking a whole bottle or more of cough medicine produces severe intoxication. Because dextromethorphan is available as an OTC medication, it lacks the stigma of being drug abuse. There are numerous internet sites promoting dextromethorphan abuse and providing instructions on how much to take to get high. Most alarming, instructions for making the base form of DM called "crystal DEX" are easily obtained and forensic cases confirm this emerging form of OTC drug abuse.[14] The danger of crystal DEX is that this formulation of DM makes the drug more potent and increases drug availability. The change in abuse patterns of cocaine powder compared to crack cocaine (a base form) is the classic example of increased drug abuse due to a change in drug formulation.

Benadryl® and the Brain

The second commonly abused OTC drug is diphenhydramine. Diphenhydramine, an antihistamine, is the active ingredient in various Benadryl® and other OTC products.[15] Antihistamines work by blocking the receptors for the natural brain neurotransmitter, histamine. Diphenhydramine is an example of a drug that works by blocking the activity of an endogenous neurotransmitter. These types of blocking drugs are generally called *antagonists*. Again, using the lock-and-key model of a drug-receptor interaction, an antagonist can be thought of as a key broken off in the lock. Antihistamines, or any antagonists for that matter, don't activate drug receptors like agonist drugs (e.g., opioid analgesics), but rather prevent receptor activation by doing nothing. An antagonist does nothing except preventing any other drug to turn on the receptor.

Diphenhydramine is an old drug and was the first prescription antihistamine approved by the Food and Drug Administration (FDA) in 1946.[16] Diphenhydramine was made by Parke-Davis Company, in Detroit, Michigan.[17] It is now sold over-the-counter by the Parke-Davis subsidiary of Pfizer. Diphenhydramine is an example of one of the first drugs approved as a prescription-only medication that later switched to OTC status, although prescription-only formulations of diphenhydramine still exist. Originally marketed to treat allergies, newer antihistamines with fewer side effects have largely supplanted diphenhydramine's use as an antiallergy drug. Benadryl® with diphenhydramine remains on the OTC market, along with other nonbranded products. Prescription diphenhydramine is formulated in a solution for injection. Injectable diphenhydramine is administered alongside epinephrine (from an EpiPen®) for the treatment of anaphylaxis, a serious medical condition produced by deadly allergies to such things including bee stings, peanuts, or latex.[18]

Diphenhydramine is mainly found as a sedative-hypnotic agent in OTC sleep aids and "PM" forms of cold medicine. Diphenhydramine is essential to brands such as Unisom® and Sominex® marketed for treatment of insomnia, and numerous pain and sleep formulations such as Advil PM®, Excedrin PM®, Midol PM®, Motrin PM®, and Tylenol PM®. Diphenhydramine is also found in an even larger number of cold and cough OTC drugs, including the heavily marketed Nyquil®, Robitussin Night Time Cough and Cold®, Coricidin®, and PediaCare Children's Allergy and Cold®. After years of OTC drug abuse of Nyquil® for sedation and its sleep-inducing effects, the makers of Nyquil®, Vicks® and its parent company, Proctor and Gamble, launched a new OTC product called ZzzQuil® in 2012 for inducing sleep.[19] Its active ingredient is diphenhydramine, basically Nyquil® without any cold or cough medicine. This diphenhydramine-containing new OTC product will be helpful if it decreases the use of more powerful and addictive prescription sleep-inducers (like benzodiazepines) but harmful if it increases OTC drug abuse in youth.

Diphenhydramine abuse

The propensity for certain individuals to alter their brains with mind-altering substances is not restricted to adults and in many individuals begins with adolescent experimentation. As discussed before, abuse with OTC products is especially prevalent in young people. Abuse of diphenhydramine is typically carried out by taking higher than recommended oral doses of diphenhydramine-containing allergy or cough and cold medicines. At normal doses, diphenhydramine, like other "first generation" antihistamines, blocks brain histamine receptors and produces drowsiness and sedation, impairment of

[14] Hendrickson RG, Cloutier RL (2007) "Crystal DEX": Free-base dextromethorphan. J. Emerg. Med. 32:393–396.

[15] Benadryl® Information (McNeil Consumer Healthcare) at *www.benadryl.com.*

[16] Grugzit O et al. (1947) A toxicologic study of two histamine antagonists of the benzhydryl alkamine ether group. J. Pharmacol. Exp. Ther. 89:227–235.

[17] Parke-Davis was once the most successful pharmaceutical company in the world and created the first modern techniques for standardization of pharmaceutical products. See Hoefle ML (2000) The early history of Parke-Davis and company. Bull. Hist. Chem. 25:28–34.

[18] Diphenhydramine Hydrochloride Injection Prescribing Information (Becton, Dickinson and Company) at bdrxinc.com.

[19] Landor was the branding firm hired by P&G to develop a design solution that debunked social stigmas about sleep aids, assuring consumers it is only natural to want to get some sleep. Within the first six weeks of the national launch, ZzzQuil® hit the number one position in dollar and unit sales for OTC sleeping aids. See *landor.com/#!/work/case-studies/zzzquil.*

cognitive function, and decrements in psychomotor performance.[20] These brain effects are sought by abusers of diphenhydramine. At high doses, diphenhydramine loses its selectivity for blocking histamine receptors and blocks the activity of other neurotransmitter-receptor systems in the brain. Most prominently, diphenhydramine at high doses blocks acetylcholine receptors, producing an anticholinergic effect.[21] Acetylcholine is a brain neurotransmitter like histamine, and antagonism at acetylcholine receptors produces the high dose effects of diphenhydramine abuse. The anticholinergic effect of diphenhydramine produces delirium, severe confusion, and hallucinations. The anticholinergic delirium caused by high doses of diphenhydramine is often misdiagnosed as schizophrenic psychosis.[22] Epileptic seizures and status epilepticus, the condition of nonstop seizures that can quickly be fatal, can also occur with high dose diphenhydramine.[23]

Normal therapeutic levels after acute dosage of diphenhydramine in the blood range from about 50 to 100 ng/mL. Forensic studies examining postmortem blood samples showed that lethal levels of diphenhydramine ranged from 3000 to 100,000 ng/mL, with concentrations greater than 5000 ng/mL considered potentially lethal.[24]

Testing for Drug Use in the Recently Dead

The dead tell no tales and are notoriously reluctant to speak of their recent drug use. However, the recently dead are often the only sample source for detecting drug use. In many cases, it is crucial to compare postmortem concentrations of the drug in the decedent with normal therapeutic concentrations of the drug and drug concentrations in forensic cases. Blood samples obtained after death are not as good as blood draws from a living person, but can be informative regarding suspected drug use, especially at the extremes. For example, even considering passage of time from death until postmortem sampling, postmortem redistribution of the drug,[25] and numerous other factors, a blood sample obtained from the recently dead that yields a drug concentration 100 times greater than the peak therapeutic drug concentration suggests drug abuse in the decedent. High postmortem concentrations literally suggest that the decedent was taking greater amounts of the medicine than directed, that is drug abuse. At the other extreme, when a zero concentration of drug is found, the lack of detected drug will conclusively rule-out drug-taking by the deceased.

There are five main bodily emanations that are routinely used to determine drug use: breath, saliva, blood, urine, and hair. Breath testing is, at this time, limited to alcohol detection and if confirmatory, can provide evidentiary findings as to the level of alcohol intoxication.[26] Breath testing is most convenient and easily done at the roadside, and its use to detect alcohol in driving with intoxication cases is well accepted. Devices and methods of breath testing for detection of other drugs are under active development. For example, breath tests for the detection of recent marijuana use in drivers are a burning issue in the states that legalized recreational and medical marijuana use. Breath testing is definitely not an option for detecting drug use in the recently dead.

Saliva or spit samples, known formally as oral fluids, can detect drug use from a broad window of time. Depending on the drug, oral fluids can be informative when sampled as soon as immediately after drug use and up to 3 or 4 days later.[27] Conventional drug testing using urine samples is not as accurate as saliva in detecting usage in the first few hours after drug use. This makes drug testing using oral fluids superior to urine testing in some time-dependent situations, like immediately after a motor vehicle accident. However, urine is one of the best bodily fluids to assay for drugs of abuse.[28] Urine is easily obtained, painless to get, and risk-free to the tester. With supervised procedures, urine drug testing is resistant to scamming by urine substitution or urine adulteration. Urine can be used as a postmortem sample in the recently dead but urine is most commonly obtained for employment hires and compliance testing in individuals under court order.

The best method for estimating drug use in both the living and recently deceased individuals is to assay a peripheral blood sample. Blood samples yielding drug concentrations are the gold standard of pharmacokinetic data and the overwhelming majority of medical and pharmacological studies use blood samples to measure drug concentration. Obtaining a blood sample and assaying drug concentration makes it possible to opine on what drugs and how much drug was taken

[20] Romanelli F, Smith KM (2009) Dextromethophan abuse: clinical effects and management. J. Am. Pharm. Assoc. 49:20–25.

[21] Orzechowski RF et al. (2005) Comparative anticholinergic activities of 10 histamine H1 receptor antagonists in two functional models. Eur. J. Pharmacol. 506:257–264.

[22] Christensen RC (1995) Misdiagnosis of anticholinergic delirium as schizophrenic psychosis. Amer. J. Emerg. Med. 13:117–118.

[23] Radovanovic D et al. (2000) Dose-dependent toxicity of diphenhydramine overdose. Human Exp. Toxicol. 19:489–495.

[24] Pragst F et al. (2006) Poisonings with diphenhydramine-a survey of 68 clinical cases and 55 deaths. Forensic Sci. Internat. 161:189–197.

[25] See Chapter 19 for a more erudite and complete discussion of postmortem redistribution (PMR) of drugs.

[26] Kelly AT, Mozayani A (2012) An overview of alcohol testing and interpretation in the 21st century. J Pharm Pract. 25:30–36.

[27] Bosker WM, Huestis MA (2009) Oral fluid testing for drugs of abuse. Clin Chem. 55:1910–1931.

[28] Schwartz RH (1988) Urine testing in the detection of drugs of abuse. Arch Intern Med. 148:2407–2412.

by a person or by the deceased. The motto that most aptly adorns the drug testing laboratory is not the well-known *in vino veritas* but *in sanguis veritas; "*in blood [there is] truth."

In the living, a blood draw is usually made from the antecubital vein in the crook of the arm; from the dead, a more precise procedure is done by drawing blood from the femoral vein in the groin or upper-thigh. The blood-getter in the case of the recently dead has an advantage over the phlebotomist in the living as the recently dead feel no pain so the femoral vein can be laid bare by a cut-down dissection. The actual drug toxicological test involves two steps to be considered valid in scientific and legal terms.[29] The first test or assay ran on the sample is a preliminary screening test. This test contains antibodies to specific drugs and simply tells whether the drug or a member of its drug class is present. The results of the screening test, sometimes called the preliminary test, is *qualitative*, a simple yes or no to the drug's presence in the sample. The second drug test performed on a sample is called a GC-MS[30] test, which can yield *quantitative* results in terms of the drug concentration in the sample. The GC-MS test is confirmatory of a positive screening test. In some cases, the preliminary screening test does not pick up a particular drug molecule and a GC-MS test is performed first if an uncommon or new drug is suspected.

Finding a Drug Expert

Most referrals for litigation consulting and expert witnesses come from word-of-mouth recommendations between attorneys. Lawyers are a talkative bunch and interact often at the courthouse and at legal conferences. Adversarial relationships in the courtroom become collegial conversations at the conference hotel bar. State bar associations and other law groups maintain email discussion lists which are queried for drug expert referrals. There are also a number of business services that can locate an expert witness in Pharmacology for a fee. These services are the results that show up first in an online search for drug experts and are first in the ads promoted by Google. Conversely, there are free online listings of expert witnesses in Pharmacology in which the expert witness has paid a listing fee. Either of these online methods for finding an expert may yield a competent and knowledgeable drug expert. However, these listings are mainly of forensic psychiatrists and other clinicians who are not drug experts per se. A perusal of these online listings reveals that most drug experts are full-time professionals who are generalists, mostly retired clinicians, or those that do not hold a current academic or institutional appointment. They may not have had complete training in Pharmacology which is needed to be a true drug expert. Such heavily advertised and exorbitantly expensive professionals may be considered by the judge or the jury as "hired guns."[31]

The best drug experts are those with a Ph.D. degree in Pharmacology. This is not a personal bias but a logical conclusion based on graduate training in Pharmacology, which is the study of drugs. There is no other professional training program that exposes the budding drug expert to a more comprehensive knowledge of drugs. A doctorate in Pharmacology is awarded after 2–4 years of coursework and another 2–4 years of drug research. Medical students receive a single course in Pharmacology, often a watered-down version of the Pharmacology course taught to graduate students. After medical students become physicians, their updated knowledge of drugs primarily comes from pharmaceutical representatives or industry-sponsored continuing education conferences.[32] Unfortunately, studies show that many physicians are often unfamiliar with the FDA-approved indications for the drugs they prescribe.[33] Physicians simply do not have the broad and deep knowledge of drug principles and drug action held by a Pharmacologist.[34] There are also some professionals with a Ph.D. in Toxicology, a subdiscipline of Pharmacology, or a Pharm.D. degree from a pharmacy school that are broadly trained

---

[29] From the Federal Workplace Drug Testing Mandatory Guidelines as implemented by the Substance Abuse and Mental Health Services Administration (SAMHSA), a division within the U.S. Department of Health & Human Services. See Phan HM et al. (2012) Drug testing in the workplace. Pharmacother. 32:649–656.

[30] GC-MS stands for gas chromatography-mass spectrophotometry which is a sophisticated method that ionizes drug molecules and identifies chemical structure by retention times in the machine and quantifies the amount of drug present by the height of the peaks on the chromatogram. This can be made clearer to the jury or judge by analogies and further testimony provided by the drug expert.

[31] There are many experts that only work as expert witnesses, advertising on slick websites, and charging exorbitant fees which contributes to the notion of a "hired gun." This book suggests that attorneys use academic Pharmacology professors, or equivalent professionals, employed at a public or private medical or pharmacy schools as their drug expert for reasons of fiscal containment and drug expert credibility.

[32] For example, a 2009 survey found that that 57% of new drugs are first learned of by physicians from pharmaceutical reps and 66% of physicians almost always or often use reps to help make prescribing decisions. Anderson BL (2009) Factors associated with physicians' reliance on pharmaceutical sales representatives. Acad. Med. 84:994–1002.

[33] Chen DT et al. (2009) U.S. physician knowledge of the FDA-approved indications and evidence base for commonly prescribed drugs: results of a national survey. Pharmacoepidemiol. Drug Saf. 18:1094–1100.

[34] No slight intended to my physician colleagues; I couldn't diagnose most diseases or take out an appendix if my life depended on it.

in pharmacological principles with a medical focus that would also serve as excellent drug experts. We will see in a later chapter that there is case law supporting the admissibility of pharmacologists vis-à-vis pharmacists (see Chapter 14).

The simplest and quickest way to find a drug expert is by calling the Department of Pharmacology, or a similarly named entity, at the closest medical school. The head of the Pharmacology department, the Chair, will often be willing to take on a case or may know someone in the department who has experience as a ligation consultant or expert witness. Pharmacology faculty wishing to pursue an avocation as a drug expert should convey this desire to their Chairs. Lawyers can initiate their search for a drug expert by calling the general number of the medical school and will be patched through to the Pharmacology department. Even easier, the reader may consult Appendix A at the end of this book which contains a listing of contact information for pharmacology departments in all U.S. medical schools. Attorneys can also find drug experts by searching pharmacology faculty webpages of these listed medical schools. The pharmacology faculty webpage will often include a CV and list legal consulting activities. The CV stands for curriculum *vitae*, Latin for "course of life." The CV is often a "padded" document used in academia and medicine instead of the more reasonable and common *résumé* used in other occupations.

On occasion, the attorney may need to encourage a first-time litigation consultant or coax a drug expert out of the ivory towers of academia and medicine. Academic scientists live in a world of futile grant applications, long delays in publication, repetitive committee meetings, and constant deadlines. The last thing they may want to do is to spend their precious time working with and for an attorney. However, many will be lured to the task by the intellectual challenge of the case, a sense of civic duty to participate in the legal system, or the potential for a hefty extra paycheck. Most academic faculty contacted by an attorney will be amazed that someone actually called them on the phone and knew who they were.

The Drug Expert's Initial Contact With an Attorney

The average Pharmacology faculty member is not generally known to the public and will be surprised to get a call from an attorney. It is one of the goals of this book that prosecutors, defense attorneys, and public defenders will utilize more drug experts in their cases and that pharmacologists will end up getting more phone calls.

On the phone, the attorney will lay out the general details of the case and possible drug issues, and ask the drug expert for his or her thoughts on the case. If the case revolves around a common drug-legal issue, like wrongful death due to opioid overdose, the expert may reply with preliminary thoughts or a hypothesis, but quickly adds that current research into any drug issue needs to be done before a final opinion can be rendered. The drug expert is not a real-time expert on every aspect of all drugs or any specific drug issue. The river of knowledge moves swiftly past us and each draw of its waters gives a new taste.[35] Drug expertise comes from a solid foundation in pharmacology and continued education in the field, and an up-to-date research and reading of the pertinent medical and pharmacology journals. Before that is accomplished, a drug expert is not drug expert enough to offer a solid opinion.

To put it another way, the attorney does not engage a drug expert fully formed. The drug expert only becomes a drug expert for the issue at hand after completion of his or her research on the particular drug issue. Attorneys hire a "future" drug expert if you will. The attorney should tread cautiously when encountering a drug expert who appears to be able to expound fully upon any drug issue at first mention. There is simply too much information coming in on every scientific front for anyone to be fully up to date in pharmacology and toxicology knowledge until the actual research and reading dozens of journal articles and reviews is done. The goal of the drug expert's testimony is that every statement and finding is based on the best evidence from a thorough research into the drug issues at hand.

The drug expert should be watchful for an overly protracted initial phone call. While the drug expert can and should offer enough scientific expertise to assure the lawyer of the value of a potential consultation, there are two reasons why the initial phone call should be short and sweet. Firstly, as mentioned above, there are few pharmacologists that are current on all the medical and forensic research that may be pertinent to the drug issues at hand. Pharmacologists have special areas of expertise, by nature of their specific research and scholarly areas of interest, but it is not likely that the lawyer will find or need the one or two people in the nation with the special area of expertise that is perfectly aligned with the drug issue brought to bear in the case at hand. For example, the lawyer in a case involving opioid overdose in a wrongful death suit does not need to employ the most expert pharmacologist in the nation that has actually done the clinical research on opioid overdose in humans. An academic or medical school pharmacologist is well versed in the research methods to gain the special expertise needed in the current case.

---

[35] In other words, science in general advances at a rapid pace and new information about drug use and abuse and drug effects are constantly being published in the scientific journals and no expert is up to date without researching the latest findings.

The second reason why the initial phone call should be short is that a small minority of lawyers will want free expert advice during the case assessment phase. While drug experts will extend professional courtesy to speak with an attorney to rule out cases that clearly may not be fruitful,[36] at some point in the conversation the drug expert may need to tell the attorney that he or she believes that they can be helpful on the case and offer to send a letter of engagement to get the ball rolling.

[Narrative continued]
The medical examiner obtained a postmortem peripheral blood sample from Jimmy Cattoni in the morgue. Preliminary screening revealed a presumptive positive test for cannabinoids and confirmatory testing using GC/MS gave a THC blood concentration of 2.2 ng/mL. The drug expert noted that THC concentrations was lower than usually found after recent marijuana smoking. Smoking marijuana results in rapid absorption with peak THC blood reaching 80–160 ng/mL during smoking and fall below 5 ng/mL by 2 h after smoking marijuana.[37] Marijuana use in the past was likely, but the low levels of THC in the decedent's blood sample suggested that marijuana intoxication was not present at the time of the shooting. Because a half-empty bottle of Benadryl® was found at the crime scene, additional tests specific for diphenhydramine were ran. Diphenhydramine showed a concentration of 580 ng/mL in the postmortem blood sample from the decedent. The normal therapeutic levels of diphenhydramine after taking Benadryl® range from about 50–100 ng/mL and blood concentrations of diphenhydramine greater than 5000 ng/mL are considered potentially lethal.[38] The drug expert concluded more likely than not that the decedent took 5–6 times more than the recommended doses of Benadryl® the night of his death. Furthermore, the known anticholinergic effects of high dose diphenhydramine is consistent with the agitation and psychotic behavior exhibited by Jimmy Cattoni. The findings that Jimmy Cattoni more likely than not abused Benadryl® on the night of the incident, and that the decedents psychotic behavior was more likely than not caused or exacerbated by Benadryl® abuse did not exculpate the Police Department for their lethal actions according to the jurors. The jury found recklessness, excessive force, and deliberate indifference by the Police, resulting in the case settling on appeal for damages of $680,000 awarded to the parents of Jimmy Cattoni.

---

[36] For example, an attorney once contacted me about obtaining evidentiary blood levels of oxycodone from a corpse after being in the ground for five years. I told him that there is no blood left as it was replaced by embalming fluid and that a hair sample might work better. I never heard from him again.

[37] Huestis MA et al. (1992) Blood cannabinoids. I. Absorption of THC and formation of 11-OH-THC and THCCOOH during and after smoking marijuana. J Anal Toxicol. 16:276–282.

[38] Pragst F et al. (2006) Poisonings with diphenhydramine—a survey of 68 clinical and 55 death cases. Forensic Sci Int. 161:189–197.

Chapter 3

Show Me the Money: Epilepsy drugs and the four million dollar embezzlement

Overview of the Legal Infrastructure—Movement of Drugs in the Body

Epilepsy, Antiepileptic Drugs, and the Law—Adverse Brain Effects of Phenobarbital

Drug Use and Criminal Responsibility—The Drug Expert Letter of Engagement

[Narrative]

In this criminal case, 52-year-old Elizabeth Branson was charged with embezzlement while working as a Vice-President at a local bank. Ms. Branson did not have a criminal record, was married, and a mother of two children. The U.S. Attorney had evidence that Elizabeth Branson embezzled $3,786,044 by obtaining home equity loans using her bank client's properties, then transferring the loan funds into her own private account. The trial was over in a few days with little defense offered. Ms. Branson cooperated with the prosecution to an unprecedented degree. She was found guilty on all counts and the presentencing report suggested a prison term of up to 30 years.

Medical records obtained by the public defender showed that Ms. Branson was treated with unremitting, daily doses of the antiepileptic drug, phenobarbital, since she was first diagnosed with epilepsy at the age of eight. Toxicology reports ordered by one of her new doctors documented the high concentrations of phenobarbital in blood samples from Ms. Branson. The public defender petitioned the Court for the appointment of a drug expert for the sentencing phase of trial. The public defender obtained approval from the court to hire a local pharmacologist to examine the medical records and to interpret the phenobarbital concentration in blood samples obtained from the defendant. The drug expert also researched the adverse effects of phenobarbital on the brain and behavior, especially after long-term exposure.

Overview of the Legal Infrastructure

This brief overview of the legal system is not meant to be detailed enough for the reader to pass the bar exam in any state. However, it is helpful for review or to introduce readers to the different types of courts that the drug expert may encounter. The court system in the United States is built upon a hierarchical infrastructure that recognizes the sovereign power of both federal and state governments.[1] The U.S. federal court system is the simplest, with three levels of hierarchy. The initial trial courts of the federal court system are the 94 U.S. district courts, each with their own geographic jurisdiction. Each state has at least one federal district court, some large and largely populated states have two or more. In 2018 there were 389,226 cases filed in U.S. district courts, broken down into 82,675 (21%) criminal cases and 278,721 (79%) civil cases.[2] The civil cases in U.S. district courts include contract, real property, tort, antitrust, bankruptcy, and civil rights cases. Criminal cases in U.S. district courts are mostly drug offenses, followed by immigration, property (fraud, larceny and theft, embezzlement), and firearms and explosives offenses.

Overseeing the initial trial (district) courts are the intermediate appellate courts which adjudicate any appeals handed up from the U.S. district courts. There are 13 regional intermediate appellate courts, called collectively the U.S. Circuit

---

[1] Much of the following overview comes from Baumgras (2010) The basic legal structure and organization. In Miller NS (Ed.) *Principles of Addiction and the Law*, Academic Press: Elsevier, London, Burlington, San Diego.

[2] From the US Courts government website at *www.uscourts.gov*.

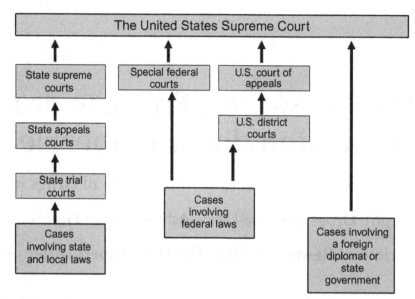

FIG. 3.1 U.S. legal infrastructure overview.

Courts of Appeals. Appeals from these intermediate appellate courts may be heard by the single highest court of the land, the Supreme Court of the United States (SCOTUS), should they deign to do so.[3]

Understanding the state court system is not as simple (see Fig. 3.1). Initial state trial courts go by a variety of different names in different states, and some states do not have an intermediate appeals court.[4] Unlike the federal court system, state court structure is not mandated by the U.S. Constitution or Congressional Law but rather by the individual state's constitution or legislation. However, most states mimic the three-tier system of the federal courts with state trial courts (county or state district courts), state intermediate appeals courts, and state supreme courts. California follows the federal model of courts closely, changing only the names of the courts with their California trial courts called Superior Courts, followed by the California Courts of Appeal, and finally the California Supreme Court. Other states, such as Oklahoma, have two courts of last resort, one for civil appeals (Oklahoma Supreme Court) and one for criminal appeals (Oklahoma Court of Criminal Appeals). Eight states have no intermediate appellate courts and appeals from initial trial courts go directly to the state supreme court. Appeals from the highest court of any state may be taken up by SCOTUS, should they choose to do so.

There are 15,916 initial trial courts at the state and local level in the United States.[5] More than half of these courts are special jurisdiction courts, like municipal courts ("traffic courts" but they also handle city ordinances and fines), tax courts, probate and estate courts, juvenile and family courts, and other specialized types of courts. Drug courts are a type of special jurisdiction court and serve to apply a treatment model to an otherwise punitive legal system.[6] A defendant under drug court supervision forms the narrative basis for a chapter case later in the book.[7]

Four states have special administrative courts with the narrow jurisdiction of adjudicating workmen's compensation claims. The state of Montana has one, and Colorado has seven, Water Courts exclusively mandated to handle water-rights claims and adjustments. The state of Maryland has the only so-named Orphan's Court, which is the state's probate court and also has jurisdiction over the guardianships of minors.[8] The remaining state trial courts are general jurisdiction trial courts, variously known as circuit, district, county, justice of the peace, or superior courts depending on the state. These initial state trial courts number about 5000.

---

[3] SCOTUS gets thousands of appeals (*Petitions for Writ of Certiorari*) sent to it each year and accepts only a small fraction of them (around 1%). Additionally, even that small fraction has decreased dramatically (58% reduction) since the 1980s which can be traced to a new crop of justices appointed between 1986 and 1993. See Stras DR (2009) The supreme court's declining plenary docket: a membership-based explanation, Constitutional Commentary, Minnesota Legal Studies, Research Paper No. 09–39.

[4] Much of the following information comes from the National Center for State Courts at *www.ncsc.org.*

[5] National Center for State Courts at *www.ncsc.org.*

[6] See Hora PF, Stalcup T (2008) Drug treatment courts in the twenty-first century. Georgia Law Review 42:719–811.

[7] See Chapter 5 *Wrong Place at the Wrong Time.*

[8] The Orphan's Court was established before statehood and its name derives from the old City of London's Court for Widows and Orphans. Lord Baltimore recapitulated this court system with the founding of his colony in the New World. It is one of the oldest continuously operating courts in the United States today. From Judge Lawler, "About the Orphans' Court" at *mdcourts.gov.*

Over the last few generations, growth in the reach of the federal criminal code created a huge overlap between federal and state criminal justice, especially in the areas of drug and gun laws. Federal prosecution of criminal cases increased 25% in the last decade. The rate of federal prison incarceration, largely due to drug offenses, increased nearly 300% in the last twenty years, while state prison incarceration rate "only" increased about 130% in the same time period.[9] According to legal scholars, this growth in federal caseload results from the U.S. political system such that lawmakers place great symbolic value in hardening criminal legislation, with the expanding federal criminal docket having little impact on the federal budget.[10] Illegal drugs and legal controlled substances are regulated by both federal and state drug laws. For the drug defendant, the same conduct could lead to criminal charges in federal court, in state court, or both. Federal drug prosecution often follows state prosecution and leads to significantly longer prison sentencing. Federal enhancements to drug sentences, such as prior drug convictions, can produce mandatory life sentences for small amounts of seized drugs.[11] Such drug offenses prosecuted in state courts may yield less draconian sentences.

Because of the "dual sovereign" clause in the U.S. Constitution pertaining to the "double jeopardy" protection, both the state and the federal government can try and convict a defendant for the same criminal act. This apparent "double jeopardy" violation is justified by the rationale that the criminal act is wrong against two distinct entities: the people of the state and the people of the nation.[12] In drug cases, both state and federal authorities may file charges, then decide who will pursue the case and who will wait. Or they may agree in advance that only one will file charges. If no agreement is reached and both state and federal prosecutors file charges, federal law requires state prosecutions to be suspended while a federal case arising from the same incident is pending, even if the charges differ. However, in 2018 there were about 389,226 criminal and civil cases filed in federal district courts but about 84 million cases filed in all the state trial courts across the nation.[13] Unlike the federal trial courts, state trial courts see roughly an equal number of civil and criminal cases. As a whole, more than 99% of all criminal and civil litigation in the United States occurs in state trial courts. The drug expert will become most familiar with state trial courts and appear before state trial court judges; however, drug experts will occasionally find themselves in federal district courts.[14]

Movement of Drugs in the Body

This section could more formally be titled "Pharmacokinetics" as this one word sums up the principles of the movement of drugs in the body (Greek derivation: *pharmaco*, drug, and *kinesis*, movement).[15] After administration of a drug, say by swallowing a pill, the drug molecules first dissolve out of the pill, move across the wall of the gut, get transported into the liver, move out of the liver and into the main bloodstream, make numerous circulations around the body and brain, and finally move out through the kidneys into the urine. Most drugs or drug metabolites ultimately move out from the bladder into the water system of the municipality. There is now such a vast consumption of drugs that assaying drug levels in municipal water systems is a way to determine the prevalence of legal and illegal drug use among city populations.[16]

The following four aspects of drug movement in the body, pharmacokinetics, are considered independently, but in reality may be occurring at the same time after drug administration: absorption, distribution, metabolism, and elimination.

Absorption of a drug refers to the process of a drug getting into the bloodstream. As most drugs are swallowed, it is easy to imagine absorption when the drug molecules cross the gut wall and are sucked into the bloodstream in small blood vessels just behind the gut cells. Other ways of taking drugs, or routes of administration, include an intramuscular shot with a needle, usually given into the deltoid muscle of the shoulder or the *gluteus maximus* of the buttocks. Absorption in this case is visualized as the

---

[9] Wright RF (2006) Federal or state? Sorting as a sentencing choice. Criminal Justice, Summer issue, pp. 16–21.

[10] See Gray J (2014) Why Our Drug Laws Have Failed and What We Can Do about It: A Judicial Indictment of the War on Drugs (2nd Edition). Temple University Press, Philadelphia.

[11] See Chapter 11 for details on Federal Drug Sentencing Guidelines.

[12] In *Bartkus v. Illinois*, 359 U.S. 121 (1959), SCOTUS affirmed that serial federal and state trials were not unconstitutional under the "double jeopardy" clause. However, later cases such as *Rinaldi v. United States*, 434 U.S. 22 (1977) and *Petite v. United States*, 361 U.S. 529 (1960) established guidelines for the exercise of discretion by the Department of Justice in federal prosecution based on substantially the same act(s) involved in a prior state or federal proceeding (U.S. Attorneys' Manual §9–2.031).

[13] State trial court caseload numbers were from 2016, the latest data available at: *www.courtstatistics.org*.

[14] There are slightly different sets of rules regarding discovery, litigation reports, and expert witness qualifications among federal and state trial courts, discussed in later chapters.

[15] See generally Brenner GM, Stevens CW (2018) *Brenner and Stevens' Pharmacology, 5th Ed.*, Elsevier: Philadelphia, PA.

[16] For example, studies of the 50 largest wastewater treatment plants serving cities across the United States detected over 60 active pharmaceutical drugs. The prescription opioid analgesics, hydrocodone and oxycodone, were detected in all city water systems surveyed. From Kostich MS, Batt AL, Lazorchak JM (2014) Concentrations of prioritized pharmaceuticals in effluents from 50 large wastewater treatment plants in the US. Environ. Poll. 184:354–9.

drug leaving the muscle tissue and sucked up into the bloodstream of the small vessels supplying the muscles. Other routes, such as snorting (known officially as *insufflation*) deliver the drug molecules onto moist nasal membranes which are then absorbed into underlying blood vessels. Ditto the route of drug administration by smoking, which presents the large surface area of the lungs for drug absorption. Many illegal drugs are shot up directly into blood vessels, by the IV or intravenous route, initially in the arm and, as vessels contract from repeated needling, eventually smaller veins between the toes and in more private parts. With the IV route of administration, there is no drug absorption phase as the drug enters the bloodstream directly.

The distribution phase of the drug is the process of getting the drug from the bloodstream out to the drug's site of action or the rest of the body. For drugs acting on the brain, this means getting the drug into the blood vessels of the brain and onto the brain neurons. The brain is a privileged organ, surrounded by a line of defense called the blood-brain barrier. It is not easy to get drugs into the brain, and the development of many CNS-active medications often comes to a grinding halt in the pharmaceutical industry when a test drug does not cross the blood-brain barrier.[17] The various CNS drugs that are abused have no problems crossing the blood-brain barrier and targeting reward pathways and pleasure centers in the brain.

Drug metabolism is based on a complex system of metabolic enzymes, primarily located in the great detoxifier organ, the liver. The parent drug, that is the original drug taken or administered, is changed to different chemical molecules during metabolism, called drug metabolites. In general, drug metabolism produces drug metabolites that are more water soluble so that they can easily pass into the urine and be excreted. In some cases, drug metabolites, instead of the parent drug, are tested in drug use cases as they may persist in the body much longer. Some drug metabolites may be more active at the target drug receptor than the parent drugs, the so-named active metabolites, and contribute to the overall drug effect. Drug metabolism is variable according to each individual's genetic makeup, as many studies show that drug effects differ in people with different drug metabolic enzymes. A common gene-based phenomenon is the different rate of drug metabolism due to genetic makeup, which spawned the whole field of pharmacogenomics.[18]

Elimination of drug is the final step in the movement of drugs throughout the body. Most drugs and their metabolites are excreted in the urine and eliminated by that route. Other drugs exit through the other, more primitive fecal waste system. A few drugs are famous by their elimination route, namely ethanol, which partially leaves the body though expired air and is detectable by an external Breathalyzer-type instrument.[19]

The drug expert should review the established literature and current research about the movement of the drug in the body for each drug in a particular case. It is essential and foundational knowledge for every drug, legal or illegal, that should be considered and compared to the specific drug information of the case in hand.

Epilepsy, Antiepileptic Drugs, and the Law

Epilepsy is a serious brain disease that is characterized by the onset of various seizures and convulsions. The brain event that triggers the onset of a seizure is unknown in many types of epilepsy.[20] However, the trigger is known in rarer types of seizure disorders called "reflex epilepsies." For example, persons with strobe-induced epilepsy begin seizing and convulsing while riding in a car watching the sunlight flicker through the trees. A personal favorite is "hot water epilepsy," most prevalent in Mid-Eastern and Asian populations, which causes seizures by pouring hot water over the head, like in a bathtub or shower.[21]

The seizures that jerk the arms and legs of the untreated epileptic are the outward signs of aberrant brain function. Epilepsy is caused by the misfiring of millions of neurons and the outward effects of such brain dysfunction depend on which part of the brain is misfiring. When neurons in the part of the brain that control muscle activity in the limbs are involved in the seizure, loss of voluntary motor control occurs sometimes accompanied by a loss of consciousness. With no great surprise, the drugs used to treat epilepsy are drugs that reduce the stimulation of brain neurons, generally classified as CNS depressants. The drugs used to treat epilepsy are called antiepileptic drugs or AEDs, and include older, classic drugs like phenytoin (Dilantin®) and carbamazepine (Tegretol®), and a surprising number of new AEDs in the last decade.[22] Another class of CNS depressant drugs used to treat epilepsy are the sedative-hypnotic agents. Sedative-hypnotics

---

[17] Pardridge WM (2005) The Blood-Brain Barrier: Bottleneck in Brain Drug Development, NeuroRx 2:3–14.

[18] Wang L, McLeod HL, Weinshilboum RM (2011) Genomics and drug response, N Engl J Med 364:1144–53.

[19] Breathalyzer is a trade-marked name but due to its popularity is also used more generically for any alcohol breath-testing device. Prof. Robert Borkenstein of Indiana University invented the first truly practical and reliable breath-testing instrument, the Breathalyzer, in 1954. Swartz J (2004) Breath Testing for Prosecutors: Targeting Hardcore Impaired Drivers. American Prosecutors Research Institute, Alexandria, VA.

[20] Xu D, Miller SD, Koh S (2013) Immune mechanisms in epileptogenesis. Front Cell Neurosci 7:1–8.

[21] Patel M, Satishchandra P, et al. (2014) Hot water epilepsy: Phenotype and single photon emission computed tomography observations. Ann Indian Acad Neurol 17:470–2.

[22] The surge recently in newer seizure medications may also be related to increase markets of these drugs for other nonseizure indications. For a review of new AEDs and drug development, see Löscher W, Klitgaard H et al. (2014) New avenues for anti-epileptic drug discovery and development. Curr Treat Options Neurol 16:757–76.

include benzodiazepines, like diazepam (Valium®) and alprazolam (Xanax®), and older barbiturate drugs, like thiopental (Pentothal®) and phenobarbital (Luminal®). Sedative-hypnotic agents used to treat epilepsy include diazepam (Valium®), lorazepam (Ativan®), and phenobarbital (Luminal®).

Antiepileptic drugs are one of the more dangerous drug classes used for therapeutic benefit. AEDs produce a number of adverse effects on the body and the brain, although newer AEDs have less side effects and are better tolerated than older drugs.[23] The adverse effects of AEDs are not limited to epileptic patients. There is strong preclinical evidence and human epidemiological data that show AED use during pregnancy leads to increased fetal malformations.[24]

Epilepsy, automatism, and the law

Common law is based on the assumption that all behavior of an individual is voluntary and that the individual is consciously aware of the act.[25] This basic assumption of voluntary behavior and consciousness is then whittled-down in special cases of the intellectually disabled, children, and those suffering from mental illness. More specifically, for criminal liability to be asserted, the prosecution needs to prove beyond a reasonable doubt two conditions: that the criminal act was voluntary (*actus reus*) and that there was intent to commit the crime (*mens rea*).[26]

Epilepsy is noted by seizures that can occur spontaneously and sometimes at inopportune moments, like when driving a car. If such a driver has a seizure and swerves off the roadway onto the sidewalk and kills a pedestrian, the criminal charge of vehicular homicide would rightly be fought with a defense of *automatism*. Automatism occurs when automatic behavior is generated without conscious control or the will to do so.[27] The seizure itself produced the erratic driving behavior and therefore it was not a voluntary act by the driver, likewise there was no mental intent of the epileptic driver to kill a pedestrian. The defense of automatism is also used in crimes committed during sleepwalking (somnambulism), which can include violent assault and homicide.[28] A close ally of the automatism defense is the "diminished capacity" defense where all or some part of conscious intent and/or voluntary behavior is compromised.[29]

Adverse Brain Effects of Phenobarbital

Phenobarbital is a prominent member of the barbiturate class of sedative-hypnotic drugs and is used clinically as an antiepileptic (a.k.a. anticonvulsant or antiseizure) drug. Phenobarbital produces its antiepileptic effect by quieting the brain cells (neurons) that are abnormally active during an epileptic seizure. Phenobarbital is a second-line or third-line drug for use in treating epilepsy and is the oldest of all currently used antiepileptic medicines. A "second-line" drug means that doctors should first consider another antiepileptic agent for treating epilepsy before using phenobarbital; "third-line" means that other drugs and drug combinations should be tried before use of phenobarbital.

Phenobarbital was first marketed by the Bayer Company as Luminal® in 1912 but lost exclusive patent rights long ago and is available from various manufacturers as a generic drug.[30] Its use in the United States and other developed countries has declined due to its well-known toxic effects, but in poorer nations and most of the world, it is still the most commonly used antiepileptic drug.[31] Phenobarbital is supplied in various formulations such as tablets (pills), elixirs (syrups), and injectable forms. The pills are the most common formulation and come in dosage strengths from 15 to 100 mg per tablet. Phenobarbital, like other sedative-hypnotic drugs, is often abused and therefore available by prescription only. As discussed further in the ultimate chapter of this book, phenobarbital is a member of the barbiturate family and a close cousin to thiopental and pentobarbital, drugs famous for their use in lethal drug executions.

The recommended dosage range for the treatment of epilepsy is 50–100 mg given two or three times daily.[32] Phenobarbital is an extremely long-acting drug with a 5–7 day elimination half-life, the time it takes until half the amount of given drug

---

[23] Bialer M, White HS (2010) Key factors in the discovery and development of new antiepileptic drugs. Nat Rev Drug Discov 9:68–82.

[24] Etemad L, Moshiri M, Moallem SA (2012) Epilepsy drugs and effects on fetal development: Potential mechanisms. J Res Med Sci 17:876–81.

[25] Denno D (2009) Consciousness and culpability in American criminal law. Waseda Proc Comp Law 14:115–126.

[26] *Actus reus* and *mens rea* are Latin terms that translate to "guilty act" and "guilty mind," respectively. In "strict liability" crimes, like statutory rape, the *mens rea* condition or intent does not need to be proved to convict. See Edersheim JG, Brendel RW, Price BH (2012) Neuroimaging, diminished capacity and mitigation. In Simpson JR, *Neuroimaging in Forensic Psychiatry: From the Clinic to the Courtroom*, John Wiley & Sons, Ltd: Hoboken, NJ.

[27] McLeod HJ, Byrne MK, Aitken R (2004) Automatism and dissociation: Disturbances of consciousness and volition from a psychological perspective. Int. J. Law Psych. 27:471–487.

[28] Rolnick J, Parvizi J (2011) Automatisms: bridging clinical neurology with criminal law. Epilepsy Behav. 20:423–427.

[29] Morse SJ (1979) Diminished capacity: a moral and legal conundrum. Int. J. Law Psych. 2:271–298.

[30] López-Muñoz F, Ucha-Udabe R, Alamo C (2005) The history of barbiturates a century after their clinical introduction. Neuropsych. Dis. Treat. 1: 329–343.

[31] Kwan P, Brodie MJ (2004) Phenobarbital for the treatment of epilepsy in the 21st century: a critical review. Epilepsia 45:1141–1149.

[32] Phenobarbital Prescribing Information, available from generic manufacturer West-Ward Pharmaceuticals at *www.west-ward.com*.

is metabolized and removed from the body. The target therapeutic level in the blood for phenobarbital is 15–40 μg/mL (micrograms per milliliter) and concentrations above 30 μg/mL are associated with severe adverse and toxic effects.[33]

It is well known from the medical literature that the adverse or toxic effects of phenobarbital for the treatment of epilepsy severely limit the use of this drug. This is the reason that phenobarbital is considered a second- or third-line drug for epilepsy treatment. In fact, one report states that phenobarbital "is almost never used now, except for people with mental retardation."[34] The likelihood of toxic effects is greater at higher doses of phenobarbital. Acute adverse effects of phenobarbital include central nervous system (CNS) depression, sedation, drowsiness, dizziness, and lethargy. When phenobarbital is given on a long-term or chronic regimen, the toxic effects include clinical depression and changes in cognitive behavior, including memory problems, motor performance, and impaired attention and concentration.[35] In this regard, phenobarbital has been noted to have the greatest effects on cognitive behavior and be worse than other antiepileptic agents in producing these toxic cognitive effects.[36]

The cognitive effects of long-term therapy with phenobarbital for the treatment of epilepsy were noted as early at 1983 when it is was stated that phenobarbital may cause hyperactivity, behavioral problems, sedation, and even dementia.[37] An additional paper from this time noted that phenobarbital and other antiepileptic medications produce adverse effects on the brain that include all categories of psychiatric symptomatology, including disturbances of consciousness (delirium, confusion), psychotic state (schizophrenia-like psychosis, affective disorder), neurotic state, behavior, and character disorder.[38] There is evidence that chronic use of older antiepileptic drugs like phenobarbital can produce structural changes in the brain leading to cognitive deficits.[39] Other chronic adverse effects of phenobarbital include problems with connective tissue, especially in the shoulders and hands, and a unique hand ligament problem called Dupuytren's contracture.

Drug Use and Criminal Responsibility

Prescription and illegal drugs are new technology. Like the latest iPhone® model, each new blockbuster drug is heavily marketed, may have only slight improvements to previous versions, and usually costs more. Like new technology, drugs are part of the mainstream culture, a part of everyday life. The concept of a "drug subculture" is dead, there remains just drug culture which is American culture. The surge of legal and illegal drug use to the status of an entrenched cultural phenomenon was not foreseen by Congress or the U.S. Sentencing Commission, or state and local governments. There are many instances where the law has not caught up to scientific knowledge, including the effects of drugs on brain and behavior. The topic of drug use and diminished capacity is introduced here and will be taken up in greater depth in future chapters.

Drug use as diminished capacity

At one extreme, no one is held responsible for altered behavior due to involuntary intoxication from a drug.[40] If someone surreptitiously slips a sedative-hypnotic drug into your drink, and after you finish it you get into a vehicle, run off the road and kill someone, you would not be guilty of a crime. Like automatism discussed before, involuntary intoxication is an affirmative defense in this case. Similar reasoning applies in individuals diagnosed with auto-brewery syndrome, a rare but real medical condition where overgrowth of yeast in the gut creates enough endogenous ethanol that the person becomes intoxicated without drinking anything.[41] There is also a rare psychiatric phenomenon called pathological intoxication, where extremely low doses of drugs can produce an overwhelming intoxication. Pathological intoxication is most known in cases of alcohol use, but could also occur with other drugs.[42]

---

[33] Tolman JA, Faulkner MA (2011) Treatment options for refractory and difficult to treat seizures: focus on vigabatrin. Ther. Clin. Risk Manag. 7: 367–75.

[34] The preferred term now is intellectually disabled. The quoted author is probably referring to those with Lennox-Gastaut syndrome, a severe brain disorder noted by intellectual disability and seizures. From Poindexter AR (2000) Phenobarbital, propranolol, and aggression. J. Neuropsychiatry Clin. Neurosci. 12:413.

[35] Schmidt D (2009) Drug treatment of epilepsy: options and limitations. Epilep.Behav. 15: 56–65.

[36] Eddy CM, Rickards HE, Cavanna AE (2011) The cognitive impact of antiepileptic drugs. Ther. Adv. Neuro. Dis. 4: 385–407.

[37] Iivanainen M, Savolainen H (1983) Side effects of phenobarbital and phenytoin during long-term treatment of epilepsy. Acta Neurol. Scand. Supplement 97: 49–67.

[38] Kato H (1983) Antiepileptic drugs and psychiatric disorders: mechanism involved in manifestation of psychic symptoms of high blood level of antiepileptics. Folia Psych. Neurol. Japan 37: 283–289.

[39] Bortz JJ (2003) Neuropsychiatric and memory issues in epilepsy. Mayo Clinic Proc. 78: 781–787.

[40] Involuntary intoxication is discussed more fully in Chapter 14.

[41] Kaji H, Asanuma Y et al. (1976) The auto-brewery syndrome-the repeated attacks of alcoholic intoxication due to the overgrowth of *Candida* (*albicans*) in the gastrointestinal tract. Mater Med Pol 8:429–35.

[42] Pathological intoxication with alcohol was brought to the public's attention by the 1992 movie "Final Analysis" starring Richard Gere and Kim Basinger. Although the defense of pathological intoxication was used by Kim Basinger's lawyer to get her off the hook for a murder charge, some experts disagree if the condition really exists. See Tiffany LP, Tiffany M (1990) Nosologic objections to the criminal defense of pathological intoxication. Int J Law Pysch 13:49–75.

Defense of altered brain and behavior leading to civil or criminal charges that are due to everyday drug use is not as clear. The "drug made me do it" defense is a type of *diminished capacity* defense, which harkens back to the keystone concept of *means rea*, or the mental capacity, for one to be culpable for a criminal offense or civil action.[43] Diminished capacity due to drug use, or sometimes called diminished responsibility, is different from an all-out insanity defense.[44]

The Drug Expert Letter of Engagement

Once the attorney and his or her client decide to solicit the opinion or testimony of a drug expert, the first step for the drug expert is to draft a letter of engagement. The letter of engagement is a contract between the attorney and the drug expert, signed by both parties.

Two issues are essential to the letter of engagement: the nature of the work and an hourly rate schedule. The letter of engagement first spells out the nature of consultancy and stresses that trials and depositions need to be scheduled by joint arrangement. A sample of this language is given here; a complete letter of engagement is provided in Appendix B.

> *The purpose of this letter is to confirm my engagement as a Pharmacology expert witness/litigation consultant for you and the firm. I will act in the capacity of a consultant in performing the services that you request of me on matters relevant to the above-mentioned case, including phone consultations and office meetings, research, analysis, litigation reports, and other consulting services as you deem necessary. In addition, I will also be available, at your request and in accordance to our joint arrangement and schedules, to testify as an expert witness at a deposition, hearing and/or trial in a civil or criminal action or in any arbitration should such services be needed.*

Secondly, a rate schedule is included in the letter of engagement. The suggested starting rate for drug experts at a public university or medical school is $150–$250 per hour for research, analysis, and preparation of litigation reports. The hourly rate increases to $250–$400 an hour for giving depositions or testifying in court. This rate is dependent on the expert's experience and is conservative, reflecting the innate public service aspect of a drug expert employed by the state university or otherwise publicly funded institution.[45] Reasonable rates also serve to distinguish between a professional who moonlights as a drug expert from the full-time expert witness who does nothing else but seek employment as an expert witness. A retainer is a payment sometimes made by the attorney when engaging the services of an expert witness.[46] It is not needed contractually to establish the attorney-drug expert relationship; that is accomplished by the duly signed letter of engagement. Retainers are usually not needed, except perhaps in large, complex cases involving numerous drugs and drug issues that will take a lot of nights and weekends to complete, or if the drug expert should find that a particular firm is consistently late in providing payments.

It is important to keep track of drug expert cases; a master spreadsheet file in Excel serves that function well and is easily updated. Suggested column headings include case number, attorney name and contact info, date of engagement, case information and filing number, drug issue, invoice date and amount, and date payment received. Most importantly, keeping track of the consulting income is needed for the filing of income taxes. A section in the drug expert's professional CV could list expert witness cases under the subheading of Expert Witness/Litigation Consulting and updated as needed. Under the Federal Rules of Evidence, which we will get to later, the drug expert's CV is submitted during discovery along with a list of previous expert witness cases.[47] Because both the CV and the listing of previous litigation consulting cases are often needed by the court, including the list of drug expert cases in the CV nicely provides a single document. Additionally, consulting as a drug expert is an accomplishment worthy of including on the pharmacologist's professional CV.

---

[43] Huckabee HM (1988) Avoiding the insanity defense strait jacket: the *mens rea* route. Pepp. Law Rev. 15:1–32.

[44] Lack of legal knowledge and fortitude prevents further consideration of "the insanity defense" and drug-induced states. Even though drugs and mental disease can overlap phenotypically (e.g., LSD and schizophrenia both produce hallucinations) and altered behaviors may arise from the same molecular causes in the brain, there is no reason to merge drug-induced diminished capacity into a type of insanity defense as it can advance on its own merit.

[45] Conservative meaning cheap; the average rates for expert witnesses according to a SEAK survey of 1931 experts in 2014 was $333/h for file review and research, and $451/h for depositions and in-court testimony; *www.seak.com/expert-witness-fee-data-form/*. SEAK is a continuing education, publishing, and consulting company for expert witnesses. See Chapter 16 for a fuller description of SEAK and other expert witness training.

[46] In over 80 cases, I have not asked for a retainer and had no problems getting paid after the job was over, even though the check sometimes took a while to arrive. However, I was once given a hefty retainer check from one colorful attorney at an initial meeting in my office; he also purchased the latest edition of my *Pharmacology* textbook right off my bookshelf. Check it out: Brenner GM, Stevens CW (2018) *Pharmacology, 5th Ed.*, Elsevier, Philadelphia PA, USA.

[47] Federal Rules of Civil Procedure implement the Federal Rules of Evidence (FRE) for expert witnesses with the requirement of providing "a list of all other cases in which, during the previous 4 years, the witness testified as an expert at trial or by deposition" among other things. The emphasis on Federal rules and laws here and throughout the book provides a general template for state courts as well, however some states differ in their adherence to the Federal model.

Depending on the timeline, which in some cases can be quite acute, work as a drug expert may begin immediately after receiving the signed letter of engagement and copies of medical records, prescription records, medical examiner's report, toxicology report, or whatever files are provided to the drug expert from the client attorney. The drug expert may also be consulted on what files or records are needed; the basic *modus operandi* is to provide to the drug expert everything the attorney has. Only having the pharmacy records, without the medical records, provides no sure-proof indication of the medical condition that prompted the doctor to write a prescription. Only having the toxicology report without additional pharmacy records provides no indication of how often prescriptions were filled. There are also a number of instances when a statement in an incident report or a clinical note among a mountain of medical records will be essential to the issue at hand. The progress of the drug expert, in some cases, will be held in stasis until complete records are obtained from the client attorney by subpoena or otherwise.

As the drug expert works on the case, careful records of start times and job tasks should be kept on an invoice. This invoice should be updated as the case progresses; it is problematic to wait until the end of the job to compete the invoice, as many months often pass between beginning a case and the end of the drug expert's involvement. The drug expert's invoice may not be as detailed as the typical attorney's invoice with charges broken down to tenths of an hour and including tasks such as reading emails and short phone calls. The drug expert may want to provide such time-limited services for free (*gratis*). A sample of a final billing invoice from a drug expert is included in Appendix C. The invoice notes that payment should be made within 30 days; however, the need to send a second invoice after that time is not unusual.

As a point of clarification, there is a certification program for police officers that leads to a title of Drug Recognition Expert, or DRE.[48] The DRE should not be confused with a drug expert as used in this book. A drug recognition expert is a law enforcement officer who has successfully completed all phases of the Drug Evaluation and Classification (DEC) program training requirements for certification. The DRE is trained to detect persons under the influence of drugs and to identify the category or categories of drugs causing the impairment. Further consideration of DRE and DRE reports are detailed in Chapter 17.

[Narrative continued]

Elizabeth Branson's public defender submitted the drug expert's litigation report to the court for consideration during the sentencing phase of the trial. The drug expert's report highlighted the finding that at the time of defendant's criminal activity, she had taken over 42 years of constant, high dose phenobarbital under the direction of various health care professionals. The drug expert documented the toxic blood levels of phenobarbital present in blood tests ordered by her physician, and the adverse cognitive and behavioral effects of long-term phenobarbital. The drug expert also noted that the medical records contained documented memory and other cognitive deficits of the defendant and that the defendant's hand ligament pathology, called Dupuytren's contracture, is associated with long-term phenobarbital treatment.

The findings reported by the drug expert were considered mitigating factors by the Court and Ms. Forthwright was sentenced to only 4.5 years in the regional Federal penitentiary, with the stipulation that she never work in the banking or finance field again. She was ordered to pay more than $3 million in restitution to the bank's insurer as well as $859,474 to the Internal Revenue Service for unpaid taxes on the embezzled funds.

---

[48] Talpins SK (2004) The Drug Evaluation and Classification (DEC) Program: Targeting Hardcore Impaired Drivers. Americans Prosecutors Research Institute, Alexandria, VA.

Chapter 4

The Power of the Poppy: Opioid overdose in the treatment of pain

Treatment of Cancer Pain With Opioids

Official Prescribing Information for Drugs

Medical Malpractice Due to the Prescribing of Opioids

Federal Rules of Evidence and the Expert—The Drug Expert Litigation Report

[Narrative]

Ms. Wilma Jackson was diagnosed with stage 1 pancreatic cancer in the summer and received two outpatient chemotherapy treatments. In the fall, complaining of increased pain, she returned to the cancer care hospital with her husband. Ms. Jackson also suffered from asthma and chronic obstructive pulmonary disease (COPD). At the hospital, the pain specialist gave her two IV morphine injections for her pain. Later the same day the pain specialist returned and gave Ms. Jackson a fentanyl oral transmucosal lozenge (an opioid "lollipop"). The pain specialist also applied a 75 mg fentanyl transdermal patch to Ms. Jackson, which was removed and replaced with a fresh 75 mg fentanyl patch after 12 h. The physician prescribed two more fentanyl lollipops and ten more fentanyl patches which were filled at the hospital pharmacy when the couple left for home. The couple returned to their home on the edge of town and went to bed.

The next morning, Wilma Jackson was found in her bed unresponsive by her husband with no respiratory movements. Her husband called emergency services, and after attempts to resuscitate her, Ms. Jackson was pronounced dead at the scene. Later, the husband of the deceased filed a civil suit naming the pain specialist and the cancer care hospital corporation for medical malpractice and the wrongful death of his wife.

Treatment of Cancer Pain With Opioids

Opioid drugs maintain their status as the number one "painkillers" or analgesic drugs since their discovery and use over 5000 years ago.[1] Early civilizations knew that the juice obtained from the seed pod of the poppy plant, a sticky white exudate called *opium*, produced potent relief of pain. But it was not until 1806 that morphine was isolated as the main active ingredient in opium. There are a number of well-known opioid analgesic drugs besides morphine including codeine, methadone, hydrocodone (in Lortab®, Norco®, Vicodin®, and others), oxycodone (OxyContin®), and hydromorphone (Dilaudid®).

Heroin is also an opioid drug and activates the same *opioid receptors* as morphine. The heroin molecule is simply morphine with two simple acetyl group additions. Not many realize that Heroin was a brand name drug that was discovered and heavily marketed by the Bayer Corporation. Heroin was freely available at the corner drugstore at the turn of the last century and was widely used as an analgesic and cough suppressant. Due to its high propensity for opioid abuse and dependence, it is now an illegal drug in the United States and most of the world.

Cancer pain is one of the main indications for chronic or long-term use of opioid analgesic drugs.[2] While opioid analgesics are presently the best agents to treat pain and do so quite effectively, they are also a dangerous group of medicines that

---

[1] Brownstein MJ (1993) A brief history of opiates, opioid peptides, and opioid receptors. Proc. Natl. Acad. Sci. USA 90:5391-5393; Trescot AM et al. (2008) Opioid pharmacology. Pain physician 11:S133-S153.

[2] Mayyas F et al. (2010) A systematic review of oxymorphone in the management of chronic pain. Pain Symptom Manag. 39:296-308.

are responsible for many intentional and unintentional fatalities. Opioid analgesics work by inhibiting pain transmission in the brain and spinal cord and by binding to *opioid receptors* on pain neurons.

Morphine and other opioids also bind and activate opioid receptors on other tissues. For example, the presence of opioid receptors on neurons that control the GI tract leads to opioid-induced constipation, a common problem among chronic pain patients treated with opioids. A more deadly problem is that opioids also bind to opioid receptors on brain neurons that control breathing so that opioids produce respiratory depression.[3] With high doses of opioids, breathing ceases and cardiac arrest and brain death ensues. This pharmacological fact underlies the present opioid overdose epidemic.

In the last few decades, there has been a mounting epidemic of overdose deaths due to prescription opioids and fatal respiratory depression.[4] The number of opioid overdose fatalities rapidly increased from 2007 (18,515) to 2017 (47,600) leading to a 2.5-fold increase in annual deaths over 10 years.[5] In many cases, a new formulation of an existing opioid analgesic drug spurred the growth of prescription opioids and increased fatalities. For example, oxycodone is an opioid analgesic that has become one of the most commonly prescribed opioids for cancer pain in the United States mainly due to the aggressive marketing of OxyContin®, a long-acting, controlled release formulation of oxycodone.[6]

Fentanyl transmucosal lozenges (Actiq®) and fentanyl transdermal patches (Duragesic®)

Fentanyl is a synthetic opioid analgesic that is 80-100 times more potent than morphine.[7] Fentanyl is a highly lipophilic, or fat-loving, drug molecule that can be rapidly absorbed through the mouth lining (called the mucosa) or the skin and get into the bloodstream. Actiq® is the trade name of a fentanyl formulation that consists of a lozenge imbued with fentanyl and an attached handle.[8] It is a solid drug lozenge that comes in 200, 400, 600, 800, 1200, and 1600 μg (microgram) of fentanyl dosages. Actiq® is indicated for management of breakthrough pain in cancer patients. Breakthrough pain is reoccurring pain that arises intermittently during the course of chronic pain treatment using a long-acting opioid analgesic formulation. For example, a patient taking one OxyContin® at morning and one at night (providing 24-h opioid coverage) who reports pain at 2 pm is having breakthrough pain.

Duragesic® is the trade name for a transdermal patch of fentanyl that slowly releases fentanyl onto and through the skin, and into the blood to provide continuous analgesia for 3 days.[9] The Duragesic® patch is formulated in 12, 25, 50, 75, and 100 μg/h fentanyl dosages. The fentanyl doses are in μg/h units, micrograms per hour, so this is the amount of fentanyl released onto the skin every hour from the patch, like the grains of sand in an hourglass. Except in this case, the grains of sand are potent fentanyl drug molecules. Duragesic® is indicated for the management of pain in opioid-tolerant patients that is severe enough to require daily, around-the-clock, long-term opioid treatment and for which alternative treatment options are inadequate. Both Actiq® and Duragesic® fentanyl preparations have "Black Box" warnings stating that serious, life-threatening, or fatal respiratory depression may occur with use of these products.

The FDA regulates the approval and safety of prescription drugs marketed in the United States. In reaction to the increasing opioid overdose fatalities, the FDA attempted to curtail the rising opioid overdose epidemic by issuing public health advisories and letters to health care professionals. For example, in the case of fentanyl patches, in July, 2005 the FDA sent out letters to health care providers and the public stressing that the directions on the product label and package insert should be followed exactly in order to avoid overdose.[10] However, the FDA continued to receive reports of deaths and life-threatening side effects after doctors inappropriately prescribed the fentanyl patches or patients incorrectly used them. A second round of public health advisories and FDA alerts sent to health care professionals highlighting the deaths from respiratory depression from the use of fentanyl patches was sent out in December of 2007.[11]

In spite of these repeated warnings and others to health care providers, there was not a drop in in the number of opioid-related fatalities across the nation. This impact of opioid analgesic use and other drugs already on the market, led to

---

[3] White JM, Irvine RJ (1999) Mechanisms of fatal opioid overdose. Addiction 94:961-972.

[4] Bohnert AS et al. (2011) Association between opioid prescribing patterns and opioid overdose-related deaths. J. American Med Assoc 305:1315-1321.

[5] National Institute on Drug Abuse (2019) Overdose death rates, revised January, 2019 at: *www.drugabuse.gov/related-topics/trends-statistics/overdose-death-rates*.

[6] Lexchin J, Kohler JC (2011) The danger of imperfect regulation: OxyContin® use in the United States and Canada. Int J Risk Saf Med. 23:233-40.

[7] Grond S et al. (2000) Clinical pharmacokinetics of transdermal opioids: focus on transdermal fentanyl. Clin Pharmacokinet. 38:59-89.

[8] Actiq® Full Prescribing Information, available at *www.actiq.com*.

[9] Duragesic® Full Prescribing Information, available at *www.duragesic.com*.

[10] FDA Public Health Advisory: Safety Warnings Regarding Use of Fentanyl Transdermal (Skin) Patches, July 15, 2005; and FDA Alert: Narcotic Overdose and Death, Information for Healthcare Professionals: Fentanyl Transdermal System (marketed as Duragesic® and generics), July 15, 2005.

[11] FDA Public Health Advisory: Important Information for the Safe Use of Fentanyl Transdermal System (Patch), December 21, 2007; FDA Alert: Narcotic Overdose and Death, Information for Healthcare Professionals: Fentanyl Transdermal System (marketed as Duragesic® and generics), Update, December 21, 2007.

considerable strengthening of the FDA's regulation of high-risk pharmaceutical products through a provision in the *FDA Amendments Act of 2007* (Public Law 110-85, Title IX) called *Risk Evaluation and Mitigation Strategies* (REMS).[12] REMS are treatment plans designed to minimize the harm done when using high-risk drugs or agents in high-risk drug classes. REMS may contain a medication guide for patients to be given with each prescription at the pharmacy, a specialized patient package insert, a communication plan if training is needed by physicians and/or pharmacists, and a registration database if deemed necessary. However, most REMS contain only educational information for patients, which may be ineffective in educating patients about drug harms.[13]

Both transdermal and transmucosal formulations of fentanyl are regulated by REMS. Transdermal fentanyl (Duragesic®) is covered by one of the first REMS approved by the FDA, called *ER/LA (Extended-Release/Long-Acting) Opioids REMS*.[14] Transmucosal fentanyl (e.g., Actiq®) is regulated by the newer and stronger *Transmucosal Immediate-Release Fentanyl (TIRF)* REMS.

For the drug expert, the use of FDA Full Prescribing Information provides key background data for the forming of expert opinion. Much of the background information about drugs in the litigation report will come from restating or citing the FDA prescribing information. The additional regulations and requirements provided by the FDA in the form of REMS for some drugs, such as opioid analgesics, add considerable weight against the errant physician who does not follow the prescription guidelines in the Full Prescribing Information. The physician who does not obtain the additional certification and training that may be required by the REMS for a particular drug or drug class is also at risk.

Official Prescribing Information for Drugs

The *U.S. Food and Drug Administration* (FDA) is the federal agency responsible for approving and regulating the use of nonprescription and prescription drugs.[15] One tangible outcome of FDA drug regulation is the *Full Prescribing Information* (FPI) that is available for each marketed drug. This FPI document, also known as the *FDA label*, is written by the drug manufacturers with feedback and approval by the FDA.

The FPI contains mandated paragraph sections for organizing the information needed for the prescriber.[16] These sections include *Boxed Warnings, Indications and Usage, Dosage and Administration, Dosage Forms and Strengths, Contraindications, Warnings and Precautions, Adverse Reactions, Drug Interactions, Use in Specific Populations, Drug Abuse and Dependence, Over-Dosage*, and others. Because the FPI is a document approved by the FDA, the information found on these documents is foundational to the drug issues of the case at hand. The FPI is the first document the drug expert downloads for each drug in the case. Getting the FPI, reading it, and relating any information to the case is the first step in the research process for a drug expert.

Because the FPI for each drug is FDA approved and widely available to all physicians, any deviation from clear and unambiguous prescription guidelines may be considered *prima facie* evidence of negligence.[17] More commonly, the FDA label alone does not establish deviation of the "standard of care" leading to medical malpractice without the concurrent testimony of an expert witness.[18] The use of the FDA label, along with scientific studies that support its warnings and precautions, provides a strong basis for a drug expert's testimony in cases where an apparent deviation from approved prescribing practices led to injury or death of the plaintiff.

The FPI can be obtained rather nicely from the FDA label depository[19] or from the drug manufacturer website. A Google search of a drug's brand name, like OxyContin® (oxycodone) or Duragesic® (fentanyl), usually topcasts the drug website posted by the makers of the drug. The official full prescribing information (FPI) can be downloaded from this slick website.

---

[12] Leiderman DB (2009) Risk management of drug products and the U.S. Food and Drug Administration: evolution and context. Drug Alcohol Depend. 105 Suppl 1:S9-S13.

[13] Current medication guides are of little value to patients due to complexity and length. The average guide for patients was over 1900 words or about 4 single-spaced typed pages. Nelson LS et al. (2014) Assuring safety of inherently unsafe medications: the FDA risk evaluation and mitigation strategies. J Med Toxicol. 10:165-172.

[14] Brooks MJ (2014) Mitigating the safety risks of drugs with a focus on opioids: are risk evaluation and mitigation strategies the answer? Mayo Clin Proc. 89:1673-1684.

[15] See Chapter 15 *Snake Eyes* for a fuller discussion of FDA drug regulation and approval process.

[16] FDA drug labeling rules are contained in the document "Labeling for Human Prescription Drug and Biological Products—Implementing the PLR Content and Format Requirements" available from the FDA website at: *www.fda.gov/downloads/drugs/guidancecomplianceregulatoryinformation/guidances/ucm075082.pdf.*

[17] The Minnesota Supreme Court case that is most often cited for this ruling is *Mulder v. Parke, Davis & Co.*, 288 Minn. 332, 181 N.W.2d 882 (1970). See Cooney M (2010) Medical malpractice. In Miller NS, Principles of Addictions and the Law, Elsevier: London, Burlington, San Diego.

[18] The Supreme Court of New Jersey upholds this ruling: *Morlino v. Medical Center of Ocean City*, 152 N.J. 563, 706 A.2d 721 (1998).

[19] *www.accessdata.fda.gov/scripts/cder/drugsatfda/index.cfm.*

Major pharmaceutical manufacturers have wisely bought up their products' website domain names (e.g., www.oxycontin.com). Entering a brand name drug as a dot-com domain name directly into the URL address box of a web browser in the format of "brandname.com" often links directly to the drug manufacturer's website where the FPI can be obtained for that drug.[20]

The Physician's Desk Reference (PDR) is a free resource available to all doctors and contains the complete set of FPI documents for all FDA-approved prescription drugs.[21] There are only FDA labels for approved prescription drugs, such a tidy and well-organized federally approved compendia for illegal drugs does not exist. Once a hefty book occupying a good chunk of real estate on the physician's desk, the PDR is now available online or by phone app for easy access to the FDA labels.

Medical Malpractice Due to the Prescribing of Opioids

Considering the rising epidemic of prescription opioid overdose deaths in the United States, it is not unforeseen that physicians will come under increasing scrutiny with regard to prescribing opioid analgesics (although some would say not enough scrutiny, see later). After all, except for the relatively minor cases of prescription opioid theft from pharmacies and health care offices, people are dying from opioid drugs that ultimately come from a prescription written by a physician.[22] The pharmacologist who moonlights as a litigation consultant/expert witness will likely be involved in a medical malpractice case involving an overdose death from prescription opioids.

Besides being named as a defendant in a civil suit involving improper prescribing of opioids and medical malpractice, a physician can be indicted with criminal drug offenses including drug trafficking, conspiracy to engage in drug trafficking, health care fraud, continuing criminal enterprise, drug trafficking resulting in serious bodily injury (if patient survives but is injured), and drug trafficking resulting in death (if patient dies).[23] Law enforcement officers often become aware of improper opioid prescribing from patients arrested for selling their prescription opioids and during the investigation of opioid overdose deaths. There are a few cases of physicians charged with murder when a patient dies of opioid overdose, although surprisingly few physicians are sanctioned or punished for improper opioid prescriptions by their State Medical Boards.[24]

State prosecutors or district attorneys are reluctant to indict and pursue criminal charges against physicians for overprescribing of opioid medications. A research survey of prosecuting attorneys discovered underlying attitudes and beliefs regarding physician treatment of chronic pain with opioids.[25] In this unique study, 112 state prosecutors across four states were presented with a case where a physician was clearly overprescribing opioids to a patient for treatment of noncancer pain and the prosecutors were asked to return a survey based on what they would do. Only 49% of state prosecutors stated that they would recommend a law enforcement investigation. Prosecutors were more likely to refer the case to the State Medical Boards, however many professed that they do not trust the medical boards to "police their own." Few prosecutors were likely to involve the DEA in an investigation of the physician's overprescribing of an opioid analgesic. It appears that tighter regulation of opioid prescribing by physicians is badly needed and provides the justification for mandatory Prescription Monitoring Programs (PMP) now springing up in numerous states across the country.[26] Additionally, in 2017, many states passed laws limiting the prescribing of opioids by physicians.[27] There are now 26 states that impose mandatory limits on prescribing and dispensing of opioids for acute pain.

---

[20] Examples: Typing *Oxycontin.com* into the URL address box of any internet browser brings one directly to its manufacturer's website at "*www.purduehcp.com*." Typing "*Valium.com*" redirects to "*www.roche.com*" and entering "*Xanax.com*" redirects one quite nicely directly to the Xanax® FPI at the Upjohn website.

[21] The Physician's Desk Reference (PDR) is available online to doctors by registering at *www.pdr.net*.

[22] In one survey, college students reported that about 60% of their pain medication used for prescription drug abuse came from peers (friends mostly, roommates, boyfriends, and girlfriends also) and about 12% from family members. Interestingly, illegal pain drugs are about three times more likely to be obtained from mothers than fathers. See McCabe SE, Boyd CJ (2005) Sources of prescription drugs for illicit use. Addict Behav. 30:1342-1350. The simple fact that diversion primarily comes from unused supplies is *prima facie* evidence that there is overprescribing of opioid analgesics; otherwise there would not be so many "extra" and unused pills laying around.

[23] Benjamin DM (2007) Prosecution of physicians for prescribing opioids to patients. Clin Pharmacol Ther. 81:797-798.

[24] Or "virtually non-existent" according to one study. Richard J, Reidenberg MM (2005) The risk of disciplinary action by state medical boards against physicians prescribing opioids. J Pain Symptom Manag. 29:206-212.

[25] Ziegler SJ, Lovrich NP (2003). Pain relief, prescription drugs, and prosecution: a four-state survey of chief prosecutors. J Law Med Ethics 31:75-100.

[26] Prescription monitoring programs (PMPs) are statewide databases containing prescriber and patient-level prescription data on controlled substances. Oklahoma was the first state to set up a real-time PMP database. PMPs are shown to decrease state trends in opioid-related abuse and misuse. Reifler LM et al. (2012) Do prescription monitoring programs impact state trends in opioid abuse/misuse? Pain Med. 13:434-442.

[27] Davis CS et al. (2019) Laws limiting the prescribing or dispensing of opioids for acute pain in the United States: A national systematic legal review. Drug Alcohol Depend. 194:166-172.

Federal Rules of Evidence and the Expert

The testimony of a drug expert is governed by procedural laws for expert witnesses at the federal and state level. Although the *Federal Rules of Evidence* (FRE) are presented here, more than forty states have adopted evidence codes that are nearly the same, in language and numbering, as in the FRE.[28] The FRE and its associated committee infrastructure were created when President Ford signed *An Act to Establish Rules of Evidence for Certain Courts and Proceedings* on January 2, 1975.[29] The FRE is an evolving document with the most recent amendments made in 2016.[30]

The definition of a drug expert and drug expert testimony, which applies to all expert witnesses, is addressed in six *Rules*.

Rule 701. Opinion testimony by lay witnesses

If a witness is not testifying as an expert, testimony in the form of an opinion is limited to one that is: (a) rationally based on the witness's perception; (b) helpful to clearly understanding the witness's testimony or to determining a fact in issue; and (c) not based on scientific, technical, or other specialized knowledge within the scope of Rule 702.

Rule 701 serves to steer any potential lay testimony that is actually expert witness testimony to *Rule 702* (later). According to the *Committee Notes for Rule 701*, this rule prevents the practice of "sneaking in" expert witness testimony by presenting them as a lay witness.[31] The rule also ensures that a party will not skirt the expert witness disclosure requirements.[32] The remaining five *Rules* directly address the qualifications and testimony of an expert.

Rule 702. Testimony by expert witnesses

A witness who is qualified as an expert by knowledge, skill, experience, training, or education may testify in the form of an opinion or otherwise if:

(a) the expert's scientific, technical, or other specialized knowledge will help the trier of fact to understand the evidence or to determine a fact in issue;

(b) the testimony is based on sufficient facts or data;

(c) the testimony is the product of reliable principles and methods; and

(d) the expert has reliably applied the principles and methods to the facts of the case.

As stated in *Rule 702*, the drug expert must first be qualified by "knowledge, skill, experience, training, or education" to testify on drug issues. Without doubt, a pharmacologist with a Ph.D. in Pharmacology is best qualified to serve as a drug expert considering these criteria as a whole. For example, a physician might have experience in administering a drug, or even skill in putting in an IV line, but does not have the requisite knowledge, training, or education focused on the study of drugs like a pharmacologist. Clause 702 *(a)* pertains to the drug issue at hand and the drug expert *ipso facto* will assist the *trier of fact* (judge in a bench trial or a jury). A drug expert doing research on a particular drug issue and sharing the results with the Court will always be of assistance to the fact finder.

That the drug expert's testimony is *(b) based on sufficient facts and data* is satisfied by the extensive research the drug expert carries out before the development of an expert opinion. For clause *(c) reliable principles and methods*, the drug expert, a Ph.D.-trained scientist, would know no other method to arrive at a summary and conclusion of the findings. The *modus operandi* of the drug expert is the scientific method, which has the *most* reliable principles and methods. Resources researched by the expert are based on sound principles and methodology as primary literature is searched. These resources include peer-reviewed research studies and clinical trials designed with double-blind methodology, which meet the criteria of *reliable principles and methods*.

---

[28] Merritt DJ, Simmons R (2014) *Learning Evidence: From the Federal Rules to the Courtroom.* West Academic Publishing: St. Paul.

[29] Information from the U.S. Courts website at: *www.uscourts.gov.*

[30] FRE is amended each year by the United States Supreme Court in March, taking effect the following December if Congress does not intervene. The full text of the FRE is available at the FRE organizational website: *www.rulesofevidence.org.*

[31] *www.law.cornell.edu/rules/fre/rule_701.*

[32] Set forth in Fed.R.Civ.P. 26 and Fed.R.Crim.P. 16.

The last aspect listed of the expert's opinion, *(d) applying the principles and methods to the facts of the case at hand,* is the most difficult part of the drug expert's job and the area of testimony most open to challenge during cross-examination. Clinical studies in the literature give population data, e.g. the incidence of daytime drowsiness in a large group of clinical trial participants. The results that are obtained are *general* to the population of *Homo sapiens* targeted by the clinical study. The particular individual in the case at hand that was under the influence of a drug is just that—one particular individual. Legal proceedings are done to right the wrong, or reverse a wrong charge if innocent, of a single *specific* individual. The application of pharmacological data arising from clinical studies applied to a drug issue in a particular plaintiff or defendant is a crucial link in every drug expert's case.[33]

Rule 703. Bases of an expert's opinion testimony

An expert may base an opinion on facts or data in the case that the expert has been made aware of or personally observed. If experts in the particular field would reasonably rely on those kinds of facts or data in forming an opinion on the subject, they need not be admissible for the opinion to be admitted. But if the facts or data would otherwise be inadmissible, the proponent of the opinion may disclose them to the jury only if their probative value in helping the jury evaluate the opinion substantially outweighs their prejudicial effect.

Without going into the legal underpinnings of this rule, suffice it to say that this rule allows experts to use *hearsay* evidence, which is usually inadmissible.[34] The first clause of *Rule 703* empowers experts to rely on inadmissible facts or data as long as the facts or data are commonly used to form opinions by other experts in the same field of expertise.[35] For example, the drug expert is often provided a toxicology report from the Medical Examiner's office and then testifies on the interpretation of the drug levels found in the blood. The drug expert can use the information from the toxicology report as the basis for testimony under *Rule 703*. The actual lab technician who ran the blood sample and produced the toxicology report need not testify, but the drug expert acts as a surrogate and legitimately uses the toxicology report to support expert opinion. The second clause in *Rule 703* is met by the drug expert's use of the toxicology report because it has "probative value in helping the jury evaluate the opinion" of the drug expert.

With regard to *Rule 703*, there is a trilogy of recent SCOTUS decisions that attempt to better define the interaction between the defendant's right to confront a witness and the many forms of forensic evidence that provide the foundation of a prosecutor's case.[36] *Rule 703* was controversial since it was instated, and much of the current argument centers on testimonial evidence that is not cross-examined by the opposing party. This can be construed to interfere with the defendant's right to confront the witness, a constitutional right known as the *Confrontation Clause of the Sixth Amendment.*[37]

The remaining Rules pertaining to the drug expert, *Rule 704 Opinion on an Ultimate Issue, Rule 705 Disclosing the Facts or Data Underlying an Expert's Opinion,* and *Rule 706 Court-Appointed Expert Witnesses,*[38] will be saved for a later chapter in this book.[39]

The Drug Expert Litigation Report

Not all cases in the drug expert's portfolio will include a formal litigation report. In Federal and state trial courts, discovery rules are such that much pretrial consulting can be done without a formal litigation report produced. Initially, an attorney may hire a drug expert to help evaluate the case and the drug expert will provide an opinion not subject to the rules of

---

[33] One simple approach to counter the challenge of using average values obtained in a clinical study applied to a specific case in hand is to assert that the defendant (or plaintiff) is no more than an average person, that is there is no reason to suspect that the defendant is an outlier (less than 5 out of 100) with respect to some aspect of drug use without further evidence.

[34] As with other discussion of all legal matters, readers who desire to explore this topic further will need to look elsewhere, like in a book written by an actual lawyer.

[35] Perrin LT (1997) Expert witnesses under Rules 703 and 803(4) of the Federal Rules of Evidence: Separating the wheat from the chaff. Indiana Law J. 72:939-1014.

[36] These cases are *Melendez-Diaz v Massachusetts,* 557 US 305 (2009); *Bullcoming v New Mexico,* 131 S Ct 2705, 2716 (2011); and *Williams v Illinois,* 132 S Ct 2221 (2012) as provided by: Mnookin J, Kaye D (2013) Supreme Court Review, Vol. 2012.

[37] Gianelli PC (2012) Confrontation, experts, and Rule 703. J. Law Policy 20:443-456.

[38] The full text of the FRE is available from the Legal Information Institute run by Cornell University Law School at: *www.law.cornell.edu.*

[39] See Chapter 7 *Firewater,* under the section *Junk Science and the Drug Expert.*

discovery, much like the work product protected under the attorney/client privilege.[40] In some cases, one drug expert may only serve during the pretrial period (strictly as a litigation consultant) and another drug expert (the expert witness per se) during the trial. In cases played out in federal district courts, a written litigation report from the expert is mandatory under federal discovery rules. However, because consistency of opinions is key to sound expert testimony, writing at least a preliminary draft of a litigation report on the drug issues is useful. This draft report will also contain the medical and pharmacological journal references used in supporting the drug expert's opinion and will be needed if a formal report is submitted to the Court later. As noted before, draft reports are considered privileged attorney work product and may not be discoverable if the expert witness does not testify.

The drug expert litigation report is a formal written statement of the drug expert's opinion and conclusion. Typical sections include a cover page with a descriptive title, court and case styling information, date prepared, for whom the report was prepared, and a byline of the drug expert who prepared the report. The body of the report is organized in sections which may include sections such as Resources Available, Case Narrative, Background on Drugs, Adverse Effects of Drugs, Timeline of Medications Prescribed, Drugs Detected Postmortem, Summary and Conclusions, and References Cited.

The supporting documents for a drug litigation report include both complete medical and pharmacy records and additional records or items received from the attorney (case documents). The drug expert will research the drug issues and obtain the numerous medical, pharmacological, and forensic reports to read and ponder before providing an opinion.[41] Case documents may include results of drug screening tests, medical examiners records and toxicology lab reports, police records, EMT/ambulance crew reports, hospital reports, and any other documents that may be pertinent to the case. There may be a tendency for the attorney to dole out case documents slowly or only in response to repeated requests from the drug expert. However, experience shows that the attorney should scan into PDFs (or make physical hardcopies if still paper-bound) of all available case documents for the perusal of the drug expert. Many times a statement in the emergency services report, or a physician's note in the medical records, or a police note from the crime scene report provides a crucial piece of data that strengthens the opinion of the drug expert.

A sample of a litigation report prepared by the author is included as Appendix D. It is a redacted and shortened copy of the actual ligation report used in the medical malpractice case presented in this chapter case.

[Narrative continued]

The legal team representing the widower husband contacted a drug expert to examine the medical records and the use of opioid medications. The drug expert researched the use of fentanyl in the treatment of cancer pain by extensive searching of the medical and pharmacological journals using PubMed. Key to this research was the Full Prescribing Information for both fentanyl transmucosal lozenges (Actiq®) and fentanyl transdermal patches (Duragesic®). A number of irregularities were found: 1. The pain specialist (physician) did not assess Mrs. Jackson for the presence of opioid tolerance (resistance to chronic opioids); both fentanyl products are indicated only in patients that are opioid-tolerant. 2. Mrs. Jackson had a history of asthma and COPD, which is a contraindication for the use of fentanyl patches and strongly cautioned against use for fentanyl lozenges according to FDA Labels. 3. The fentanyl lozenge is indicated for use in breakthrough cancer pain in patients already taking around-the-clock (long-acting) opioid medications according to FDA label. Mrs. Jackson was not on long-acting opioid formulations but was taking oral morphine sulfate immediate-release as needed (PRN). 4. The initial dose of fentanyl lozenge should also be 200 μg according to the FDA Label. Mrs. Jackson was started with the initial dose of 1000 μg. 5. Likewise, the FDA guidelines for the initial fentanyl skin patch dosage strength were lower than the 75 mcg/h fentanyl patch given to Mrs. Jackson. After the drug expert's litigation report was submitted to the opposing party and the expert's deposition taken, the case went to mediation and was settled for an undisclosed amount.

---

[40] Miller NS (2010) Expert witness in civil and criminal testimony. In Miller NS (Ed.) *Principles of Addiction and the Law*, Academic Press: Elsevier, London, Burlington, San Diego.

[41] The research methods of the drug expert are elaborated in the next chapter.

Chapter 5

Wrong Place at the Wrong Time: Meth manufacture and urine drug tests

The Drug Treatment Court Alternative—A Profile of Methamphetamine

Environmental Exposure When Making Meth

The Detection of Methamphetamine in Urine

Rules of Discovery for the Drug Expert—Deposition of the Drug Expert

[Narrative]
Gary Winfield was a 24-year old male with a history of methamphetamine use and a record of prior arrest for methamphetamine possession. Instead of the traditional criminal court proceedings, his meth possession case was went through the Drug Treatment Court. Mr. Winfield's weekly urine samples were tested for illicit drugs as part of the Drug Court ruling. With the help of a job assistance program, Mr. Winfield found work as a welder at an auto junkyard just outside the city. After he worked there for about 6 months, the junkyard was raided by the police and a clandestine meth lab was discovered in an outbuilding. Mr. Winfield was charged in Federal District Court with the manufacture of methamphetamine along with everyone else on the premises. A public defender was assigned to his case by the court from a pool of local lawyers. The public defender argued that a drug expert was needed to interpret and analyze the urine drug tests to see if their results were consistent with someone cooking meth. The public defender obtained approval from the Court for the use of federal funds to hire a drug expert.

The Drug Treatment Court Alternative

In the late 1980s, a movement began within the justice system to establish an alternative to the traditional criminal courts system for low-level drug offenders, called drug treatment courts. These drug courts were a response to a justice system overburdened with drug crimes. The first adult drug court was established in 1989 in Miami, Florida, an area synonymous with rampant cocaine use and drug arrests at that time.[1] Drug courts are specialized court-based treatment programs designed for low-level criminal drug offenders, and parents in child welfare cases who have alcohol and other substance abuse problems.

As of June, 2015, there were over 3000 drug courts operating in the United States, with all but 27 located in state jurisdictions.[2] More than half of the drug courts are for nonviolent drug and adult alcohol dependent offenders; others are designed to address juvenile drug offenders, drug use and child welfare, veteran drug courts, and drug courts for offenders charged with DWI. There are also 138 tribal drug courts for Native American offenders and a handful of Campus Drug Courts for college students charged with drug offenses. Nationwide, there are 306 veteran drug courts to serve those who served.

Arrestees of drug-related crimes are eligible for the drug court alternative if they meet certain offense categories and if a drug court is available in their jurisdiction. The drug court system emphasizes a public health approach with treatment, with drug testing and court supervision available as an alternative to incarceration. Studies show that drug offenders who successfully complete the drug court alternative remain in drug treatment programs longer, have lower rates of drug use,

---

[1] Hora PF, Stalcup T (2008) Drug treatment courts in the twenty-first century: the evolution of the revolution in problem-solving courts. Georgia Law Rev. 42:717–811. See also the TV series *Miami Vice*.
[2] Latest data from the National Institute of Justice, U.S. Dept. of Justice, at: *www.nij.gov/topics/courts/drug-courts*.

The Drug Expert. https://doi.org/10.1016/B978-0-12-800048-9.00005-5

higher rates of employment, and lower rates of recidivism. Drug courts also are successful on a cost-benefit basis with a societal savings of $5680 per participant.[3]

Successful drug court clients may have their drug charges expunged in pre-plea drug court hearings or avoid a sentence in post-plea drug court. Drug offenders who fail the drug court mandates by positive drug tests and skipping court appointments are convicted and sentenced to intensive probationary supervision or incarcerated.[4] There is strong evidence that drug offenders are persons better handled as those in need of medical and drug treatment programs that the drug court alternative provides. Otherwise, the low-level drug offender is treated as a wrongdoer and enters the vastly overcrowded criminal justice system associated with terribly poor outcomes.

Drug experts may be involved in drug court cases, especially with regard to the interpretation and analysis of drug testing that is mandated as part of the drug court treatment program. The drug expert's testimony may be important for the drug court participant if he is charged with a drug-related crime during the drug court probationary period, as occurred in the present case.

A Profile of Methamphetamine

Methamphetamine is a good drug that went bad. Amphetamines, when properly used, are fairly safe and effective agents for the treatment of attention deficit-hyperactivity disorder (ADHD), narcolepsy, and obesity.[5] The structure of methamphetamine looks like the drug amphetamine, with an additional simple chemical modification. The reader should be aware that the term *amphetamine* is used both as a specific drug and as a class of CNS stimulants.[6] To make matters even more confusing, amphetamine is also an active metabolite of methamphetamine. To summarize, methamphetamine itself is a member of the amphetamine drug class, it has a structure similar to the specific drug amphetamine, and methamphetamine is metabolized to amphetamine in the body.

Amphetamine use in large numbers began during World War II, with the U.S. military issuing amphetamine pills to troops for them to remain alert and stay awake during battle.[7] Pilots on long bombing missions were among the greatest users of amphetamines. Reports from veterans who took amphetamines during WWII state that amphetamine had "morale-elevating" effects and increased their confidence and aggression.[8] In the decade after the war, amphetamine production increased in the United States with the aggressive marketing of amphetamine as Benzedrine®, followed by dextroamphetamine as Dexedrine®.[9] Amphetamine use was touted as a remedy for fatigue and "melancholy" (depression). In fact, amphetamines were the first type of drugs marketed as antidepressants. Amphetamine and methamphetamine were also among the first blockbuster drugs for Smith, Kline and French, a drug company with roots in Philadelphia dating back to 1929. The Smith, Kline and French company survives today as part of the large pharmaceutical firm, GlaxoSmithKline (GSK).[10]

Methamphetamine, besides being a type of amphetamine drug, belongs to the larger class of drugs called CNS stimulants. CNS stimulants generally "ramp-up" the brain, fight fatigue, and increase mental acuity. Coffee and tea are mild CNS stimulants, whereas methamphetamine and cocaine are potent CNS stimulants. For this reason, amphetamine drugs including methamphetamine are among the most abused and dangerous drugs in this country and around the world. The danger of amphetamines comes from the changes in behavior that amphetamine use produces on an acute basis and the long-term

---

[3] Drug court participants were compared to similar nondrug court probationers. Cost-benefit analysis included crime and victimization costs. Downey PM, Roman JK (2014) Cost-benefit analysis: a guide for drug courts and other criminal justice programs. National Institute of Justice, U.S. Dept. of Justice, Washington, DC.

[4] Franco C (2010) Drug courts: background, effectiveness, and policy issues for Congress. Congressional Research Service, Washington, DC.

[5] Brenner GM, Stevens CW (2017) *Brenner and Stevens' Pharmacology*, 5th Ed. Elsevier: Philadelphia. ADHD is Attention Deficit-Hyperactive Disorder, also called attention deficit disorder (ADD), though this is considered an outdated term. Approximately 10% of children 4–17 years of age (6.1 million) were diagnosed with ADHD as of 2016 according to the CDC (*www.cdc.gov/ncbddd/adhd/data.html*).

[6] CNS equals Central Nervous System, which is the brain and spinal cord. CNS stimulants activate the neurons in the brain and include drugs such as amphetamines, cocaine, caffeine, and nicotine, among others.

[7] German troops took the more powerful drug, methamphetamine, and their method of making methamphetamine survives today as the "Nazi" method. See Vearrier D et al. (2012) Methamphetamine: history, pathophysiology, adverse health effects, current trends, and hazards associated with the clandestine manufacture of methamphetamine. Disease Mon. 58:38-89.

[8] Rasmussen N (2011) Medical science and the military: the Allies' use of amphetamine during World War II. J Interdiscip Hist. 42:205-233.

[9] Rasmussen N (2008) America's first amphetamine epidemic 1929-1971. Amer J Public Health 98:974-985.

[10] In 2012 GSK pleaded guilty to criminal charges and paid $3 billion to the US government to keep its top executives out of prison. It was the largest fine for drug law violations by a drug manufacturer at the time. Criminal charges against GSK ranged from promoting its headliner antidepressants, Paxil® and Wellbutrin®, for uses that were not FDA approved, to hiding safety data about the blockbuster diabetes drug Avandia®, and for paying kickbacks to physicians to prescribe their drugs over competitors. In spite of this action and other corporate cases of criminal activity, according to Sidney Wolfe of Public Citizen, even large fines have little impact on BigPharma corporate behavior. See Wollfe SM (2014) Escalating criminal and civil violations: Pharma has corporate integrity? Not really. British Med. Journal 348:f7507.

effects of chronic amphetamine use which includes brain damage and psychosis. Methamphetamine-induced murder and drug expert testimony on amphetamine-induced aggression and psychosis are visited in a later chapter.

Amphetamines are CNS stimulants and mimic the surge of hormones and neurotransmitters that are released during a "fight or flee" situation. This is the classic sympathetic nervous system response that is noted also by the release of adrenaline (also called epinephrine) from the adrenal glands into the bloodstream. There is good reason to suspect that one can become "addicted" to this innate sympathetic nervous system reaction and its release of adrenaline. Individuals characterized as "adrenaline junkies" go bungee-cord jumping, skydiving, hang-gliding, base-jumping, surfing, or rock climbing (or testify as an expert witness in court) to excite their own sympathetic nervous systems. At low doses, methamphetamine increases arousal, cardiac stimulation, and improves attention and psychomotor coordination. At the higher doses typically used by drug abusers, methamphetamine can produce psychosis and hypertensive crisis leading to heart attack and death.[11] Methamphetamine strongly activates the dopamine reward pathways in the brain, the mechanism of all addictive drugs and addictive behavior.

Methamphetamine is easy to make. Compared to cocaine, meth gives the user a stronger and longer-lasting "high."[12] Recipes for homemade meth manufacture are found on the internet and can be done with methods involving little expense and equipment. In terms of numbers, illegal methamphetamine use is second only to the illegal use of marijuana in the United States and around the world.[13] However, alcohol is still the number one abused drug in the world.

Environmental Exposure When Making Meth

The active drug expert will likely encounter cases involving the manufacture of methamphetamine. Methamphetamine manufacture is cheap and easy, albeit extremely dangerous to the individual manufacturer, family members, and others present at the site of the "meth lab." Recipes for making methamphetamine are found on the internet and the precursor ingredients are readily available, although somewhat harder to obtain now since the passage of precursor drug laws limiting the amount of pseudoephedrine-containing medicines that are available in over-the-counter preparations. Precursor laws, increased awareness of clandestine meth labs, and efforts to prosecute home meth cookers, caused a shift in the meth manufacturing business to larger "superlabs" in Mexico and elsewhere producing crystal meth and smuggling the product into the United States.[14] In response to increasing methamphetamine seized at the U.S. border, Mexican drug cartels are now smuggling liquid methamphetamine (meth dissolved in a solvent and crystallized out later) into the United States in windshield wiper fluid reservoirs, concealed in gasoline tanks, liquor bottles, laundry and antifreeze containers, and flavored water bottles.[15] Meanwhile domestic small clandestine meth labs continue to adapt their methods, now using the "one-pot" or "shake and bake" method to produce small batches of a single gram or milligram quantities of methamphetamine using an empty 2-L soda bottle as the chemical reaction chamber.

The domestic methods for making meth create a toxic hazard for the meth manufacturer, significant others or spouses, and any children or other family members living in the same space. Manufacturing methamphetamine contaminates the surrounding area of the manufacturing site. In controlled "cooks" done in residential settings to simulate meth labs, methamphetamine persisted for as long as 24 h in the carpet fibers and other exposed surfaces.[16] Illicit methamphetamine manufacture was associated with a high degree of aerosolized particles that were deposited on these surfaces and concentrations of methamphetamine particles increased with more traffic through the house.

As children are often present in such homes, much research has focused on methamphetamine in these innocent subjects. In one study, half of the children suspected of living in a home where methamphetamine was manufactured tested positive for meth by hair analysis.[17] A more direct evaluation of children removed from a meth lab home showed that of 83 children tested, over half (52%) had a positive urine sample for the presence of methamphetamine.[18] Most surprisingly,

[11] Cruickshank CC, Dyer KR (2009) A review of the clinical pharmacology of methamphetamine. Addiction 104: 1085–1099.

[12] Lineberry TW, Bostwick JM (2006) Methamphetamine abuse: a perfect storm of complications. Mayo Clin Proc. 81:77-84.

[13] Vearrier D et al. (2012) Methamphetamine: history, pathophysiology, adverse health effects, current trends, and hazards associated with the clandestine manufacture of methamphetamine. Dis Mon 2012;58:38-89.

[14] Mawwell JC, Rutkowski BA (2008) The prevalence of methamphetamine and amphetamine abuse in North America: a review of the indicators, 1992-2007. Drug Alcohol Res 27:229-235. Maxwell JC, Brecht M-L (2011) Methamphetamine: Here we go again? Addict Behav. 36:1168-1173.

[15] DEA (2014) National drug threat assessment summary (unclassified version). Available from the DEA at: www.dea.gov/resource-center/dir-ndta-unclass.pdf.

[16] VanDyke M, Erb N, Arbuckle S, Martyny J (2009) A 24-hour study to investigate persistent chemical exposures associated with clandestine methamphetamine laboratories. J Occup Environ Hygiene 6:82-89.

[17] Farst K et al. (2011) Hair drug testing of children suspected of exposure to the manufacture of methamphetamine. J Forensic Legal Med 18:110-114.

[18] Grant P (2006) Evaluation of children removed from a clandestine methamphetamine laboratory. Clin Ped Emerg Med 7:170-180.

drug testing of 50 individuals who use methamphetamine packets in sealed canisters to train drug-sniffing dogs for federal agencies yielded positive urine tests for methamphetamine in 32 individuals the following day.[19] These individuals were wearing gloves, inhalation masks, and lab coats during the training of the canine drug-detection units. And to repeat, the methamphetamine was in a *sealed container.*

Not surprisingly, there is strong evidence linking the manufacture of methamphetamine to the simultaneous use of methamphetamine by the person making meth. In one study of 31 burn patients that tested positive for methamphetamine in urine drug tests, all but three were also identified as methamphetamine manufacturers.[20] It is clear that a person manufacturing methamphetamine would yield a positive urine drug test for methamphetamine either from snorting or smoking meth, or from environmental contamination as part of the meth manufacturing process.

The Detection of Methamphetamine in Urine

After methamphetamine enters the body, metabolic processes occur to break it down and remove it from the body. The methamphetamine molecule is metabolized in the liver primarily to hydroxy-methamphetamine and amphetamine; however, as much as 50% of methamphetamine is not metabolized and is excreted directly in the urine.[21] The metabolites hydroxy-methamphetamine and amphetamine make up the rest of the original methamphetamine dose and are also excreted in the urine. Methamphetamine accumulates in the urine with repeated meth use and has a urinary terminal half-life of 25 h,[22] meaning it takes about a day for half of the original dose to be excreted in the urine. Methamphetamine has been detected in the urine from 2 to 4 days[23] or as long as 7 days after stopping 4 days of methamphetamine use.[24]

The validity of an initial drug screen using urine can be affected by other drugs taken by the subject, especially in the case of methamphetamine and amphetamines. For example, urine drug screens using the initial preliminary immunoassay test show false positives for amphetamine/methamphetamine with the following prescription and over-the-counter drugs: amantadine, brompheniramine, bupropion, chlorpromazine, desipramine, dextroamphetamine, ephedrine, isometheptene, labetalol, methylene dioxymethamphetamine, methylphenidate, phentermine, phenylephrine, phenylpropanolamine, promethazine, pseudoephedrine, ranitidine, selegiline, thioridazine, trazodone, trimethobenzamide, and trimipramine.[25]

In a study examining urine initial drug screens in chronic pain patients, almost 10% of tests that were presumptive positive amphetamines were subsequently found to be negative for amphetamines (i.e., *false positives*) after a second confirmatory test.[26] For this reason, presumptive positive drug tests using an immunoassay need to be followed by confirmatory drug tests using gas chromatography-mass spectrophotometry (GC-MS) tests. GC-MS tests are more expensive and time consuming, but more accurate than initial immunoassay tests. In GC-MS tests, the drug molecules are separated by the gas chromatograph and analyzed by the mass spectrometer. Each molecule is broken down into ionized fragments and identified by its mass-to-charge ratio. The accuracy of this method, as well as the ability to determine the quantity of the drug in question, makes GC-MS the forensic and legal standard for drug testing.[27]

Detection of drugs in the urine is an ideal bodily fluid to assay for drug use. Urine is easily obtained, painless to obtain, and basically risk-free to the collector. With supervised procedures and additional tests for other proteins normally found in urine, urine samples are also resistant to scamming by urine substitution or chemical alteration. For drug court enrollees, urine drug testing is the standard method for testing compliance with drug court mandates prohibiting drug use.

---

[19] Stout PR et al. (2006) Occupational exposure to methamphetamine in workers preparing training aids for drug detection dogs. J Anal Toxic 30:551-554, 2006.

[20] Burke BA et al. (2008) Methamphetamine-related burns in the cornbelt. J Burn Care Res 29:574-579; Danks RR et al. (2004) Methamphetamine-associated burn injuries: a retrospective analysis. J Burn Care Rehabil 25:425-429.

[21] Courtney KE, Ray LA (2014) Methamphetamine: an update on epidemiology, pharmacology, clinical phenomenology, and treatment literature. Drug Alcohol Depend. 143:11-21. There is also secretion of methamphetamine and its metabolite, amphetamine in the sweat and can be detected in users' clothes. See Al-Dirbashi OY et al. (2001) Drugs of abuse in a non-conventional sample; detection of methamphetamine and its main metabolite, amphetamine in abusers' clothes by HPLC with UV and fluorescence detection. Biomed Chromatogr. 15:457-463.

[22] Elimination half-life, abbreviated $t_{1/2}$, is the time it takes a drug to reach half the concentration of its initial concentration and usually refers to the decrease of drug levels in the blood.

[23] Huestis MA, Cone EJ (2007) Methamphetamine disposition in oral fluid, plasma, and urine. Ann N Y Acad Sci. 1098:104-121.

[24] Oyler JM et al. (2002) Duration of detectable methamphetamine and amphetamine excretion in urine after controlled oral administration of methamphetamine to humans. Clin Chem 48:1703-1714.

[25] Congrats if you mentally verbalized each of those drug names. I promise it will not happen again. The drug list is from: Markway EC, Baker SN (2011) A review of the methods, interpretation, and limitations of the urine drug screen. Orthopedics 34:877-881.

[26] Melanson SE et al. (2013) Optimizing urine drug testing for monitoring medication compliance in pain management. Pain Med. 14:1813-1820.

[27] Standridge JB et al. (2010) Urine drug screening: a valuable office procedure. Am Fam Physician 81:635-640.

Rules of Discovery for the Drug Expert

Information is power. The power of information to affect human lives is greatest in the courtroom. Information in the form of testimony, documents, reports, pictures, and video can set an innocent person free or convict a hardened criminal. In the adversarial process of legal proceedings, there is an innate tension between the self-interest of each side in keeping some information secret (at least until the trial) and the equal sharing of information. Discovery is the pretrial procedure by which one party in a legal proceeding gains information held by the other party.[28] One party can obtain testimony and evidence from the other party by discovery motions made to request responses to interrogatories, production of documents, and depositions. Medical and pharmacy reports are discovered in cases of medical malpractice ("medmal," see Chapter 4, above). *Subpoenas* are used to obtain discovery information in the form of a deposition from nonparties, such as expert witnesses.[29] However, in many cases, a formal *subpoena* to a deposition or trial is not issued to the drug expert. In all cases, the contracting attorney and the opposing attorney should work with the drug expert to schedule a mutually agreeable time and place to take the deposition and schedule the trail.

The drug expert will follow the advice of the contracting attorney in all matters of discovery but a brief review of discovery rules may help to understand this crucial aspect of the legal system. In real-life experience, the drug expert will find hiring attorneys that act quite differently under the same rules of discovery in a single jurisdiction. Some lawyers appear overly concerned with discovery matters and keep all communications with the drug expert limited to phone calls. One attorney only sends case documents by post or hands them over to me in person during an unannounced visit.[30] Additionally, like all of the laws of the land, there can be significant differences in the rules of discovery between federal and state jurisdictions, and between the states themselves.[31]

The issue of discovery arises in every case with the creation or not of a litigation report. Such a report from an expert is then shared with the opposing attorney in a timely manner as dictated by the court's scheduling orders. If the case is in Federal Court, a written litigation report is mandatory. In most cases, the drug expert should produce a litigation report, nicely organized and referenced, that will be provided to the opposing party by the rules of discovery. This of course is an important document that will be used as a foundation for the drug expert's further testimony.

In a lesser number of cases, the hiring attorney may still be deciding whether to take the case and needs a preliminary opinion. This is often accomplished with a phone call from the attorney to the drug expert. Such preliminary (and nonbinding) opinions, usually given *pro bono* by the drug expert, are informal and not subject to discovery. The danger lies in providing a preliminary opinion without at least some research. Even the most mainstream pharmacological issue pertaining to a drug impacting a legal case needs to be researched for the latest research results and a more detailed understanding before a sound opinion can be made. Such pretrial consulting that does not result in a formal litigation report is not discoverable.[32] Likewise, notes can be kept that are nondiscoverable but if the drug expert becomes a testifying witness, the drug expert's complete file may be discoverable.

The rules of discovery for expert witnesses are embodied in the Federal Rules for Civil Procedures, an evolving codebook that is produced by the Judicial Committee of the U.S. Supreme Court and approved by the U.S. Congress.[33] There is also a complementary codebook for criminal cases entitled Federal Rules for Criminal Procedures that mirrors discovery rules in the Civil Procedures codebook. Most states follow the federal rules in their own codes for civil and criminal procedures concerning discovery issues with expert witnesses.[34]

While the force and interpretation of these rules is left to the hiring attorney and the Court, the drug expert should be aware of Rule 26 (a)(2) entitled "Disclosure of Expert Testimony."

Rule 26 (a)(2) disclosure of expert testimony.

(A) In General. In addition to the disclosures required by Rule 26(a)(1), a party must disclose to the other parties the identity of any witness it may use at trial to present evidence under Federal Rule of Evidence 702, 703, or 705.

(B) Witnesses Who Must Provide a Written Report. Unless otherwise stipulated or ordered by the court, this disclosure must be accompanied by a written report—prepared and signed by the witness—if the witness is one retained or

---

[28] Gifis SH (2003) Discovery, Barron's Law Dictionary, 5th Edition, page 149. Barron's Educational Series, Inc. Hauppauge, NY.

[29] *Subpoena* (Latin: "under penalty") served to the drug expert may also be called *subpoena duces tecum* ("under penalty to bring with you") which orders the expert to bring along certain documents or supporting references.

[30] I am waiting for the first lawyer to communicate only by Morse code.

[31] See Appendix B in: Bergman P, Moore A (2014) Nolo's deposition handbook. Nolo Publishers, Berkeley CA, USA.

[32] And covered by "attorney work product" rules.

[33] The latest version of the Federal Rules for Civil Procedures is at: *www.federalrulesofcivilprocedure.org/frcp/.*

[34] For example, the Oklahoma Discovery Code appears to mimic the Federal code in most sections.

specially employed to provide expert testimony in the case or one whose duties as the party's employee regularly involve giving expert testimony. The report must contain:

(i) a complete statement of all opinions the witness will express and the basis and reasons for them;
(ii) the facts or data considered by the witness in forming them;
(iii) any exhibits that will be used to summarize or support them;
(iv) the witness's qualifications, including a list of all publications authored in the previous 10 years;
(v) a list of all other cases in which, during the previous 4 years, the witness testified as an expert at trial or by deposition; and
(vi) a statement of the compensation to be paid for the study and testimony in the case.

The litigation report format was detailed in Chapter 4 and will include items (i), (ii), and (iii) (see sample in Appendix D). Item (iv) the witness's qualifications and publications are covered by the drug expert's CV (curriculum vitae) usually provided to the hiring attorney either before or with a letter of engagement. A list of all other testimonial cases during the last 4 years (v) should be available when needed by a federal court. Item (vi) is the invoice billed to the hiring attorney for work up to the present, and hopefully paid before the drug expert takes the stand.[35]

Deposition of the Drug Expert

After submitting the litigation report, it is not uncommon for the attorney of the opposing party to schedule a deposition with the drug expert. The time and place are mutually agreed by the drug expert and the hiring attorney. The opposing attorney pays the drug expert for the time it takes to complete the deposition or by some other arrangement agreed to by the attorneys. Depositions taken on behalf of the opposing attorney's clients are optional and many times the drug expert will go to trial without being deposed first by the other side. The procedures for a case in federal court for depositions are contained within the Federal Rules of Civil Procedure (FRCP), primarily Rule 30 "Depositions by Oral Examination."[36] Each state has its own discovery and deposition rules, with most states similar to the rules of deposition in the FRCP.[31]

Sometimes the drug expert will be asked to arrive 30 min or an hour earlier to meet in the hiring attorney's office to go over the depo and the likely lines of questioning. Do not be surprised if a stuffed gazelle and a mountain lion are eye-balling you from the vast savanna of the attorney's high-rise office.[37] While you may be glancing at your watch as the appointed time arrives, the hiring attorney may wave you back in your chair and make his opponent wait a few more minutes.

The conference room that the depo takes place in will offers a vantage point of the city unknown to the drug expert. The table will likely be made of a rare wood, perhaps with inlaid tile or stone around the borders. Coffee, soft drinks, and water will be offered and served to the drug expert, who should drink something to keep hydrated.[38] After cordial greetings around the table and a quick introduction to the court reporter, the reporter switches on a recording machine and administers the oath to the drug expert. The oath here will be the same as in the courtroom. The court reporter will first ask the deponent his or her name and its spelling for the record.[39] Next the court reporter will ask the attorneys if the usual stipulations are invoked. These stipulations are agreements between the parties that govern the procedures of the deposition such as the duration of the deposition, rules for objections, and numbering of exhibits.[40]

---

[35] After initial research and production of a litigation report, the drug expert should submit an invoice and receive payment before testifying at trial. The expert will be asked during cross-examination what the hourly rate charged is and the total payment made to the expert. As considerable time usually passes between the litigation report and eventual trial or deposition testimony, there is plenty of time to submit an invoice before trial and another final invoice after trial.

[36] The Federal Rules of Civil Procedures (FRCP) govern civil proceedings in the United States district courts. Their purpose is "to secure the just, speedy, and inexpensive determination of every action and proceeding." The rules were first adopted by order of the Supreme Court on December 20, 1937, transmitted to Congress on January 3, 1938, and effective September 16, 1938. From the US Courts website at: *www.uscourts.gov/rules-policies/ current-rules-practice-procedure/federal-rules-civil-procedure.*

[37] This is a true story; it was the finest taxidermy ever seen outside of a museum.

[38] It may be the longest time the drug expert is ever confined in a room. However, FRCP *Rule 30 "Depositions by Oral Examination"* limits duration of the deposition to 1 day of 7 h unless otherwise stipulated or ordered by the court.

[39] See Appendix E for an excerpt of a drug expert's deposition.

[40] Bergman P, Moore A (2014) *op. cit.*

Standard of care limits for a drug expert

A common ploy to discredit a drug expert by the opposing attorney is to elicit testimony outside of the drug expert's expertise. This is most likely encountered during the deposition of the drug expert by the opposing attorney where a greater degree of badgering can occur and without the benefit of the judge to keep order and sustain objections.[41] Likewise, the drug expert walks a thin line when forming an expert opinion in a particular case where prescription drugs are used by a physician in treating a patient. The drug expert is not a physician and does not see patients, which the opposing attorney will make abundantly clear. The drug expert is not qualified to opine on the general standard of care for treating pain in cancer patients, for example. But the drug expert is qualified in the proper use, pharmacological effects, and dangers of opioid analgesics in treating cancer pain. Indeed, one of the main themes of this book is that the best expert by training, research, and experience to testify on questions of drug use, drug effects, and drug adverse effects is a Ph.D. in Pharmacology.

The drug expert can successfully defend challenges to their expertise in general standard of care issues by arguing a unique and well-supported expertise in pharmacology; a more narrow "standard of care" expertise focused on the use of drugs. This is easier said than done, as most drug experts also have a great deal of medical knowledge and the opposing attorney would love to hear the drug expert's ideas on general medicine and treating a patient. The drug expert must only give deposition testimony on what can be supported by scientific evidence and remain silent about everything else.

[Narrative continued]

From records provided from the hiring attorney, the drug expert created a timeline of the defendant's UA test dates and results. For the last 2 years, Mr. Winfield had 94 weekly urine drug tests. There were only 4 days when the defendant tested positive for methamphetamine. The most recent positive UA for methamphetamine was nearly 9 months before the meth lab raid. The defendant was positive only on 4.26% of the days tested and therefore methamphetamine-free on 95.74% of the time over the last 2 years. After researching scientific studies of the environmental impact of meth lab homes on children and adults, as well as persons handling methamphetamine, it was clear that the defendant would have tested positive for methamphetamine in more than 4% of the time if he was making or handling meth. In the preliminary hearing, the drug expert's testimony reviewed the findings of his litigation report and concluded upon direct examination that Gary Winfield was not involved in meth manufacture, due to the finding of repeated negative urine tests. The consensus of the research showed that contamination of the "cooker" with detectable methamphetamine is a part of meth lab manufacture and it is more likely than not that the defendant would test positive for meth if he was involved in meth manufacture. On cross-examination, the drug expert was questioned about a few studies cited in the literature that did not show detectable levels of methamphetamine after meth manufacture, but the drug expert pointed out that these studies were noted in his report and that his testimony reflected the scientific consensus. Upon redirect, the drug expert verified that the vast majority of studies cited in his report showed positive meth UAs in meth lab personnel and other occupants, and in persons handling methamphetamine. The defendant went to trial and was found guilty of methamphetamine possession but charges of methamphetamine manufacture were dropped. This felony conviction violated the conditions of his drug court program and the defendant was incarcerated. He is currently serving time in prison.

---

[41] As noted above, the hiring attorney can raise objections to questions asked of the drug expert by the opposing attorney at the depo to get them on record, but the drug expert is still expected to answer the question in most instances.

Chapter 6

Hairs of the Innocent: Detection of marijuana in a child custody case

A Profile of Marijuana—Drug Use in Pregnancy

Drug Use by Parents and Child Maltreatment—Testing for Drugs in Hair Samples

Drug Expert Testimony in Court

[Narrative]

Nothing was going right for Mr. Julian Andrews. After a failed career as a musician, he was now employed as a barista at a massively-franchised coffee shop chain. He was recently divorced from his wife of 8 years, and had alternate-weekend custody of their 6 year-old daughter. Mr. Andrews enjoyed his weekends with his daughter, which usually involved outside activities at the park and pizza with movies on Saturday night. On a recent Sunday night, the mother caught the scent of marijuana on the father when he brought their daughter home. She noticed that her daughter appeared sleepy and "out of it." She was extremely upset and accused the father of feeding their daughter marijuana brownies. He denied the accusation. The next day the mother hired an attorney, who arranged for the daughter's hair to be tested for the presence of THC, the active ingredient of marijuana. The daughter's hair sample came back positive for THC. The mother claimed that this proved the father is giving marijuana to their child. She petitioned the Family Court to grant her sole custody. The father, Mr. Andrews, hired a lawyer who tells him they need a drug expert to interpret the results of the drug tests from the daughter's hair samples. The lawyer submitted a query to an email listserver run by the state bar association and got several recommendations for a local university pharmacologist, who agreed to take the case.

A Profile of Marijuana[1]

The marijuana plant, *Cannabis sativa*, is a common weed that grows in the wild in many parts of the world.[2] Marijuana is a plant whose leaves and flowers are dried and smoked, or eaten in baked goods, for the action of its main psychoactive ingredient, *delta*-9-tetrahydrocannabinol, abbreviated as THC.[3] The marijuana plant, like many other plant species, produces various chemicals that it uses as defense substances so it won't get eaten. The natural role of THC and other chemicals may also be to prevent desiccation, as the amount of THC-containing resins is greatest in plants from hot, arid regions of the world.[4] While alcohol is the most used and abused *legal* drug, marijuana is the most used and abused *illegal* drug in the United States and across the world.[5]

Smoking marijuana, usually in the form of a cigarette ("joint" or "blunt") or in the bowl of a pipe, produces subjective effects of a "high" in less than 10 min.[6] The pharmacological effects of THC are most prominent for about 1–3 h after

---

[1] "Marijuana" with a "j" is the most popular spelling of the plant. It is also spelled as "Marihuana" with an "h" in some federal statutes and documents, although this spelling is considered archaic and is used infrequently.

[2] *Cannabis sativa* is the genus and species name of the marijuana plant; subspecies or strains also exist.

[3] Brenner GM, Stevens CW (2018) *Brenner and Stevens' Pharmacology, 5th edition*. Pharmacology textbook for medical and health professional students, Saunders/Elsevier, Philadelphia/London.

[4] Pate DW (1994) Chemical ecology of *Cannabis*. J. Int. Hemp Soc. 2:32–37.

[5] Desrosiers NA et al. (2014) Phase I and II cannabinoid disposition in blood and plasma of occasional and frequent smokers following controlled smoked cannabis. Clin Chem. 60:631–643.

[6] Smoking marijuana is the most common route of administration for THC. THC is also abundantly available in medicinal and/or recreational marijuana states in oral forms like cookies, candy, and gummy bears, collectively called "edibles." Liquid THC in gelatin capsules is also available as a pharmaceutical product called dronabinol (Marinol®) indicated for the anorexia associated with weight loss in patients with AIDS and for nausea and vomiting associated with cancer chemotherapy in patients who have failed to respond adequately to conventional antiemetic treatments.

smoking a marijuana cigarette.[7,8] Users report a feeling of euphoria (high), increased loquaciousness, and mild perceptual alterations (e.g., a sense of time slowing down). Acute cardiovascular effects of marijuana are transient and include tachycardia, systemic vasodilation, and increased blood pressure.[9]

Adverse effects of marijuana smoking include reduction in performance on tests of memory, reaction time, attention, tracking, and motor function.[10] These adverse effects of marijuana are dependent on the dose of THC which is delivered into the bloodstream and are greatest during the first hour after smoking marijuana. The adverse effects of marijuana, including impairment of driving, dissipate by 3–4 h after smoking and are usually undetectable after this time,[11] but there are some exceptions.[12]

Mechanism of action of marijuana

As mentioned before, the major psychoactive ingredient in the marijuana plant is THC. THC was isolated from marijuana flowers and leaves in 1964, coming rather late in the game compared to the isolation of other medicinal plant substances.[13] It wasn't until the late 1980s that specific THC drug binding sites, called cannabinoid receptors, were identified in the brain.[14] The genetic code of the proteins comprising these THC binding sites was obtained by cloning the first cannabinoid receptor in 1990.

Obtaining the gene that codes for the cannabinoid receptor by cloning means that the actual sequence of DNA that codes for the protein receptor is known. That the cannabinoid receptor gene is encoded in our human genome is strong evidence for a natural endogenous substance in the brain whose purpose is to interact with the cannabinoid receptor. After an extensive search of endogenous chemicals extracted from pig brains, a lipid chemical was isolated that bound to the cannabinoid receptor and acted like exogenous THC.[15] The endogenous THC-like substance was named *anandamide*, a portmanteau of the Sanskrit word for bliss (*Ānanda*) and the chemical descriptor "amide."[16]

Pharmacokinetics of marijuana

The psychoactive ingredient of marijuana, THC, is metabolized by enzymes in the liver and forms one weakly active metabolite, THC-OH, and one inactive metabolite, THC-COOH.[17] The THC molecule and the THC-COOH inactive metabolite are the drug molecules that are routinely detected and quantified in forensic toxicology and clinical studies. Importantly, THC could be detected with a second-hand smoke exposure but detection of the THC-COOH metabolite only occurs following ingestion or smoking of the marijuana product.

Pharmacokinetic studies examine the time course of the drug concentration in the bloodstream after drug administration. Peak levels of THC in the bloodstream occur about 5 min after smoking and can range from 50 to 120 ng/mL in clinical studies.[18] The time it takes for the metabolism and excretion of a drug is quantified as the elimination half-life of a drug. The

---

[7] Kelly P, Jones RT (1992) Metabolism of tetrahydrocannabinol in frequent and infrequent marijuana users. J Anal Toxicol. 16:228–235.

[8] Huestis MA et al. (2005) Estimating the time of last cannabis use from plasma delta 9-tetrahydrocannabinol and 11-nor-9-carboxy-delta9-tetrahydrocannabinol concentrations. Clin Chem. 51:2289–2295.

[9] Tachycardia is fast heart rate, about 10-20 beats per minute over baseline. Vasodilation in the vessels of the eye leads to the "red-eye" seen after marijuana use. Sachs et al. (2015) Safety and toxicology of cannabinoids. Neurotherapeutics 12:735–746.

[10] Kramer JL (2015) Medical marijuana for cancer. CA Cancer J Clin. 65:109-122; Ramaekers et al. (2004) Dose related risk of motor vehicle crashes after cannabis use. Drug Alcohol Depend. 7:109–119.

[11] Grotenhermen F et al. (2007) Developing limits for driving under cannabis. Addiction 102:1910–1917.

[12] Performance deficits have been noted for longer than 4 hours in chronic heavy users of marijuana during a controlled abstinence period. See Bondallaz P et al. (2016) Cannabis and its effects on driving skills. Forensic Sci Int. 268:92–102.

[13] Morphine was isolated from the raw opium juice of the poppy plant by Sertürner about 160 years earlier when he reported the discovery of a sleep-inducing molecule isolated from opium in a letter to the editor of the *Trommsdorffs Journal der Pharmacie* in 1805. He named it morphine after *Morpheus*, the Greek god of sleep.

[14] Atakan Z (2012) Cannabis, a complex plant: different compounds and different effects on individuals. Ther Adv Psychopharmacol. 2:241–254.

[15] Felder CC et al. (1993) Anandamide, an endogenous cannabimimetic eicosanoid, binds to the cloned human cannabinoid receptor and stimulates receptor-mediated signal transduction. Proc Natl Acad Sci USA 90: 7656–7660.

[16] This path from a drug's binding site, to a cloned receptor, to an endogenous substance differs from the discovery of endorphins two decades earlier. In that case, the endogenous substance (endorphin) that bound to opioid binding sites was discovered first and the opioid receptors cloned later.

[17] Schwope DM et al. (2011) Identification of recent cannabis use: whole-blood and plasma free and glucuronidated cannabinoid pharmacokinetics following controlled smoked cannabis administration. Clin Chem. 57:1406–1414.

[18] Ramaekers JG et al. (2006) Cognition and motor control as a function of Delta9-THC concentration in serum and oral fluid: limits of impairment. Drug Alcohol Depend. 85:114-122; Toennes SW, Ramaekers JG, Theunissen EL, Moeller MR, Kauert GF (2008) Comparison of cannabinoid pharmacokinetic properties in occasional and heavy users smoking a marijuana or placebo joint. J Anal Toxicol. 32:470–477.

elimination half-life is usually measured in the blood and is the time in hours or minutes that is takes to decrease the blood concentration by half. Because the active ingredient in marijuana, THC, is fat soluble, it can be detected in the bodily fluids for long periods of time—days or weeks after it is used. In the blood, the elimination half-life of THC and its metabolites ranges from 4 to 6 days.[19] These studies show that the active ingredient of marijuana, THC, and inactive THC metabolites, can be detected in the blood for many days after it is used and long after any pharmacological effects of marijuana have worn off.

The marijuana plant contains a vast array of chemical substances, with THC as the primary psychoactive ingredient in marijuana. Another active chemical found at high concentrations in the marijuana plant is cannabidiol (CBD).[20] CBD is also psychoactive and can produce sedation, but has gained most acclaim as a potential antiseizure agent. CBD is approved for medical use in some states, even though medical marijuana is still illegal in the same state.[21]

Bedsides the chemicals (drugs) found in the marijuana plant, known as natural cannabinoids, there are other THC-like chemicals entirely synthesized in the laboratory. The use and abuse of these potent and dangerous synthetic cannabinoids are further discussed in Chapter 11.

Drug Use in Pregnancy

As detailed in Chapter 1, we live in a drugged society with soaring rates of prescription drug use, over-the-counter (OTC) drug use, alcohol use, and illegal drug use. In the overwhelming majority of cases, we do not know the ill effects of a particular drug, if any, on the growing fetus. Research suggests that less than 10% of new drugs approved by the U.S. Food and Drug Administration (FDA) have determined if there is a risk for fetal malformations or birth defects.[22] Additionally, online information of drugs to avoid during pregnancy are unreliable and inconsistent.[23] After marketing and use of certain types of prescription drugs for many years, patterns of adverse effects on pregnancy sometimes emerge. For example, drugs for the treatment of epilepsy and other seizure disorders, called antiepileptic drugs (AED) emerged as drugs that may be unsafe to use during pregnancy.[24]

Not surprisingly, there is more research done on the ill effects of alcohol and illegal drug use during pregnancy than prescription drug use in pregnancy. There is an alarmingly high use of alcohol by women during pregnancy. Alcohol use in pregnancy has a prevalence rate of 1 in 13 or about 8% of pregnant mothers.[25] Alcohol use is associated with serious damage to the fetus, sometimes leading to fetal alcohol spectrum disorder (FASD)[26] diagnosis in newborns. It is the leading cause of cognitive disability (mental retardation) in the United States. Children with full FASD are characterized physically by craniofacial deformities and functionally by mental retardation and other neurodevelopmental disabilities.[27] It is estimated that 2000–8000 infants are born each year with FASD caused by the intrauterine exposure to alcohol.[28] Children with FASD grow up to be adolescents and adults with FASD, with persistent disability plaguing them since birth.

Exposure to alcohol in utero produces brain damage that may cause difficulty in living a productive life. Persons with FASD are overrepresented in the criminal justice system and among the incarcerated. Research shows that mental illness is present in 94% of individuals with FASD, 50% of FASD adolescents and adults display inappropriate sexual

---

[19] Johansson E et al. (1989) Terminal elimination plasma half-life of delta 1-tetrahydrocannabinol (delta 1-THC) in heavy users of marijuana. Eur J Clin Pharmacol. 37:273-277; Kelly P, Jones RT (1992) Metabolism of tetrahydrocannabinol in frequent and infrequent marijuana users. J Anal Toxicol. 16:228-235; Schwilke EW et al. (2009) Delta9-tetrahydrocannabinol (THC), 11-hydroxy-THC, and 11-nor-9-carboxy-THC plasma pharmacokinetics during and after continuous high-dose oral THC. Clin Chem. 55:2180–2189.

[20] Pate DW (1994) *Op cit.*

[21] For example, even some of the most conservative states in the South (e.g., Mississippi, Alabama, and Georgia) have passed a Compassionate Use of Cannabidiol law for treating intractable epilepsy in children. See *norml.org/states.*

[22] Adam MP et al. (2011) Evolving knowledge of the teratogenicity of medications in human pregnancy. Am J Med Genet Part C. 157:175–182.

[23] Peters SL et al. (2013) Safe lists for medications in pregnancy: inadequate evidence base and inconsistent guidance from Web-based information. Pharmacoepidemiol Drug Saf. 22:324–328.

[24] See Chapter 3, *"Show Me the Money: Epilepsy Drugs and the Four Million Dollar Embezzlement."*

[25] Centers for Disease Control Prevention (2012) Alcohol use and binge drinking among women of childbearing age—United States, 2006–2010. Morbidity and Mortality Weekly Report 61:534–538.

[26] Fetal alcohol syndrome (FAS) is now called fetal alcohol spectrum disorder (FASD) to recognize the continuum of adverse effects. See CDC website on this topic at: *www.cdc.gov/ncbddd/fasd/index.html.*

[27] Riley EP et al. (2011) Fetal alcohol spectrum disorders: an overview. Neuropsychol Rev. 21:73–80.

[28] Cannon MJ et al. (2015) Prevalence and characteristics of women at risk for an alcohol-exposed pregnancy (AEP) in the United States: Estimates from the national survey of family growth. Matern Child Health J. 19:776–782.

behavior at some times in their life, 60% of individuals diagnosed with FASD have "trouble with the law," and some 50% of FASD-afflicted persons have a record of confinement in a jail, prison, residential drug treatment facility, or psychiatric hospital.[29]

The American Bar Association (ABA) recently released a detailed guide for attorneys concerning representation of FASD clients.[30] This ABA guide also lists case law concerning legal issues that may arise for clients with FASD such as the right to expert witnesses (a drug expert would be useful here), a hands-on expert for examination of the FASD defendant, mitigation for sentencing, false confessions, testimony by victims or witnesses with FASD, competency to waive Miranda rights, plea bargain, or stand trial; and drug-induced diminished capacity.

Besides alcohol, studies have found that children born to mothers used abused drugs during pregnancy are at a higher risk of child maltreatment than children from the general population.[31] A woman who abuses drugs during pregnancy is likely to continue to abuse drugs as a new mother and her parenting abilities may be serious impaired.

During the cocaine "crack epidemic" of the 1980s and the upsurge of pregnant women delivering infants addicted cocaine (crack babies) various state jurisdictions criminalized drug-abusing pregnant women.[32] Much of drug testing on pregnant women was done without their informed consent, with criminal charges and forced confinement. At the Medical University of South Carolina (MUSC) in Charleston, hospital administrators worked with city police to develop a policy of arresting pregnant women who tested positive for illegal drug use. Thirty women were arrested; Ferguson and 9 other women brought suit claiming that MUSC policy was a violation of right against unreasonable searches, stated in the Fourth Amendment. This case eventually found its way to the Supreme Court of the United States, leading to the landmark decision in *Ferguson v. City of Charleston, 2002*. In a majority opinion, the Court found that drug testing in pregnant women did not fall within the "special needs exception" of obtaining a warrant as guaranteed by the Fourth Amendment. Recognizing the conflict with the adverse effects of prenatal drug use, the Court held that "the governmental interest did not justify violating a patient's constitutional right to privacy. As a result, the drug tests were unconstitutional searches in violation of the Fourth Amendment."[33]

In light of this ruling, hospitals and health care professionals obtain urine samples after informed consent from all of their prenatal patients. Each clinic or hospital appears to have different policies with regards to drug testing, most will do so under the treating physician's orders whereas others may test all potential mothers for drug use.[34] As of 2019, about half of the states and the District of Columbia deem maternal drug use during pregnancy to be child abuse under civil child welfare laws, and three states consider it grounds for civil commitment in prison or mandatory stays in drug rehabilitation facilities.[35] Half of the states and DC mandate that health care professionals report suspected prenatal drug use, and eight states require them to test neonates for drug exposure if they suspect substance abuse.

Drug Use by Parents and Child Maltreatment

The arrival of a newborn into a single- or dual-parent environment often produces abrupt changes in the parent's lifestyle, especially with the first-born child. Ideally, a newborn provides an impetus to curb substance use in drug-using parents. However, in the United States where more than half of all pregnancies are unintended and dwindling options available to obtain a medical abortion,[36] parents with a substance abuse disorder may find themselves with an unwanted child and little incentive to maintain sobriety.

An early study found that about 25% of all cases of child abuse or maltreatment involved at least one parent or caretaker abusing alcohol and/or illegal drugs.[37] Among these drug-using caretakers, 77% used alcohol, 37% abused crack or powder cocaine, 32% marijuana, and only 4% of caretakers used heroin. After the crack epidemic came the meth epidemic. By the year 2005, data from the National Drug Intelligence Center's National Drug Threat Survey showed that state and local enforcement agencies now identify methamphetamine as their greatest drug threat (39.6%), a greater problem than cocaine,

[29] Streissguth AP et al. (2004) Risk factors for adverse life outcomes in fetal alcohol syndrome and fetal alcohol effects. J Develop Behav Ped. 25:228–238.

[30] American Bar Association (2011) Fetal alcohol spectrum disorders (FASD): what you need to know to help your clients. Available at: *www.americanbar.org*.

[31] Jaudes PK et al. (1995) Association of drug abuse and child abuse. Child Abuse Negl. 19:1065–1075.

[32] Toll (2001) For My Doctor's Eyes Only: *Ferguson v. City of Charleston*. Loyola Univ Chicago Law J. 33:267–319.

[33] Toll (2001) *Ibid*.

[34] Personal communication from OB/GYN colleagues.

[35] These three states are Minnesota, South Dakota, and Wisconsin. See *www.guttmacher.org/state-policy/explore/substance-use-during-pregnancy*.

[36] Roberts SC et al. (2014) Alcohol use before and during unwanted pregnancy. Alcohol Clin Exp Res. 38:2844–2852.

[37] Magura S, Laudet AB (1996) Parental substance abuse and child maltreatment: Review and implications for intervention. Child Youth Serv Rev. 18:193–220.

marijuana, heroin, or 3,4-methylenedioxymethamphetamine (MDMA, a.k.a. "X" or "Ecstasy").[38] Children exposed to methamphetamine manufacture suffer a much worse fate than other drugs, with known fatalities and long-term adverse effects. This unfortunate topic was discussed in Chapter 5, under the section on exposure of children to meth manufacturing.

Besides parental neglect and physical abuse, children of drug using parents in worst-case scenarios are recruited to help in the drug distribution ring or prostituted to obtain money for drugs.[37] Very recent data includes an alarming rate of adolescent homicides in Philadelphia correlated with drug-using parents and caretakers.[39]

In a study of 3023 respondents to a telephone survey carried out in 50 mid-sized cities in California, current marijuana used by one or more parents was positively related to frequency of child physical abuse.[40] As the State of California legalized recreational marijuana, additional studies showed a positive correlation between the density of marijuana retail stores and the number of child abuse cases.[40] Marijuana use in parents also affects later characteristics in their offspring.[41] For example, marijuana use in parents is positively correlated with impulsivity in their children.

Besides parental maltreatment, marijuana in the child's environment carries some risk of poisoning. Children are especially susceptible to marijuana that may be present in an oral formulation, such as cookies, candy, or gummy bears (called "edibles"). In Colorado, the rate of children presenting to the Children's Hospital with acute marijuana exposure more than doubled from the 2 years before recreational marijuana legalization compared to the 2 years after legalization.[42] There are cases in the literature of infants and toddlers presenting to the hospital in a coma from eating marijuana cookies or marijuana resin (hash).[43] Fortunately, no overdose fatalities occurred and most of the poisoned children recovered after a day in the hospital.

Child custody and marijuana use

Family court and custody cases often depend on issues of drug-using parents. Studies show that 65% of judicial officers adjudicating custody and visitation disputes reported that alcohol and drug use issues were raised "often" or "very often."[44] The use of marijuana by a parent does not automatically deem that parent unable to maintain custody or joint custody[45] of a child. If there is no evidence of impairment or use of marijuana in the presence of the child, it is likely that custody will be maintained, even in states where marijuana use is illegal.[46] Family courts generally decide child custody disputes on the basis of what is in the child's best interests. Most courts consider it in the child's best interests to have regular contact with both parents.

Testing for Drugs in Hair Samples

Hair is a keratin protein matrix at the molecular level. Within this interlocking matrix are other substances that were in the bloodstream at the time the hair strand was formed. These other substances in the blood get "frozen" in time as they are deposited along the growing hair strand. Drugs and drug metabolites are among the many molecules in the bloodstream that get frozen into the hair strand as it grows.[47] As an analogy, a strand of hair is like a licorice stick[48] dropped on the beach. The grains of sand adhered to the licorice are like the drug molecules, drug metabolites, and other substances floating around in the blood when the hair strand, the licorice stick, was formed.

[38] Grant P (2007) Evaluation of children removed from a clandestine methamphetamine laboratory. J Emerg Nurs. 33:31–41.

[39] Hohl BC et al. (2017) Association of Drug and Alcohol Use With Adolescent Firearm Homicide at Individual, Family, and Neighborhood Levels. JAMA Intern Med. 177:317–324.

[40] Freisthler B et al. (2015) Examining the relationship between marijuana use, medical marijuana dispensaries, and abusive and neglectful parenting. Child Abuse Negl. 48:170–178.

[41] Riggs NR (2009) Protecting against intergenerational problem behavior: mediational effects of prevented marijuana use on second-generation parent-child relationships and child impulsivity. Drug Alcohol Depend. 100:153–160.

[42] Wang GS et al. (2016) Unintentional Pediatric Exposures to Marijuana in Colorado, 2009-2015. JAMA Pediatr. 170(9):e160971.

[43] Appelbaum A, Oades PJ (2006) Coma due to cannabis toxicity in an infant. Eur J Emerg Med. 13:177–179.

[44] Judicial Council of California/Administrative Office of the Courts (2007) Drug and Alcohol Testing in Child Custody Cases: Implementation of Family Code Section 3041.5. Center for Families, Children & the Courts, San Francisco, CA.

[45] Pun unintended.

[46] This statement and much of the information in this section is from Osbeck MK, Bromberg H (2017) Marijuana law in a nutshell. West Academic Publishing, St. Paul, MN.

[47] Skopp et al. (2007) Deposition of cannabinoids in hair after long-term use of cannabis. Forensic Sci Int 170:46–50.

[48] Twizzlers® come to mind.

Testing hair for illicit use of drugs began about 60 years ago with the major advantage that hair samples yield a much longer drug detection time than urine or blood testing.[49] Once incorporated in hair, most drugs are stable within keratin protein matrix for weeks and months. Perhaps the most extreme example of a drug's stability in hair was the detection of cocaine in a hair sample from a 900-year old Peruvian mummy.[50] Pubic hair shows the same or higher concentration of abused drugs as head hair.[51] Pubic hair samples may be useful in cases when the subject to be tested but has no head hair, as in the fashionable bald or a shaved head.

Because adult human head hair grows at an average rate of 1 cm per month (*centimeter*; 2.54 cm = 1 in.), segmentation of the hair sample by cutting into 1 cm lengths can provide data on long-term drug use month to month, limited in time only by the length of the hair sample.[52] Forensic hair testing for drugs of abuse is used to monitor the abstinence of parolees or drug treatment court participants, identifying sexual assault with "date-rape" drugs, documenting in utero exposure to drugs, and proving drug use in child custody cases.[53] Drug testing is often used in determinations of child protection cases, as in this chapter's case.[54]

Testing hair samples for marijuana use

Marijuana exposure is routinely detected either by the presence of THC, the active ingredient of the marijuana plant that produces the pharmacological effects of marijuana, or a THC metabolite, which is what the THC molecule turns into after it is metabolized by the liver. Assays or methods for hair drug analysis can be used to either detect the THC molecule or the THC-COOH molecule or both. Importantly, as shown in this chapter's drug expert case, hair samples can be analyzed with or without washing of the sample.

Marijuana is used by many routes of administration including smoking ("joints" and "blunts") and eating dessert products baked with marijuana or hashish[55] added (e.g., "hash brownies"). Marijuana can also have direct effects on nonusers in the environment. "Contact high" refers to nonsmokers feeling the effects of marijuana when in the same room with *chronic smokers* of marijuana.[56] Nonusers may get high from second-hand exposure or passive smoking of marijuana, and importantly for the present chapter case, their hair may get contaminated with THC. When this happens, the hair absorbs the THC molecule directly from the air and is not deposited from within onto the growing hair follicle. However, THC from environmental exposure is not usually detected in a washed hair sample. The finding of the THC molecule in an unwashed hair sample could be either from environmental exposure or by consumption (smoking or eating) of a marijuana product. The finding of the THC-COOH metabolite in either unwashed or washed hair is consistent only with direct consumption by smoking or eating marijuana. For a metabolite of THC to be present, the original THC molecule itself had to be in the blood first in order to get to the liver and be metabolized to the THC metabolite (THC-COOH).

Drug Expert Testimony in Court

The courtroom is often portrayed in movies and other media as a tense environment, which it is. The expert will often be sequestered in a small room or outside the courtroom in the hallway, or if not sequestered, sitting in the courtroom galley observing the proceedings. The contracting attorney will call the expert to the witness stand, where the swearing in will occur before the expert sits down.[57] The novice drug expert may initially feel quite uncomfortable in the witness box, but

---

[49] Huestis et al. (2007) Cannabinoid concentrations in hair from documented cannabis users. Forensic Sci Int 169:129–136.

[50] Springfield AC et al. (1993) Cocaine and metabolites in the hair of ancient Peruvian coca leaf chewers. Forensic Sci Int 63:269–275.

[51] Musshoff et al. (2006) Results of hair analyses for drugs of abuse and comparison with self-reports and urine tests. Forensic Sci Int 156:118–123.

[52] Wang X, Drummer OH (2015) Review: Interpretation of drug presence in the hair of children. Forensic Sci Int. 257:458–472.

[53] Huestis et al. (2007) *op. cit.*

[54] Lewis et al. (1977) Determination of drug exposure using hair: application to child protective cases. Forensic Sci Int. 84:123–128.

[55] Hashish is a concentrated form of marijuana plant resin. In countries like Nepal where hash is a major product, villagers rub the leaves of marijuana plants and scrape the sticky hash resin from their hands into round balls for sale to the tourists.

[56] Or *smoking chronic*. Perhaps because marijuana is so widely used, there are more slang or street names for marijuana than any other drug. According to the National Institute on Drug Abuse (NIDA), these are some common street names for marijuana: "pot," "grass," "herb," "weed," "Mary Jane," "reefer," "blunt", "skunk," "boom," "gangster," "chronic," and "ganja." See list at *www.drugabuse.gov/drugs-abuse/commonly-abused-drugs-charts#marijuana-cannabis*.

[57] Unlike in the movies, I've never had to place my hand on the Bible during the swearing in. For true atheists, however, the oath "Do you swear to tell the whole truth and nothing but the truth, so help you God?" can be replaced with an affirmation (replacing "swear" with "affirm" and removing the "so help you God") if the expert so requests. This is not advisable as it may bias the judge and jury against the expert, especially in Bible belt states. See Jonassen FB (2014) 'So Help Me?' Religious expression and artifacts in the oath of office and the courtroom oath. Cardozo Pub Law Policy Ethics J. 12:303–373.

will soon be put at ease by the direct examination led by the hiring attorney, who has prepped him or her with the lines of questioning.[58] The drug expert should also exert some brainpower during preparation by thinking about questions that may arise during cross-examination. It may console timorous drug experts that they do not have to worry about being sued by the represented party, except in very rare cases.[59]

Not every drug case will bring the drug expert into the courtroom; most cases will not. Some litigation consulting jobs are relatively short, with a few hours of research and a preliminary conclusion of the drug issue at hand transmitted verbally in a phone call with the hiring attorney. Other cases lead to a much greater degree of research and a formal litigation report emailed in an attachment to the attorney. After submitting a litigation report to the contracting attorney, the opposing attorney may want to take the deposition of the drug expert.[60] Both parties will work with the drug expert to agree on a mutual time and place for the deposition, usually in a conference room at one of the law firms in the case. Occasionally, a formal subpoena will be mailed to the drug expert, or more rarely, the expert will be served a subpoena at the workplace.[61] After a deposition, many cases will end up with the drug expert testifying in court, either in a preliminary hearing or in the actual trial.[62]

There is a bit of research on the characteristics of a successful expert witness in court. Researchers found that four measurable characteristics correlate to courtroom credibility.[63] These expert witness' characteristics are *trustworthiness*, *knowledge*, *confidence*, and *likability*. Confidence is correlated to credibility in an inverse "U" shaped curve with medium levels of confidence associated with the most credibility in expert witness.[64] Even though the expert witness may be the smartest person in the courtroom in the specific area of testimony, the expert should not cross the line from confidence to arrogance. The best approach may be to go into teaching mode, like you would in a lecture to students. Teaching, after all, is ultimately the basic function of a drug expert.

Not surprisingly, research shows that the gender of the expert witness is a factor in perceived credibility of experts by the jury. These results in expert gender research yield the classic good news-bad news paradigm. The good news is that experts rated high in both knowledge and likability were correlated with high credibility and it did not matter if the expert was male or female. The bad news is that for experts rated medium or low knowledge and likability, females were rated lower than males in credibility.[65] Women experts who testify are considered less credible than male experts by judges.[66] This may be due to more intrusive questions of female experts are asked during cross-examination than are asked of men. More intrusive questioning that attempts to disparage the female expert may lead to lower credibility. The bottom line with regard to differences between male and female experts is that any expert who performs diligent research and preparation, shows confidence, and is likable will most likely be judged credible.

There are few studies examining credibility and the race and gender of expert witnesses. In a 4-way study examining race and gender (African-American or White, male or female) carried out in Dallas, Texas, the African-American female expert was found to be the most persuasive and the African-American male expert to display the best reasoning ability. As these results contradicted their hypothesis that the African-American experts would be perceived less credible than their White counterparts, the authors rather sardonically suggested that the jurors were aware of gender and race stereotypes and made intentional efforts to avoid them and therefore overcompensated for such stereotypical thinking.[67] To the present

---

[58] There is a great variation in the amount of time a drug expert may spend prepping with the hiring attorney. While the drug expert should always spend at least a couple hours or so preparing for testimony (especially reading and knowing their own litigation report), one cannot always expect smaller firms to arrange time for preparation in their offices. In many cases, the expert will be prepped by their hiring attorney at a nearby Starbucks® on the day of the trial or in the hallway outside the courtroom 15 min before taking the stand.

[59] Lawsuits against expert witness are very rare and case law has created immunity for expert witnesses except in the most egregious cases. See Jurs A (2007) The rationale for expert immunity or liability exposure and case law since Briscoe: reasserting immunity protection for friendly expert witnesses. Univ Memphis Law Rev. 38:49–96.

[60] More about depositions and what to expect was discussed in the last chapter.

[61] It was a little daunting to be served a subpoena by the Sheriff at the reception desk of the main lobby at OSU Med School in between classes. All students have a natural curiosity about their professors, and medical students are no exception. Needless to say, there were quite a few rumors flying around with the consensus being that I was served with divorce papers.

[62] Appendix F gives an excerpt of drug expert court testimony.

[63] Brodsky et at. (2009) Credibility in the courtroom: how likable should an expert witness be? J Am Acad Psych Law 37:525–532.

[64] Cramer et al. (2009) Expert witness confidence and juror personality: their impact on credibility and persuasion in the courtroom. J Am Acad Psych Law 37:63–74.

[65] Neal et al. (2012) Warmth and competence on the witness stand: implications for the credibility of male and female expert witnesses. J Am Acad Psych Law 40:488–497.

[66] Daftary-Kapur et al. (2014) Gender-intrusive questioning: a survey of expert witnesses. Beh Sci Law 32:180–194.

[67] Memon A, Shuman DW (1998) Juror perception of experts in civil suits: the role of race and gender. Law Psych Rev. 22:179–197.

author, these interpretations hoist the authors on their own petard due to *their* own personal beliefs and stereotypes of persons serving on Texas juries.

[Narrative continued]

The drug expert reviewed the toxicology report from the hair testing facility, which was positive for THC, but notices that the hair samples were unwashed before testing. Additionally, the expert notes that a drug test of the hair was done only for THC and not for any THC metabolites. The drug expert researched the topic of drug testing for marijuana in hair samples and finds that unwashed hair samples that tested only for THC may be positive as a result of second-hand marijuana smoke. The drug expert suggests to the hiring attorney that they order a second test of his daughter's hair for both THC and the main metabolite, THC-COOH, using a testing protocol where the hair sample is washed before testing. The drug expert also provided the name of a national drug testing laboratory for the attorney to contact who can provide such services. The result of the second drug test of the daughter's hair sample was negative for both THC and the metabolite, THC-COOH. This result shows that the daughter did not herself consume any marijuana product because there was no THC-COOH detected. Additionally, the lack of THC detected in the second washed hair sample indicated that the first hair test with unwashed hair samples most likely detected environmental THC from second-hand marijuana smoke. The Family Court judge agreed that the daughter wasn't fed a marijuana brownie or other type of cannabis product while in Mr. Andrews' custody. However, because the first hair test was positive for THC and the drug expert testified that this result was most likely from "sidestream" or second-hand smoke from Mr. Andrews' use of marijuana in his daughter's presence, the Court reduced Mr. Andrews' custody to alternate weekend days with supervision.

Chapter 7

Firewater: Alcohol abuse and tribal homicide

The Drug Alcohol—Alcohol Effects on the Brain and Aggression

Research Methods of the Drug Expert—Alcohol Abuse in Native Americans

Junk Science and the Drug Expert

[Narrative]

Clarence Twofeathers was a Native American living in a small Midwestern town who had a record of legal problems due to alcohol abuse. He was arrested last year for public intoxication and disturbing the peace and was known to local law enforcement for that incident and other drunken episodes. One hot summer night last year, he began drinking beer and vodka with a group of nine other Native Americans at a house party. After a few hours at the party, there was an altercation between Mr. Twofeathers and the decedent at the party. Twofeathers was mad at the decedent for "hitting on" his girlfriend. Angry words were exchanged by Twofeathers and the other male, which was corroborated by witness testimony. Around midnight a fight broke out between Mr. Twofeathers and the decedent. The decedent is killed on the street from multiple stab wounds. Police are called to the scene by bystanders. A token axe was found at the scene of the crime but no other weapons. Witness statements are taken by the police implicating Mr. Twofeathers, but he fled the scene when the police arrived. The next day, law enforcement tracked down Mr. Twofeathers to a local motel and he is arrested for homicide. The State pursued a capital murder charge punishable by death.

An autopsy of the decedent by the medical examiner revealed 21 stab wounds mainly across the back, chest, arms, face, and one in the back of the head. The token axe found at the scene was determined not to be the murder weapon. A peripheral blood sample from the decedent was drawn by the hospital ER nurse on the night of the incident. The blood sample was sent to the state crime lab for a toxicology report. The toxicology report showed that the decedent had a blood alcohol concentration (BAC) of 0.19%. No other drug tests were done. The public defender's office for capital crimes contacted a drug expert to interpret the decedent's BAC and to determine the effects of alcohol on the decedent's behavior. Additionally, the public defender sought the drug expert's opinion on the acute and chronic effects of alcohol intoxication on Mr. Twofeathers' behavior.

The Drug Alcohol

Alcohol is a drug that, while socially acceptable in moderation, is abused to a greater degree and exacts more detrimental costs on society than any other legal or illegal drug in the United States. In monetary terms, the total cost to society of excessive alcohol consumption was $249 billion in 2010 or about $2.05 per drink.[1] Alcohol consumption is a leading cause of premature death in the United States, with excessive drinking accounting for 1 in 10 deaths among working-age adults.[2] The widespread availability and cultural acceptance of alcohol masks the fact that alcohol is a neurotoxic drug with devastating effects on brain function and behavior. Alcoholism, now termed alcohol dependence, is a chronic medical disease and classified in psychiatric listings alongside other mental disorders such as schizophrenia and depression.

Alcohol's active ingredient is ethanol, an insidious drug that is exceedingly more dangerous than commonly realized. Ethanol is a simple molecule and freely distributes throughout the body water, soaking every organ and crossing into the brain with impunity. Pharmacokinetics, which literally means "movement of drug," describes what happens to a drug after

---

[1] Sacks JJ et al. (2015) 2010 National and State Costs of Excessive Alcohol Consumption. Am J Prev Med. 49:e73–9.

[2] Stahre M et al. (2014) Contribution of excessive alcohol consumption to deaths and years of potential life lost in the United States. Prev Chronic Dis. 11:E109.

it is taken. Pharmacokinetic studies show that after drinking alcohol, ethanol is well absorbed from the GI tract and quickly enters the bloodstream. Ethanol reaches a maximum (peak) concentration in the blood 45–60 min after drinking.[3]

Alcohol, or more precisely ethanol, is eliminated at a constant rate from the body due to the saturation of the liver enzymes that metabolize ethanol.[4] The precise elimination rate for ethanol differs according to nutritional status, diet, concurrent food intake, frequency of alcohol intake, gender, individual genetics, and ethnicity.[5] However, average values and ranges are known from decades of research in different populations since the time of the groundbreaking alcohol metabolism research of Widmark and colleagues in the 1930s.[6] Widmark's equations are still used today by the drug expert in alcohol cases, especially for retrograde calculations of BAC from the time of the blood test to the time of the incident, such as a motor vehicle accident.[7]

Some ethanol is broken down (metabolized) in the wall of the gut, but most reaches the liver where it is primarily metabolized.[8] More than 90% of ethanol is metabolized by the liver with 2%–5% excreted unchanged in exhaled breath, urine, and sweat.[9] Alcohol taken with food produces a lower peak blood alcohol concentration (BAC) than alcohol consumed on an empty stomach.[10]

Alcohol Effects on the Brain and Aggression

Ethanol is a drug of abuse like cocaine, heroin, and marijuana. All drugs of abuse reach the brain and become drugs of abuse because they cause the release of dopamine at pleasure and reward centers in the brain and this reinforces continued use. Alcohol affects the brain in a number of ways; some of ethanol's most devastating effects involve the disruption of normal brain function. A sampling of ethanol's effects on brain function is outlined next.

Behavioral disinhibition produced by alcohol

Alcohol use produces a state where users are not inhibited in their acts; called *behavioral disinhibition*. Alcohol and other CNS[11] depressants produce disinhibition, because the brain normally operates with the brakes on. CNS depressants first depress the smaller inhibitory neurons leaving the normally inhibited excitatory neurons unchecked. The unchecked behaviors that result are associated with high-risk behaviors (unprotected sexual activity; other drug use), criminality, violence, and aggression, as discussed later. *Behavioral disinhibition* is an umbrella term used to describe impulsive and aggressive behavior due to the adverse effects of a drug on the brain circuits that control behavior. It may be described in some texts as a "paradoxical effect" or simply "aggression" in the context of alcohol use.

Alcohol use and cognitive dysfunction

Cognitive dysfunction is a general term that encompasses all manner of brain malfunctioning due to disease pathology or drug use. One of the consequences of using alcohol is a general disruption of thought processes known as cognitive impairment or dysfunction. This can include difficulties with such cognitive processes as memory, attention (ability to concentrate), planning ahead, motor (movement) control, and visuospatial performance (locating and reacting to objects).[12] Short-term use of alcohol causes temporary cognitive impairments that disappear as soon as the drugs wear off or shortly afterward. Long-term use of alcohol can produce permanent cognitive impairments.

Much of the effects of alcohol on brain function are due to toxicity to the area of the brain known as the prefrontal cortex. This part of the brain is responsible for "executive function" which has been defined as "higher-order mental abilities, such as attention, planning, organization, abstract reasoning, self-monitoring, and the ability to use external feedback to modulate future behavior."[13] Using brain imaging, it was shown that chronic alcohol use was more detrimental to the

---

[3] Pohorecky LA and Brick J (1988) Pharmacology of ethanol. Pharmacol Ther. 36:335–427.

[4] Cederbaum AI (2012) Alcohol metabolism. Clin Liver Dis. 16:667–685.

[5] Chan LN and Anderson GD (2014) Pharmacokinetic and pharmacodynamic drug interactions with ethanol (alcohol). Clin Pharmacokinet. 53:1115–1136.

[6] Jones AW (2010) Evidence-based survey of the elimination rates of ethanol from blood with applications in forensic casework. Forensic Sci Int. 200:1–20.

[7] See Chapter 17 *A Visit to the Dram Shop*, for an example retrograde BAC calculation.

[8] Cederbaum AI (2012). *Op. cit.*

[9] Paton A (2005) Alcohol in the body. BMJ 330:85–87.

[10] Jones AW (2000) Aspects of in-vivo pharmacokinetics of ethanol. Alcohol Clin Exp Res. 24:400–402.

[11] That would be Central Nervous System; i.e. brain and spinal cord.

[12] Harper C, Matsumoto I (2005) Ethanol and brain damage. Curr Opin Pharmacol. 5:73–78.

[13] Foster J et al. (1994) The cognitive neuropsychology of attention: A frontal lobe perspective. Cog Neuropsych. 11:133–147.

prefrontal cortex than chronic cocaine use.[14] Besides chronic abuse, acute alcohol consumption also disrupts executive function in the prefrontal cortex.[15] Importantly, alcohol disruption of executive function was evidenced by increased aggression in response to provocation.

Alcohol use associated with impulsivity

Impulsivity is defined as "a predisposition toward rapid, unplanned reactions to internal or external stimuli with diminished regard to the negative consequences of these reactions to the impulsive individual or others."[16] Research focused on the detrimental effects of alcohol use and alcohol-related behaviors shows that alcohol intoxication increases impulsivity.[17] This increase in impulsive behaviors was quantified in clinical studies done in a laboratory setting with measured alcohol doses.[18] The degree of impulsivity was correlated with the amount of alcohol used, known as a *dose-dependent effect*. Other studies show that impulsivity is highly correlated with alcohol-related aggression and violent behavior.[19]

Alcohol use associated with aggression and violence

Among all psychoactive substances and drugs of abuse, alcohol is the most potent agent for eliciting aggression and reducing behavioral inhibition.[20] Disturbingly, crime statistics show that the prevalence of alcohol-related crimes has increased dramatically over the last 50 years in the United States. More than half of all violent crimes such as murder, homicide, and aggravated assaults involve alcohol in the perpetrator, victim, or both.[21] There is a direct causal relationship between aggression and alcohol use mediated by the detrimental effects of alcohol on executive function (prefrontal cortex) as noted in the previous section. Increases in aggression were most noted when blood levels of alcohol were still in the rising phase and not later during the falling phase of blood alcohol levels.

In a controlled laboratory environment, subjects who drank alcohol were more aggressive in giving shocks to a fictionalized opponent, and had greater scores on loss of inhibition, emotional control, flexible thinking, and self-monitoring aspects of executive function.[22] The adverse effects of alcohol are particularly related to decreasing anger control.[23] Additionally, in human subjects given placebo beverage or alcohol, alcohol increased the perception of the level of aggression of an attacker in a controlled laboratory environment.[24]

Research Methods of the Drug Expert

The drug expert is first and foremost a *scientist-for-hire*, plain and simple. Pharmacological scientists (pharmacologists) are well trained to do the research needed to supplement the expert's knowledge of the drug issue at hand. For the drug expert, this means undergoing an intense searching and researching of medical and pharmacological studies that shed light on a particular drug issue. This intense period of journal research is necessary even on well-worn cases like the adverse effects of zolpidem (Ambien®), and malpractice suits after a prescription opioid overdose death.[25] There may be new reports and clinical studies published since the last time a drug issue was investigated. There is an incessant flow of drug knowledge produced by the researchers in medical schools, hospitals, pharmaceutical firms, federal agencies, and other institutions in this country and across the world. This vast array of drug knowledge must be searched, sifted, sorted, and read before an expert opinion can be rendered.

---

[14] Goldstein RZ et al. (2004) Severity of neuropsychological impairment in cocaine and alcohol addiction: association with metabolism in the prefrontal cortex. Neuropsychologia 42:1447–1458.

[15] Hoaken PN et al. (1998) Executive cognitive functions as mediators of alcohol-related aggression. Alcohol Alcohol 33:47–54.

[16] Moeller FG et al. (2001) Psychiatric aspects of impulsivity. Am J Psych. 158:1783–1793; Potenza MN, de Wit H (2010) Control yourself: alcohol and impulsivity. Alcohol Clin Exp Res. 34:1303–1305.

[17] Lejuez CW et al. (2010) Behavioral and biological indicators of impulsivity in the development of alcohol use, problems, and disorders. Alcohol Clin Exp Res. 34:1334–1345.

[18] Mitchell JM et al. (2005) Impulsive responding in alcoholics. Alcohol Clin Exp Res. 29:2158–2169.

[19] Dom G et al. (2006) Differences in impulsivity and sensation seeking between early- and late-onset alcoholics. Addict Behav. 31:298–308.

[20] Heinz AJ et al. (2011) Cognitive and neurobiological mechanisms of alcohol-related aggression. Nat Rev Neurosci. 12:400–413.

[21] Miczek KA et al. (2004) Role of alcohol consumption in escalation to violence. Ann N Y Acad Sci. 1036:278–289.

[22] Giancola PR, Corman MD (2007) Alcohol and aggression: a test of the attention-allocation model. Psychol Sci. 18:649–655.

[23] Parrott DJ, Giancola PR (2004) A further examination of the relation between trait anger and alcohol-related aggression: the role of anger control. Alcohol Clin Exp Res. 28:855–864.

[24] Giancola PR et al. (2006) Perceptions of one's attacker's intentions following an aggressive interaction involving alcohol. J Gen Psychol. 133:389–400.

[25] For the former case, see Chapter 15 *Snake Eyes* and for the latter, previous Chapter 4 *The Power of the Poppy*.

The drug expert should approach the drug issue in question much like researching a topic for a review article. The first phase of research involves gathering as much information as feasible.[26] As mentioned in the opening section earlier, the FDA label for all prescription drugs pertinent in a case will be among the first documents obtained. Of course, there are no FDA-approved drug labels for alcohol and illegal drugs. Pharmacology textbooks, especially the massive authoritative tome known as *Goodman and Gilman*,[27] are also useful for general background information concerning the specific drug issues in play.

Drug issues come under the large umbrella of the medical and scientific discipline of Pharmacology, the study of drugs. Pharmacology also includes the subdiscipline of Toxicology, which is the specific study of the harmful effects of drugs and other chemical substances. The *lingua franca* of science is data, and the most reliable drug data can be found in written peer-reviewed or review articles published in medical and pharmacology journals. Access to this worldwide database of drug knowledge is gained through the portal of PubMed[28] or another science publication access site. PubMed is funded and managed by the U.S. National Library of Medicine of the National Institutes of Health, located outside the DC beltway in Bethesda, Maryland. Medical schools have full access to PubMed for its faculty and students, which includes many articles available as free full text and downloadable as Portable Document Format or PDF files. Some essential articles found after a search in PubMed may not be available for free online and charge rates as high as USD $29–$75 to download a digital PDF copy. If this is the case and the journal article isn't available as a hardcopy or interlibrary loan at the medical library, the drug expert should pay for it. The article access charges will be reimbursed after sending the invoice; or if working with a retainer, are already secured by deposited funds in the drug expert's account. The sample invoice has a line for access and printing charges (see Appendix C).

Each journal article that is obtained should be retained as a computer file in PDF format. PDF is one file format that lives up to its name; PDF files are truly portable and everyone with a computer or smartphone can read a PDF file. For documents only available as hardcopy, the drug expert should scan and save as PDF files on the computer.[29]

Organizational tendencies, or lack thereof, may be ingrained in the drug expert since birth but at a minimum, the PDFs of the references cited in the notes or litigation report for each case should be kept in a subfolder of the case subfolder. Depending on the drug expert's *modus operandi*, PDF files can remain in the digital world and read onscreen. With modern computer equipment and touchscreen displays, digital copies can be marked up and highlighted with a stylus within the PDF software, and saved as a separate file. Or if the drug expert prefers reading hardcopies, such paper references should be stored with the physical case file folder in an actual filing cabinet.[30] Keeping track of the PDF files for articles cited in the drug expert report (litigation report) is essential as these references must often be provided to the State or opposing party before the deposition or trial testimony. Physically copying references at a Xerox™ machine is suboptimal due to the likelihood of paper references being marked up with highlighting, comments, or notes which may not be prudent. Providing references is most efficiently done by placing all the PDF reference files in a *Dropbox*® folder to share with the hiring attorney.[31] The size and number of PDF reference files usually prevents attaching all of them to a single email. Multiple emails could be sent, each with a reference, but that is tedious for the drug expert and the receiving attorney. The *DropBox* solution is both elegant and saves trees. Unfortunately, any PDF files sent to an attorney will likely be printed out in their entirety even if they are not planning to use them; law firms, prosecutors, and the courts are the last refuge of the nondigital domain and its tree-killing ways.

It is not easy to use the *PubMed* database to search the world of medical and pharmacological studies. There is a lot to search and a lot to read that way. Why not just *Google* or *Wikipedia* the prescription drug name rather than struggle to find the actual FDA-approved label and appropriate studies in peer-reviewed journal articles? The answer seems obvious to most

---

26 You may have given an estimate of the time and money for the job to the client-attorney and therefore cannot go drifting off-topic too often. However, following adjacent avenues of research often leads to additional information for the drug issue at hand.

27 "The 'Bible' of Pharmacology" is often used when describing the authoritative textbook called *Goodman and Gilman's The Pharmacological Basis of Therapeutics*, published by McGraw-Hill and now in its 13th Edition (2017). It was originally published in 1941 and new editions are published about every five years. A more readable and cost-effective textbook for medical, pharmacology, and allied health students is Brenner GM, Stevens CW (2018) *Brenner and Stevens' Pharmacology, 5th Ed.*, Elsevier:Philadelphia.

28 Opening search page for PubMed at: *www.ncbi.nlm.nih.gov/pubmed*.

29 The files should also exist in multiple backup locations. For example, I use a portable hard drive that plugs into the USB port of any computer I work at. There is a wonderful free program called *Synchron* that keeps the files synchronized to the latest file version on my external hard drive, my home office computer, my OSU office computer, and when I travel, current and up to date on my Microsoft Surfacebook®.

30 See Chapter 5 *Wrong Place at the Wrong Time* under *Deposition of the Drug Expert* section with regards to the contents of the physical case file and what you might be required to bring to a deposition.

31 *Dropbox* is a free cloud storage app that allows the secure transfer of files to individuals that are too big to attach to an email; check it out at *www.dropbox.com*.

of us in that we all want to avoid "junk science" and strive for the best data to answer questions arising in our drug cases. However, there is an increasing use of *Wikipedia* citations in federal courts and elsewhere which (wrongly) form the basis for scientific opinion.[32]

Perhaps the most egregious use of an online source as a basis for the State's expert testimony is in the arena of death penalty cases involving lethal injections of clinically used drugs. Midazolam, a benzodiazepine, was substituted for pentobarbital, a barbiturate, as the first drug in a number of states' 3-drug lethal injection protocols. This switch occurred when various State Departments of Corrections ran out of pentobarbital and couldn't get anymore. In a midazolam lethal injection case from Oklahoma that went all the way to the U.S. Supreme Court, the 5-4 majority opinion of the Supreme Justices did not find the use of midazolam presenting an undue risk of pain and suffering. They ruled for midazolam use in lethal execution against the expert advice presented in an *amicus brief* from Sixteen Pharmacologists.[33] In her dissent, joined by three other justices, Justice Sonia Sotomayor clearly stated that "the district court relied on a 'single purported expert' who testified from suspect sources and in a manner that contradicts empirical data." Justice Sotomayor explained, "In contending that midazolam will work as the State intends, Dr. Evans [state's drug expert, a pharmacist] cited no studies, but instead appeared to rely primarily on the Web site www.drugs.com. Here, given the evidence before the District Court, I struggle to see how its decision to credit the testimony of a single purported expert can be supported given the substantial body of conflicting empirical and anecdotal evidence."[34]

Therefore the use of general online searches to provide information to research drug issues for the drug expert is not recommended. As we will see later in the book, one of the factors determining the admissibility of an expert's testimony is the source of data and methods used to reach an expert opinion. While *Google* and *Wikipedia* are transformative for our society in quickly bringing information to our fingertips, this information does not rise to the scientifically accepted standard needed to support an expert witness' testimony.

Drug experts are scientific experts and as such their expert opinion needs to be based on sound scientific methods. This includes expert opinions that are supported by peer-reviewed scientific papers and producing well-referenced litigation report.[35] As elaborated later in the book, there are recent Supreme Court of the United States (SCOTUS) decisions that govern the acceptability and use of scientific testimony in civil and criminal trials.[36] By using established data sources like medical and pharmacological journals and scientific research methods to arrive at their expert opinion, drug experts will more likely than not be allowed to present their testimony in court.

Alcohol Abuse in Native Americans

Firewater is a calque from the loan translation of the Indian compound word for "fire" plus "water."[37] Studies show that Native Americans have high rates of alcohol use and abuse, and increased prevalence of fetal alcohol syndrome (FAS), a devastating drug-induced malady often seen in the offspring of alcohol-using pregnant women.[38] Self-identified Native Americans show prevalence rates of alcohol dependence 4–5 times higher than the general population.[39] The elevated risk of alcohol dependence in Native Americans exists even when educational level and other socioeconomic factors are parsed out.[40] Native Americans are also more likely to engage in "binge" drinking of alcohol than other ethnic populations.[41]

---

[32] Wagner AL (2008) Wikipedia made law? The federal judicial citation of Wikipedia. J Comp Info Law 26:229–257.

[33] Available at: *www.americanbar.org/content/dam/aba/publications/supreme_court_preview/BriefsV5/14-7955_amicus_neither_pharm.authcheckdam.pdf*.

[34] See website: *glossipvgross.com*.

[35] Although such a requirement for scientifically supported statements may seem self-evident, in my experience a surprising number of experts, mostly of the retired physician type, simply spout out statements without scientific or medical factual support. Without a drug expert to oppose them, they usually get away with it.

[36] The so-called *Daubert trilogy* of SCOTUS cases governs to the use of scientific testimony in court. In this regard, the trial judge acts as the "gatekeeper" in keeping "junk science" out of the courtroom. See later this chapter.

[37] For example the Ojibwan word *iškote·wa·po·* meaning "whiskey" or other distilled liquors, was made from combining *iškote·* "fire" + *-a po·* "liquid." From a search of "firewater" on *dictionary.com*.

[38] Szlemko WJ et al. (2006) Native Americans and alcohol: past, present, and future. J Gen Psychol. 133:435–451.

[39] Actual rates of alcoholism among Native Americans were 65%–85% for men and 37%–55% for women. Gilder DA et al. (2004) Comorbidity of select anxiety and affective disorders with alcohol dependence in southwest California Indians. Alcohol Clin Exp Res. 28:1805–1813; Kunitz SJ et al. (1999) Alcohol dependence and conduct disorder among Navajo Indians. J Stud Alcohol. 60:159–167.

[40] Gilman SE et al. (2008) Education and race-ethnicity differences in the lifetime risk of alcohol dependence. J Epidemiol Community Health 62:224–230.

[41] Robin RW et al. (1998) Relationship of binge drinking to alcohol dependence, other psychiatric disorders, and behavioral problems in an American Indian tribe. Alcohol Clin Exp Res. 22:518–523.

Native Americans have a high conviction rate for violent crimes of violence with over 90% of homicides in this ethnic population related to alcohol use, while alcohol-related homicide cases in the U.S. population as a whole is about 30%–40%.[42] Native Americans as a group have the highest alcohol-related death rate of all ethnic groups in the United States.[43]

Native Americans are also called First Nation people, and for good reason. Native Americans were the first humans to inhabit this land from sea to shining sea, walking over from Asia when ocean levels were low and the Bering Strait was crossed by a land bridge.[44] Because of their ancestry from Asia, there are unique genetic differences in enzymes that metabolize alcohol in Native American populations.[45] Native Americans also have genetic differences in their GABA receptors and in their opioid receptors that may play a role in alcohol addiction.[46] While a discussion of the drug metabolizing genes (pharmacogenomics) are beyond the scope of this monograph, genetic differences provide at least a provisional basis for the high rates of alcohol use, binge drinking, and alcohol-related violence and death rates in Native American populations as noted before.[47]

Junk Science and the Drug Expert

The great tragedy of Science — the slaying of a beautiful hypothesis by an ugly fact.

Thomas H. Huxley (1825–1895)[48]

The term "junk science" was popularized by the best-seller, *Galileo's Revenge*, by Peter W. Huber.[49] Dr. Huber had the perfect background for writing this book as he earned a law degree from Harvard and a Ph.D. in mechanical engineering from MIT. The book was published in 1991 with the subtitle: *Junk Science in the Courtroom*. Huber's main thesis was that judges and juries were misled by "spurious claims by so-called expert witness."[50] He documented how questionable science and outright medical quackery proffered by expert witnesses hired by plaintiffs led to astronomical monetary judgments against corporations and individuals.

For most of its storied history, the *Supreme Court of the United States* (*SCOTUS*) did not address issues of expert testimony and scientific evidence until the *Daubert trilogy* of cases in the 1990s. In a series of cases, SCOTUS ruled that judges needed to carry out their role as gatekeeper and determine the admissibility of expert evidence as stated in Rule 702, among other issues. The *Daubert* case and its impact on whether the drug expert will be allowed to testify is discussed in a later chapter.[51] A brief overview of the *Daubert* case is given next.

In 1956 Merrell Dow made a drug called Benedictin®, which was FDA approved for combating the nausea and vomiting of morning sickness in pregnant women. Benedictin® was a combination of vitamin B_6, plus an over-the-counter antihistamine called doxylamine. Doxylamine is an older, first-generation antihistamine that is available today in sleep aids such as Unisom® and in night-time cold and flu medicines. By the late 1970s, a number of women who bore children with birth defects brought suit against Merrell Dow, claiming that Benedictin® use during pregnancy caused the birth defects in

---

[42] French A, Hornbuckle J (1990) Alcoholism among Native Americans: An analysis. Social Work, 1990; 275–280.

[43] Shalala DE et al. (1997) Regional differences in Indian health. CDC/Indian Health service annual report, Indian Health Service Office of Planning, Evaluation, and Legislation. Division of Program Statistics, Washington, DC: Indian Health Services.

[44] This happened a long time ago. Visa regulations and immigration laws are much tighter now.

[45] Ehlers CL et al. (2004) Genomic screen for loci associated with alcohol dependence in Mission Indians. Am J Med Genet B Neuropsychiatr Genet. 129B:110–115; Gizer IR et al. (2011) Association of alcohol dehydrogenase genes with alcohol-related phenotypes in a Native American community sample. Alcohol Clin Exp Res. 35:2008–2018; Liu J et al. (2011) Haplotype-based study of the association of alcohol-metabolizing genes with alcohol dependence in four independent populations. Alcohol Clin Exp Res. 35:304–16; Mulligan CJ et al. (2003) Allelic variation at alcohol metabolism genes (ADH1B, ADH1C, ALDH2) and alcohol dependence in an American Indian population. Hum Genet. 113:325–336.

[46] Ehlers CL et al. (2008) Association between single nucleotide polymorphisms in the *mu* opioid receptor gene (OPRM1) and self-reported responses to alcohol in American Indians. BMC Med Genet. 9:35; Enoch MA et al. (2016) GABBR1 and SLC6A1, two genes involved in modulation of GABA synaptic transmission, influence risk for alcoholism: results from three ethnically diverse populations. Alcohol Clin Exp Res. 40:93–101.

[47] Any genetic differences provide only one factor in the constellations of factors that contribute to high rates of alcohol dependence in native populations. This should not be construed as a type of *genetic determinism* along ethnic lines.

[48] Thomas Henry Huxley was an English biologist who established the field of comparative anatomy. He was called *"Darwin's Bulldog"* for his staunch support of Charles Darwin's theory of evolution by natural selection.

[49] Huber PW (1991) *Galileo's Revenge: Junk Science in the Courtroom.* Basic Books, New York, NY.

[50] Huber PW (1991) *ibid.*, back cover text.

[51] See Chapter 13 *Speed Kills*.

their offspring. Because of the escalating costs of litigation, Merrell Dow removed Benedictin® from the market in 1983 but one suit, *Daubert v. Merrell Dow Pharmaceuticals Inc.* made in all the way up to the Supreme Court of the United States.[52] This was the first case in SCOTUS history where the central issue was based on the admissibility of scientific evidence.[53]

As mentioned in Chapter 4, the Federal Rules of Evidence (FRE) were initially passed by Congress in 1975, following several years of drafting by SCOTUS.[54] They are a set of rules that regulate the introduction of evidence at civil and criminal trials in the United States federal trial courts. Most states adopted the FRE into their own legislative code intact; some states made minor style alterations.[55] The first three of the *Rules* concerning expert witness and expert testimony were discussed in Chapter 4 (*Rules 701, 702,* and *703*). The last three *Rules* are considered next, with the exciting details of the *Daubert* decision saved for a later chapter. *Daubert* and other decisions that arose from landmark tort cases remain extremely relevant today to the attorney and the drug expert, rearing its head occasionally as a *Daubert* motion to exclude the drug expert's testimony.[56]

Rule 704. Opinion on an ultimate issue

(a) *In General — Not Automatically Objectionable. An opinion is not objectionable just because it embraces an ultimate issue.*

(b) *Exception. In a criminal case, an expert witness must not state an opinion about whether the defendant did or did not have a mental state or condition that constitutes an element of the crime charged or of a defense. Those matters are for the trier of fact alone.*

Rule 704 impacts the drug expert's final conclusion as it would any other expert's opinion. In a civil lawsuit, the drug expert can and does render an opinion on the ultimate issue. For example, did prior drug use by the defendant driver cause the pedestrian traffic fatality? This question can be asked and answered under the latest revision of *Rule 704*. Part (b) of *Rule 704* notes the important exception in criminal cases whereby the expert must stay mum about ultimate issues. However, it is rare that the hiring attorney will not be able to get the drug expert's final conclusions at the trial, be they ultimate or *penultimate* drug issues.[57]

Rule 705. Disclosing the facts or data underlying an expert's opinion

Unless the court orders otherwise, an expert may state an opinion — and give the reasons for it — without first testifying to the underlying facts or data. But the expert may be required to disclose those facts or data on cross-examination.

Rule 705 provides for another liberalization of expert witness testimony, in that an expert may express an opinion without first relying on testimony of the underlying facts or data, that is, the foundation of the opinion. That the expert will be cross-examined on these underlying facts or data provides an opportunity for an effective cross of the opposing expert.[58]

---

[52] *Daubert v Merrell Dow Pharmaceuticals* 509 US 579 (1993).

[53] Haack S (2005) Trial and error: The Supreme Court's philosophy of science. Am J Public Health 95:S66–S73.

[54] This description and entirety of Federal Rules of Evidence (2019 edition) are available from the FRE website at *www.rulesofevidence.org*.

[55] For example, Oklahoma prefixed a "2" in numbering the FRE Rules and restyled them. Compare Oklahoma Statutes, Title 12. Civil Procedure §12-2705. Disclosure of facts or data underlying expert opinion: *"An expert may testify in terms of opinion or inference and give reasons therefor without previous disclosure of the underlying facts or data, unless the court requires otherwise. The expert may in any event be required to disclose the underlying facts or data on cross-examination"* to the wording in the main text of FRE Rule 705 in box below.

[56] See Chapter 13 *Speed Kills* for further discussion of the *Daubert* decision and other cases of expert testimony.

[57] *"The abolition of the ultimate issue rule does not lower the bars so as to admit all opinions. Under Rules 701 and 702, opinions must be helpful to the trier of fact, and Rule 403 provides for exclusion of evidence which wastes time. These provisions afford ample assurances against the admission of opinions which would merely tell the jury what result to reach, somewhat in the manner of the oath-helpers of an earlier day. They also stand ready to exclude opinions phrased in terms of inadequately explored legal criteria. Thus the question, "Did T have capacity to make a will?" would be excluded, while the question, "Did T have sufficient mental capacity to know the nature and extent of his property and the natural objects of his bounty and to formulate a rational scheme of distribution?" would be allowed."* From *Rule 704, Notes of Advisory Committee on Proposed Rules,* available at *www.law.cornell.edu/rules/fre/rule_704*.

[58] Fogarty JRS, Jeng DH (2012) Cross-examinations of expert witnesses: evolution, literature, interviews (December 22, 2012). Available at SSRN: *ssrn.com/abstract=2238670* or *dx.doi.org/10.2139/ssrn.2238670*.

For the drug expert, this means the examining attorney (under direct) is able to determine the order of presenting the expert's results with regard to the drug data. This also allows the examining attorney to select favorable results to elicit from the drug expert's testimony, and downplay unfavorable findings.[59] It is up to the opposing attorney, with the help of an opposing drug expert if so engaged, to uncover any contrary data during cross-examination.

Rule 706. Court-appointed expert witnesses

(a) *Appointment Process. On a party's motion or on its own, the court may order the parties to show cause why expert witnesses should not be appointed and may ask the parties to submit nominations. The court may appoint any expert that the parties agree on and any of its own choosing. But the court may only appoint someone who consents to act.*

(b) *Expert's Role. The court must inform the expert of the expert's duties. The court may do so in writing and have a copy filed with the clerk or may do so orally at a conference in which the parties have an opportunity to participate. The expert:*
  (1) *must advise the parties of any findings the expert makes;*
  (2) *may be deposed by any party;*
  (3) *may be called to testify by the court or any party; and*
  (4) *may be cross-examined by any party, including the party that called the expert.*

(c) *Compensation. The expert is entitled to a reasonable compensation, as set by the court. The compensation is payable as follows:*
  (1) *in a criminal case or in a civil case involving just compensation under the Fifth Amendment, from any funds that are provided by law; and*
  (2) *in any other civil case, by the parties in the proportion and at the time that the court directs — and the compensation is then charged like other costs.*

(d) *Disclosing the Appointment to the Jury. The court may authorize disclosure to the jury that the court appointed the expert.*

(e) *Parties' Choice of Their Own Experts. This rule does not limit a party in calling its own experts.*

Unlike the justice systems in nearly all other democratic countries in the world, experts in U.S. courts are hired and controlled by the litigation parties.[60] The judge is merely a referee in most proceedings. In other countries using a more inquisitorial and less adversarial system, the judge may play an active role, including the selection of experts. However, the final *Rule 706* empowers the judge to hire a *court-appointed* expert. This expert can be deposed and cross-examined by either party, and testify in court before judge and jury. Court-appointed experts would go a long way toward removing the *hired gun* reputation of experts, costs would decrease (one expert only instead of one expert from each side), and the courts would turn toward a less adversarial and more inquisitorial approach.

Rule 706 gives the ability of judges to hire nonparty expert witnesses but research shows it is rarely done.[61] Judges are part of a judicial system that values and expects an adversarial production of evidence. More specifically, research showed that judges used a court-appointed expert only in extraordinary and rare cases in which the traditional process failed to present a useful and rational assessment of the facts. It was also rare for any of the litigation parties to suggest the use of a court-appointed expert. Other factors cited for the infrequency of court-appointed experts include last-minute recognition of the need for one on the eve of a trial, and the limited or poor compensation of a court expert. In the rare instances that court-appointed experts were used however, judges reported little difficulty in finding and hiring experts due to professional or personal contacts.

For large class-action tort suits, judges may empanel scientific experts under *FRE 706* for the purposes of presenting a neutral evaluation of the evidence. This was done for the thousands of breast silicone implant cases which were consolidated in a single court.[62] A National Science Panel of four scientists concluded that there was no evidence to support leaky silicone implants and connective tissue disease. However, it was found that the scientists were not actually neutral parties as all four of them had links to defendant corporations with one scientist receiving funding for speaking at a professional conference paid by a defendant corporation while serving on the panel.

---

[59] However, the drug expert's litigation report should reflect all objective findings on the drug issue at hand, with inclusion of data and references that may be contrary to the consensus opinion. Otherwise the drug expert is guilty of "cherry-picking" only favorable studies and data.

[60] Green MD, Sanders J (2014) Admissibility versus sufficiency: controlling the quality of expert witness testimony in the United States. Wake Forest Univ. Legal Studies Paper No. 2016468; U of Houston Law Center Paper No. 2016468. Available at SSRN: *ssrn.com/abstract=2016468*.

[61] Cecil JS, Willging TE (1993) Court-appointed experts: Defining the role of experts appointed under Federal Rule of Evidence 706. Federal Judicial Center. At: *www.fjc.gov/sites/default/files/2014/13.expert.PDF*.

[62] Haack S (2015) The expert witness: lessons from the U.S. experience. Humana.Mente J Phil. Stud. 28: 39–70.

More likely than not, a drug expert will not find a position as a court-appointed expert.[63] In any case, the drug expert would produce the same, well-researched and well-referenced report and testify in the same manner as in any other drug expert case.

[Narrative continued]

A litigation report on the acute and long-term effect of alcohol on behavior was prepared by the drug expert. This report showed that there is overwhelming evidence of brain dysfunction caused by both acute and chronic alcohol abuse. Because of recent scientific data on the effects of alcohol in Native American populations, the litigation report contained a section on the research results demonstrating a genetic predisposition of alcoholism in Native Americans. Later when arriving for trial, the drug expert was informed by the public defender that the finding of the genetic predisposition for alcohol abuse in Native Americans will not be allowed in court, at the insistence of the prosecutor. Unknown to the drug expert and without a Daubert hearing, the public defender agreed to this stipulation. The drug expert testified to the other findings in the ligation report, often referring to the report during direct and cross-examination. The expert concluded that "without alcohol consumption by both parties at the time of the incident, it is unlikely that this tragic incident would have occurred." The jury accepted the drug expert's findings on the acute and chronic effects of alcohol on the defendant's behavior, and the behavior of the decedent as mitigating circumstances. The jury returned a verdict of guilty. During the sentencing phase of the trial, Mr. Twofeathers was spared the death penalty and sentenced to life imprisonment without parole.

---

[63] Free copy of this book to a drug expert that comes forward with documentation of a court-appointed case.

Chapter 8

Death at the Crossing: Trace cocaine and the denial of benefits

A Profile of Cocaine—Drug Testing in the Workplace

Postmortem Redistribution of Drugs—Criteria of a Substance Use Disorder

The Drug Expert and the Toxicology Report

[Narrative]

Charlie Wilson was employed by a home improvement store and drove a delivery truck in a small town in Oklahoma. One day, while on a delivery, Mr. Wilson approached and traveled through an ungated railroad crossing on Main Street. The locomotive of a freight train slammed into the cab of Wilson's truck. The impact threw his body halfway through the windshield. He suffered massive head trauma with blood loss and was pronounced dead on arrival. Blood samples were drawn for toxicological analysis, as is done for any fatal MVA in Oklahoma. Mr. Wilson's death left a widow and his three children without a family income. The widow applied for death benefits through the State's Workers' Compensation Commission. After months of delay, the widow was denied death benefits due to the presence of cocaine metabolites in the postmortem blood sample. The widow denied that her husband recently used cocaine and hired an experienced Workers' Compensation attorney to fight for her benefits. The attorney needed a drug expert to interpret the drug toxicology report. He consulted a local pharmacology professor recommended by a colleague.

A Profile of Cocaine

In America, two illegal drugs in recent years produced an unprecedented level of drug use, drug crimes, and incarceration for drug use. The first one is *crack* cocaine, a smokable form of cocaine that is widely available and cheap to buy. The second one is methamphetamine (*meth*), spurred on by internet recipes and the wide availability of precursor drugs and chemicals. Methamphetamine and its manufacture, as well as environmental exposure from home-based meth labs, was discussed in Chapter 5. Both amphetamine and methamphetamine are highlighted coming up in Chapter 13.

Cocaine is the active ingredient in the coca plant, *Erythroxylum coca*. It is not a synthetic drug, but a natural stimulant used by the peoples of the Andes mountain range in South America for thousands of years.[1] Indigenous peoples chew the coca leaf while working at high altitude. This method of drug intake produces a slow absorption of relatively minor amounts of cocaine. The coca leaves are used to reduce hunger and thirst, and to overcome fatigue. Coca leaves were also considered sacred by the Peruvian Incas and were used in the worship of the divine in religious ceremonies.[2]

By the 1850s, cocaine was discovered as the active ingredient in coca leaves and was marketed by American pharmaceutical companies. Dr. Sigmund Freud, of *couch analysis fame*, did some of the first research on cocaine's physiological effects and extolled the value of cocaine.[3] Freud used himself as the proverbial guinea pig and took large doses of cocaine

---

[1] Much of this information comes from an excellent recent review by Biondich AS, Joslin JD (2016) Coca: The history and medical significance of an ancient Andean tradition. Emerg Med Int. 4048764.

[2] Robinson SM, Adinoff B (2016) The classification of substance use disorders: historical, contextual, and conceptual considerations. Behav Sci. 6. pii: E18.

[3] Redman M (2011) Cocaine: What is the crack? A brief history of the use of cocaine as an anesthetic. Anesth Pain Med. 1:95-97. Freud became so enamored of the drug, from both personal and professional use, that he published the treatise called *Über Coca* ("*Über*" the German word for "over or above" now better known as a peer-to-peer ride-sharing company) which he called a "*song of praise to this magic substance.*" See Freud S (1885) *Über Coca. Centralblatt für die ges.* Therapie 2:289–314.

The Drug Expert. https://doi.org/10.1016/B978-0-12-800048-9.00008-0

and noted the drug's pharmacological effects.[4] Not recognizing cocaine's potential for producing drug dependence,[5] Freud thought that cocaine could be used to treat the morphine addict. This use for cocaine ended in abject failure. American pharmaceutical companies, well established and growing throughout the late 1800s, marketed cocaine in everything from cough drops to health tonics. The soft drink *Coca-Cola*® at this time actually contained the drug cocaine, which had a great deal to do with its popularity.[6] Now cocaine is legally available only to physicians and research pharmacologists with a DEA license. Cocaine is a Schedule II controlled substance, meaning it has a legitimate medical use. It is not used clinically as it once was, but still used occasionally in ENT procedures.[7]

As mentioned in Chapter 1, the overall abuse of any illegal drug is about 10% of the U.S. population. Of these drug abusers, ~1% are abusing cocaine, either in its powder form (*Coke Classic*) or in its solid base form, called *crack* cocaine.[8] Crack cocaine is made by a simple chemical method to convert cocaine hydrochloride powder to a smokable cocaine base form. Sold and used in the form of "rocks," crack cocaine[9] destroyed inner-city neighborhoods and hooked millions of Americans onto this new cocaine formulation during the 1980s. Congress reacted to the growing crack epidemic with the passage of the Anti-Drug Abuse Act of 1986. The law enacted new mandatory minimum sentences for most illegal drugs, including cocaine and marijuana, with harsh sentences for simple possession. There was a special emphasis on punishing users and distributors of crack cocaine, with a 100:1 sentencing ratio for crack vs. powder cocaine. This meant, for example, that the Anti-Drug Abuse Act mandated a minimum sentence of 5 years without parole for simple possession of 5 g of crack cocaine, which was the same sentence for possession of 500 g of powder cocaine. Crack cocaine users and dealers filled the prisons. The inequality of cocaine sentencing was somewhat improved when the crack to powder cocaine ratio was reduced to 18:1 by the Fair Sentencing Act of 2010.[10] Of course, to a drug expert, or any rational person for that matter, sentencing should be equal for equal amounts of cocaine, and based on the actual amount of cocaine drug molecules in possession, regardless of the particular drug formulation.

Cocaine metabolism and blood concentrations

Cocaine is a central nervous system (CNS) stimulant and shares many effects on the brain with amphetamines.[11] The most common routes of cocaine administration are insufflation (*a.k.a.* "snorting") or smoking the base form of cocaine (*crack*). Intravenous (IV) injection of cocaine is a less common route of drug abuse, but does occur. Whatever the route of getting cocaine into the bloodstream, cocaine is metabolized quickly by hydrolytic enzymes.[12] Cocaine's main metabolite is benzoylecgonine (BE), which is inactive as a CNS stimulant. Half of the cocaine in the blood is removed in 35–90 min, while the metabolite BE has an average elimination half-life in the blood of 7.5 h.[13]

Peak blood levels of cocaine from snorting it range from 100 to 500 ng/mL, and intravenous administration of cocaine produces peak blood levels of 500–1000 ng/mL.[14] In a controlled study, IV administration of 25 mg cocaine (equal to a low street dose) produced peak blood levels of cocaine in the range of 102–348 ng/mL. After 12 h, cocaine fell to the range of 0–22 ng/mL.[15] A key paper evaluated the blood levels of cocaine and its main metabolite BE in actual users who smoked crack cocaine. Users that smoked crack 8 h before blood draws had cocaine and BE levels of 125 and 948 ng/mL,

---

[4] Markel H (2001) *Über coca*: Sigmund Freud, Carl Koller, and cocaine. JAMA 305:1360–1361.

[5] Perhaps in a bit of irony, Freud himself didn't recognize the *defense mechanism* he employed to deny that he was hooked on cocaine.

[6] National Institute on Drug Abuse (NIDA) (2016) Cocaine. National Institutes of Health (NIH); U.S. Department of Health and Human Services (DHHS). Bethesda, MD.

[7] ENT specialists are physicians treating Ear, Nose, and Throat disorders. See: Long H et al (2004) Medicinal use of cocaine: a shifting paradigm over 25 years. Laryngoscope 114:1625–1629.

[8] Cocaine use from since 2009 to 2014 has remained stable with an estimated 1.5 million current cocaine users aged 12 or older in 2014, which is 0.6% of the population. From the Center for Behavioral Health Statistics and Quality (CBHSQ) (2015) Behavioral Health Trends in the United States: Results from the 2014 National Survey on Drug Use and Health. Rockville, MD: Substance Abuse and Mental Health Services Administration, HHS Publication No. SMA 15-4927, NSDUH Series H-50; cited at www.drugabuse.gov/publications/research-reports/cocaine/what-scope-cocaine-use-in-united-states.

[9] Called "crack" cocaine due to the cracking noise made when the product is heated and smoked. See the National Institute on Drug Abuse (NIDA) website at: www.drugabuse.gov/publications/drugfacts/cocaine.

[10] Efforts have been made to make this retroactive, with an Amendment by the U.S. Sentencing Commission in 2011.

[11] Brenner GM, Stevens CW (2018) Brenner and Stevens' Pharmacology, 5th Ed. Elsevier, Philadelphia PA, USA.

[12] Duer WC et al. (2006) Relationships between concentrations of cocaine and its hydrolysates in peripheral blood, heart blood, vitreous humor and urine. Forensic Sci. 51: 421–425.

[13] Moolchan ET et al. (2000) Cocaine and metabolite elimination patterns in chronic cocaine users during cessation: plasma and saliva analysis. J Anal Toxicol. 24:458–466.

[14] Jatlow P (1988) Cocaine: analysis, pharmacokinetics, and metabolic disposition. Yale J Biol Med. 61:105–113.

[15] Moolchan ET et al. (2000) *op cit.*

respectively.[16] Users that smoked crack 16h before blood draws had cocaine and BE levels of 41 and 715 ng/mL and those who smoked cocaine 24h before testing had cocaine and BE levels of 14 and 238 ng/mL, respectively. The previous studies were done in living healthy volunteers and cocaine abusers. That is not true in this chapter's case, which examined the interpretation of cocaine use and other drugs in blood samples obtained from the dead.

Drug Testing in the Workplace

Prior to the 1980s, the testing of public and private employees for the use of legal and illegal drugs was rare. That all changed when President Reagan launched the "War on Drugs" in the mid-1980s. In 1986 President Reagan fired his salvo toward a "drug-free America" with the issuance of Executive Order No. 12564 declaring a "drug-free federal workplace."

Under this order, the Secretary of Health and Human Services (HHS) was authorized to develop scientific and technical guidelines for drug testing programs. Federal agencies were required to conduct their drug testing programs in accordance to these guidelines. The *Supplemental Appropriations Act of 1987* (*Public Law 100-71, Section 503, 5 U.S.C. 7301 note*) further outlined the general provisions for Federal drug testing programs, and directed the Secretary of HHS to set comprehensive standards for all aspects of laboratory drug testing. Congress passed the *Drug-Free Workplace Act* in April 1988, which resulted in the Mandatory Guidelines for Federal Workplace Drug Testing Programs. The intent of the law was to establish a substance-free work environment at federal agencies by requiring that all federal employees pass a urine drug test before employment and at random times thereafter. Today, the authority to develop and promulgate these Mandatory Guidelines resides with the Substance Abuse and Mental Health Services Administration (SAMHSA), an operational division in HHS.[17]

Preliminary presumptive and confirmatory drug tests

Confirmation of a drug or drug metabolite in the urine or other bodily emanation of a Defendant or Decedent is done using a two-step process. The first test done for drugs in the sample is usually an enzyme-linked immunosorbent assay (ELISA) test. The ELISA is easy to understand, once you realize that drug molecules each have a specific shape and that antibodies can be made specific for a particular drug molecule. In the ELISA, when antibodies latch onto drug molecules, enzymes act to produce a color change proportional to the number of antibody-drug couplings. The ELISA comes as a dipstick apparatus or more likely a container with built-in ELISA drug tests that can be read after a urine sample. The results from the first or preliminary drug test using ELISA or other similar assays are only qualitative and presumptive. This preliminary presumptive positive test is then taken as a justification for performing the more costly and labor-intensive second confirmatory drug test using a gas chromatograph and mass spectrophotometer (GC-MS), or the older method liquid chromatography and mass spectrophotometer (LC-MS).

The GC or gas chromatograph part uses a *carrier gas* to stream by the biological sample and pick up the different molecules in the sample after certain *retention* times. Basically the GC apparatus is a separator of the mixed-up molecules in the sample to provide a nicely ordered group of the same molecules. The GC sends all the groups of molecules, some of which may be drug molecules, to the MS part in a serial fashion lined up by their weight.[18] In the MS machine, the groups of molecules are bombarded with ions and a pattern of peaks are captured that is a specific signature for that substance. The placement of the peaks along spectra is compared to a database of chemical signatures and the substance is identified by a computer. The height of the peaks gives a readout of the how much drug or substance was in the sample, in terms of a concentration.[19]

The detection of a drug or drug metabolite using GC-MS in a second drug test provides a confirmation, or not, of the results of the preliminary presumptive drug test. Most importantly for the drug expert, a positive result of the GC-MS assay also provides a numerical value of the drug concentration in the sample. Confirmatory *and quantitative*. With this value in hand, the drug expert can research the existing medical and forensic literature to find corresponding drug concentration data to help develop the drug expert's opinion.

---

[16] Schramm W et al. (1993) Cocaine and benzoylecgonine in saliva, serum, and urine. Clin Chem. 39:481–487.

[17] Bush DM (2008) The U.S. Mandatory Guidelines for Federal Workplace Drug Testing Programs: current status and future considerations. Forensic Sci Int 174:111-119; Phan HM et al. (2012) Drug testing in the workplace. Pharmacother. 32:649–656.

[18] Actually lined up by their mass, thus the name of the machine—the mass spectrophotometer (MS). Weight and mass are not the same as mass is the amount of matter in an object. Weight is what we measure as the gravitational pull on an object (how a bathroom scale works). Mass of an object on the moon is the same as on Earth; however, its weight would be less. In zero gravity, an object has no weight but has the same mass.

[19] Usually in ng/mL, which is nanograms per milliliter.

Mandated second or confirmatory drug tests

There is a consistency across federal agencies and state governments to insist that second confirmative tests be done following a preliminary presumptive positive first test. The Federal Law concerning drugs of abuse in the workplace has always been clear that the initial or preliminary drug test must be followed by a second confirmatory drug test. In President Reagan's Executive Order #12564, it clearly states:

(e) The results of a drug test and information developed by the agency in the course of the drug testing of the employee may be considered in processing any adverse action against the employee or for other administrative purposes. ***Preliminary test results may not be used in an administrative proceeding unless they are confirmed by a second analysis of the same sample*** *or unless the employee confirms the accuracy of the initial test by admitting the use of illegal drugs.*

[bold underline added][20]

Furthermore, under the Mandatory Guidelines for Federal Workplace Drug Testing (developed and promulgated by SAMHSA, see earlier) certain procedures must be followed including:

Initial Screen: The first analysis done on a sample is called an initial screen. ***This one test alone is not always accurate or reliable; there is a possibility of a false positive. Thus, in the event that the initial screen is positive, a second confirmatory test should be done.***

Confirmation Test: ***A second, confirmation test (by gas chromatography/mass spectrometry or GC/MS) is highly accurate and provides specificity to help rule out any false positives (mistakes)*** *from the initial screen.* ***For a test result to be reported as positive, the initial screen and confirmation test results must agree.***

[bold added][21]

Additionally, the rules for the Department of Transportation (DOT) also make clear the necessity of a confirmation test for presumptive positive urine drug screens:

(b) On an initial drug test, you must report a result below the cutoff concentration as negative. ***If the result is at or above the cutoff concentration, you must conduct a confirmation test.***

(c) On a confirmation drug test, you must report a result below the cutoff concentration as negative and a result at or above the cutoff concentration as confirmed positive.

[bold added]. From DOT website: 49 CFR Part 40, Subpart F, sec. 40.87 b,c

The States enacted their own laws for workplace drug testing, consistent with federal rule. For example, the State of Oklahoma enacted the "Standards for Workplace Drug and Alcohol Testing Act" in 1993. This law is codified at *Title 40 of The Oklahoma Statutes, §40-551 to §40-563 (amended 2011)*. With regard to confirmation testing of an initial presumptive positive test, the Oklahoma statutes are clear that a second GC-MS test or equivalent test needs to be performed. To wit:

8. Sample testing shall conform to scientifically accepted analytical methods and procedures. ***Testing shall include confirmation of any positive test result by gas chromatography, gas chromatography-mass spectroscopy, or an equivalent scientifically accepted method of equal or greater accuracy as approved by Board rule,*** *at the cutoff levels as determined by Board rule,* ***before the result of any test may be used as a basis for refusal to hire a job applicant or any action by an employer*** *pursuant to Section 12 of this act.*

[bold added][22]

Preliminary drug screens using immunoassays, as was done in the present chapter case, are universally accepted in the medical and scientific literature as only having presumptive value and a second confirmatory test is necessary for any evidentiary value. This is true whether it be, for example, driving under the influence, opioid use in medical settings, drug use in pregnancy, workplace drug testing, or drug doping in sports.[23]

---

[20] From President Reagan's Executive Order #12564, Sec 5 (e).

[21] From Mandatory Guidelines for Federal Workplace Drug Testing, SAMHSA website.

[22] From §40-559. "Sample collection and testing – Conditions," available from *Oklahoma.gov* website.

[23] Braithwaite RA et al. (1995) Screening for drugs of abuse. I: Opiates, amphetamines and cocaine. Ann Clin Biochem. 32:123153; Christo PJ et al. (2011) Urine drug testing in chronic pain. Pain Physician 14:123–143; Concheiro M et al. (2007) Confirmation by LC-MS of drugs in oral fluid obtained from roadside testing. Forensic Sci Int. 170:156–162; D'Avila FB et al. (2016) Cocaine and crack cocaine abuse by pregnant or lactating mothers and analysis of its biomarkers in meconium and breast milk by LC-MS-A review. Clin Biochem. 2016 Jan 28. pii: S0009-9120(16)00045-X; Goldberger BA, Cone EJ (1994) Confirmatory tests for drugs in the workplace by gas chromatography-mass spectrometry. J Chromatogr A. 674:73–86; Ingels

In spite of laws in varying jurisdictions consistently mandating a second confirmatory test in cases of workplace drug testing, the drug expert may work on a number of Workers' comp cases (and others) in which the interpretation of a single, unquantified preliminary presumptive drug test is at issue. Every effort should be made to dismiss preliminary drug test evidence when it is not confirmed by a second test. And most assuredly, there can be no conclusion on a drug's impact in a case when detection from a preliminary drug test is the only evidence of drug use. The second, confirmatory test provides not only the identity of a drug, but also the concentration of the drug in the sample. The drug concentration allows the drug expert to examine the medical and pharmacological literature and in many cases, formulate an expert opinion whether the drug had an impact on the issue at hand.

Postmortem Redistribution of Drugs

As probably clear to all readers at this point, drugs need to get into the blood stream to be distributed to their target tissues. There are a few exceptions, like drugs that are designed to treat dermatological conditions or ophthalmic drugs in eye drops, but commonly prescribed oral drugs must run the gauntlet of the intestinal tract wall and survive the onslaught of liver metabolic enzymes before reaching the blood stream of the circulatory system. Certainly drugs that make you high must get into the blood and then the brain. The great pumping muscle of the heart churns the blood, delivering drug molecules throughout the body, and if designed properly, to the brain through the blood-brain barrier.[24] The movement of the drug from the blood stream to the tissues of the body is called *drug distribution*.

Drug distribution in the dead

Except in cases of brain death with external life support, the heart ceases to pump blood in the truly dead. In the living, the blood stream flows like a river, rushing forward with every beat. In the living, obtaining blood for drug concentrations is like throwing a bucket on a rope into a rushing river. In the dead, getting a blood sample is like dipping a cup into a still pond. After death, obviously only postmortem samples can be obtained. The amount of drug in the postmortem sample is then compared to the amount of drug in blood samples from clinical studies in the living.[25] When the postmortem drug values are *in extremis*, comparing ante-mortem and postmortem drug levels helps the drug expert formulate an opinion. For example, a postmortem drug concentration 100 times higher than the peak drug concentration in clinical studies can be considered abnormally high, perhaps due to drug overdose.

Postmortem redistribution

The changes in drug distribution that occur with death are called *postmortem redistribution*, also known as PMR. Both physiological processes that change after death and drug characteristics alter the PMR of a specific drug.[26] Physiological processes include disruption of cell membranes and diffusion of drugs back from tissues into the blood. After a period of time, putrefaction and bacterial growth occurs, in some cases helping to metabolize drugs and in other cases producing substances, such as alcohol. In such cases, opinions on alcohol use from detected postmortem alcohol levels are confounded by the exogenous bacterial production of alcohol. In massively putrefied corpses, the maggots that feed on the decaying tissue may be tested to determine drug use in the decedent.[27] Other bodily structures in the dead that are amenable to drug testing include finger and toe nails, and the more common hair analysis as done in the case outlined in Chapter 6.

AS et al. (2014) Screening and confirmation methods for GHB determination in biological fluids. Anal Bioanal Chem. 406:3553–3577; Manchikanti L et al. (2010) Protocol for accuracy of point of care (POC) or in-office urine drug testing (immunoassay) in chronic pain patients: a prospective analysis of immunoassay and liquid chromatography tandem mass spectrometry (LC/MS/MS). Pain Physician 13:E1–E22; Standridge JB et al. (2010) Urine drug screening: a valuable office procedure. Am Fam Physician 81:635–640; Thevis M et al. (2015) Annual banned-substance review: analytical approaches in human sports drug testing. Drug Test Anal. 7:1–20; Walsh JM et al. (2004) Drugs and driving. Traffic Inj Prev. 5:241–253; Wasels R, Belleville F (1994) Gas chromatographic-mass spectrometric procedures used for the identification and determination of morphine, codeine and 6-monoacetylmorphine. J Chromatogr A. 674:225–234; Yuan C et al. (2015) Drug confirmation by mass spectrometry: Identification criteria and complicating factors. Clin Chim Acta. 438:119–125.

[24] The brain is a privileged organ and has specialized brain cells and capillary structures to omit much of what the rest of the body gets. This selective interface between the circulatory system and the brain is called the *blood-brain barrier*.

[25] In some cases, the drug expert may use other postmortem sample drug level data. For example, comparing the decedent's drug level to studies examining the drug levels from motor vehicle accidents (MVA) fatalities.

[26] Patel G (2012) Postmortem drug levels: innocent bystander or guilty as charged. Pharm Pract. 25:37–40.

[27] Drummer OH (2004) Postmortem toxicology of drugs of abuse. For. Sci. Int. 142:101–113.

It is clear from forensic research that postmortem blood sampling from different sites in the corpse may lead to different drug concentrations in each sample. Standard practice today draws the postmortem blood sample from the femoral vein, rather than cardiac or other central blood compartments.[28] Drugs in the peripheral blood vessels exhibit less postmortem redistribution (PMR) so the drug levels obtained are most comparable to the drug data from clinical studies in living subjects. In the present chapter case, the decedent's blood samples were obtained by the Medical Examiner within one hour of the accident. The blood samples were drawn from his right femoral vein, after a minor cut-down procedure.

Interpretation of cocaine blood levels

An additional way to interpret levels of cocaine and the cocaine metabolite, benzoylecgonine (BE) in a postmortem blood sample is to compare the obtained value with those published from cocaine victims. In *cocaine-related* deaths, postmortem femoral samples gave a cocaine blood level of 420 ng/mL and BE at 2330 ng/mL.[29] In another study, postmortem blood samples in *cocaine-only* deaths gave average values of blood levels for cocaine at 890 ng/mL and BE at 4000 ng/mL.[30] In the chapter case, the decedent's cocaine and BE levels were extremely low compared to the cocaine and BE blood levels in these published forensic cases. It can be concluded that the decedent did not have toxic levels of cocaine at the time of the fatal train-truck accident.

It is also possible to exhibit low levels of cocaine due to environmental exposure to cocaine by second-hand smoke. Low levels of cocaine and the cocaine metabolite in blood samples are consistent with second-hand exposure to an environment containing smoked cocaine but not actual self-administration of cocaine.[31] The decedent in the index case for this chapter tested positive for low blood levels of cocaine and BE. It is possible that the decedent was in the presence of cocaine prior to the accident but did not self-administer or use cocaine himself.

In any event, the pharmacological effects of cocaine do not last long. In a controlled study, most pharmacological effects and rewarding effects returned to baseline values by 30 min with a moderate dose (40 mg) of smoked cocaine. At this time point (30 min after smoking cocaine) the cocaine blood levels averaged 70 ng/mL.[32] These authors summarize the results by stating that most pharmacological effects of cocaine return to baseline in the presence of detectable levels of cocaine. This means that low blood levels of cocaine cannot predict a level of impairment or the magnitude of pharmacological effect.

Regardless of the blood levels of cocaine, the presence of this CNS stimulant does not appear to have much effect on driving. A recent study of the testing of cocaine and its relationship with clinical lab studies of driving impairment found that drivers who tested positive for cocaine showed no significant clinical impairment in measures of motor coordination, walking, speech, mood, or size of their pupils compared to drivers who did not test positive for cocaine.[33]

Criteria of a Substance Use Disorder

Psychiatrists and psychologists depend on one main resource to diagnose and classify their patients; the Diagnostic and Statistical Manual of Mental Disorders, 5th version (DSM-V). The *Manual* describes all known mental disorders and lists the criteria that need to be met to be diagnosed with a particular type and subtype of mental illness. It makes for fascinating if somewhat droll reading. Published originally in 1952 with periodical updates, revision of the DSM-IV began in 2000 and culminated 13 years later with the release of DSM-V in 2013.[34]

---

[28] Launiainen T, Ojanperä I (2014) Drug concentrations in post-mortem femoral blood compared with therapeutic concentrations in plasma. Drug Test Anal. 6:308–316.

[29] Logan BK et al. (1997) Lack of predictable site-dependent differences and time-dependent changes in postmortem concentrations of cocaine, benzoylecgonine, and cocaethylene in humans. J Anal Toxicol. 21:23–31.

[30] Jones AW, Holmgren A (2014) Concentrations of cocaine and benzoylecgonine in femoral blood from cocaine-related deaths compared with venous blood from impaired drivers. J Anal Toxicol. 38:46–51.

[31] Baselt RC et al. (1990) On the dermal absorption of cocaine. J Anal Toxicol. 14:383–384; Cone EJ et al. (1995) Passive inhalation of cocaine. J Anal Toxicol. 19:399-411; Randall T (1992) Infants, children test positive for cocaine after exposure to second-hand crack smoke. JAMA. 267:1044–1045.

[32] Jenkins AJ et al. (2002) Correlation between pharmacological effects and plasma cocaine concentrations after smoked administration. J Anal Toxicol. 26:382–392.

[33] Arroyo A et al. (2013) Drivers under the influence of drugs of abuse: quantification of cocaine and impaired driving. Med Leg J. 81:135-143. Indeed, there is data to show that use of CNS stimulants, at clinical doses, may improve driving and certainly abate driver fatigue.

[34] The DSM-V is the result of the work of over 1000 health care professionals and organized by the American Psychiatric Society: www.psychiatry.org/psychiatrists/practice/dsm. American Psychiatric Association: Diagnostic and Statistical Manual of Mental Disorders, Fifth Edition. Arlington, VA, American Psychiatric Association, 2013. The thirteen years it took to finish the DSM-IV revision is consistent with the time an average neurotic spends on a psychiatrist's couch.

Using cocaine as an example, a Substance Use Disorder is defined in the DSM-V as:

Stimulant use disorder

Diagnostic criteria

A. A pattern of amphetamine-type substance, cocaine, or other stimulant use leading to clinically significant impairment or distress, as manifested by at least two of the following, occurring within a 12-month period:

  1. The stimulant is often taken in larger amounts or over a longer period than was intended.
  2. There is a persistent desire or unsuccessful efforts to cut down or control stimulant use.
  3. A great deal of time is spent in activities necessary to obtain the stimulant, use the stimulant, or recover from its effects.
  4. Craving, or a strong desire or urge to use the stimulant.
  5. Recurrent stimulant use resulting in a failure to fulfill major role obligations at work, school, or home.
  6. Continued stimulant use despite having persistent or recurrent social or interpersonal problems caused or exacerbated by the effects of the stimulant.
  7. Important social, occupational, or recreational activities are given up or reduced because of stimulant use.
  8. Recurrent stimulant use in situations in which it is physically hazardous.
  9. Stimulant use is continued despite knowledge of having a persistent or recurrent physical or psychological problem that is likely to have been caused or exacerbated by the stimulant.

It would seem that meeting at least two of the nine criteria for a Substance Use Disorder is not a great threshold to overcome and a lot of people would end up diagnosed with a Substance Use Disorder (SUD). This is true. The latest estimate from the National Survey on Drug Use and Health (NSDUH) states that 8.4% of adults or about 20.2 million souls have a substance use disorder.[35] And that data comes from a survey and is self-reported, which means that more likely than not, a truer estimate is much higher. People are reluctant to talk about their personal drug use, especially if illicit in nature.

A clinical record of the defendant's SUD diagnosis is rarely found by the drug expert. However, a record of SUD might be used to show tolerance to the drug impact or support certain blood concentrations of drug. A defendant's record of SUD may be used in support of a death penalty mitigation, when the crime was committed under the influence of an alcohol or an illegal drug for instance.[36]

The Drug Expert and the Toxicology Report

For the drug expert, a drug toxicology report is the main document that begins the expert's investigation of the findings. In a case that does not involve a fatality, the drug toxicology report may be a separate entity whereas in cases involving a deceased party, the toxicology report will be part of the medical examiner's (ME) documents. Unfortunately, there are many times when a forensic toxicological analysis is not done even when the cause of death is listed as multiple drug toxicity. Other ME reports will come to conclusion that a certain drug was involved with a toxicology analysis, that conclusion reached with information gathered at the scene, for example, prescription pill bottles. The best ME and Police Incident reports should include medicines found at the scene including counts of remaining pills for each prescription medicine. Then, in every case of potential drug overdose, a femoral blood sample should be taken from the deceased and a full toxicology report generated.

Toxicological analysis and *toxicology* report is probably not the best name for the process of quantifying drugs in a blood sample and the name of the report with the resulting data. This is like calling the results of every biopsy a *Cancer Report*, when very few cases result in a diagnosis of cancer. Not all drugs reported in a Toxicology Report are toxic or found at toxic levels. It is just a counting up, or quantifying of drug molecules found in the blood sample. Perhaps a better way to think of the process is a *Drug Identification and Concentration Analysis (DICA)*, which results in a DICA report. Getting rid of the word "toxicology" would remove the inherent bias, left over from prerampant drug use days that *any* drug detected and reported was toxic. While there are many cases where that is certainly true, in most drug expert cases the toxicology report, err, *Drug Identification and Concentration Analysis (DICA)* report, gives a drug concentration that is within therapeutic or higher but not toxic levels.

As opposed to hospital or clinic medical records, toxicology reports are rather standardized in their format, but widely differing in the drug data that they provide. Three different examples are given in Appendix G. The first report simply

---

[35] *www.samhsa.gov/disorders.*
[36] More on drug issues and death penalty cases in the exciting concluding chapter of this book, Chapter 20 *Death Be Not Proud.*

confirms the presence of two drugs (methadone and alprazolam) by GC-MS. The second report states that the blood sample is positive for amphetamine with a concentration of >0.06 μg/mL. This report also states that methamphetamine was present at 0.13 μg/mL, but no methodology nor error variance of that number is given. The third sample toxicology report is the best. The "Not Confirmed" and "Confirmed" results are clearly marked and each methodology is noted (not confirmed tests use ELISA immunoassay and confirmed tests use GC-MS). Drug concentrations are given with a range, representing a 95% confidence interval. The length of sample retention is even given for the benefit of the defendant (see last sample report, Appendix G).

[Narrative continued]

The decedent's postmortem blood level of cocaine was undetected on a second confirmatory test. The inactive cocaine metabolite benzoylecgonine (BE), was present in a low concentration. It is possible that the cocaine and cocaine metabolites measured in the decedent's postmortem samples were from second-hand or environmental exposure. It is also possible that the decedent used cocaine 12–24 h or sometime long before the accident. Based on medical and scientific research reported in the professional literature, the drug expert concluded that cocaine use was not present as an intoxicating dose and cocaine use was not a contributory cause in the train-truck collision that took the decedent's life. The Workers' Compensation Court heard the testimony of the drug expert and concluded that the widow of the decedent should receive the full death benefit for her husband's on-the-job fatal accident.

Chapter 9

Big Little Secrets: Prescription errors, generic drugs, and drugs affecting blood alcohol

Medication Errors and Patient Injury—Generic and Brand Name Drugs

Drug Interference in Alcohol Testing—The Drug Expert and Medical Records

[Narrative]

In the first case, Betty Curtison, mother of four children and eight grandchildren, lived in a retirement home with her husband of 60 years. Like many elderly women, Betty suffered from recurrent urinary tract infection (UTI) and was prescribed a common antibiotic, levofloxacin, by her primary care physician. Two days after picking up the medication from the pharmacy store, she was brought to the ER suffering from lethargy and confusion. At that time, her blood glucose was extremely low at 36 mg/dL (milligrams per deciliter; normal range is 70–99 mg/dL). She was given dextrose by the IV route and showed improved mental status. Later the she began to develop lethargy and confusion again and was again hypoglycemic. She was given additional IV dextrose and admitted to the ICU. Despite the IV administration of dextrose, she continued to deteriorate and two days after admission, Betty Curtison died. Her daughter examined the bottle of levofloxacin and noted that the pills looked different than previous prescriptions. An online pill-identifier showed the pills to be an oral antidiabetic drug called glipizide. The daughter brought suit against the pharmacy for a prescription error which she claimed caused the death of her mother. Her attorney contacted a regional drug expert to examine the case with respect to the putative prescription error.

In the second case, Joel Orsten was injured on the job and received a judgment for medical support through the Workers' Compensation Court. Mr. Orsten was back in court demanding that his medical benefits cover brand name prescription drugs, because he says he is allergic to all generic drugs. The additional cost to his employer's health insurance company for use of only brand name prescriptions was calculated at more than a million dollars over a ten-year period. The attorney representing the insurance company contacted a local drug expert to offer an opinion as to Mr. Orsten's claim of drug allergies to all generic medicines.

In the final case of the chapter, Carl Wainwright was involved in a motor vehicle accident in which his vehicle became entrapped underneath a semitrailer truck that was making a lane change. Carl was found be pinned in his vehicle and unresponsive with visible head trauma. He was administered fentanyl, etomidate, succinylcholine, and midazolam before loaded into a Lifeflight helicopter. After arriving at the Medical Center, additional medications were administered to the Plaintiff. Blood samples were drawn by a nurse at the Medical Center. One blood sample was sent to the State Forensics lab by the State Troopers and was positive for alcohol at 0.10 BAC. Mr. Wainwright recovered after two weeks in the hospital and sought payment for his astronomical medical bills from the trucker's insurance company. The insurance company denied payment for medical bills citing the BAC of Mr. Wainwright above 0.08. He retained an attorney who hired a local drug expert to examine the BAC results and the impact of medications given to Mr. Wainwright before the blood sample was drawn.

Medication Errors and Patient Injury

Early reports from the Institute of Medicine of the National Academy of Science found that medical errors caused severe injury and even death to a large number of patients. According to their findings, medical errors injure 1 million patients a year and cause at least 44,000 deaths annually.[1] More recent studies suggest that these numbers were grossly underestimated, with more accurate numbers close to 500,000 patients per year dying due to medical error. These authors maintain that medical

---

[1] Odukoya OK et al. (2014) How do community pharmacies recover from e-prescription errors? Res Social Adm Pharm. 10: 837–852.

errors in 2016 were the *third leading cause of death*, after heart disease and cancer.[2] Part of the discrepancy is due to the lack of the proper cause of death listed on death certificates, which is used by the CDC and other organizations to capture mortality statistics. With over half a million patients dying per year due to medical error, perhaps there is no better time for attorneys, working with drug experts when needed, to exert pressure on the health care system for better outcomes through tort litigation.[3]

If medical errors in general cause about 500,000 deaths per year, medication errors account for about 16% or 80,000 deaths per year.[4] The incidence and type of dispensing errors by pharmacies was recently reviewed in the International Journal of Pharmacy Practice.[5] In the United States, *unprevented* dispensing errors, meaning medication errors that were not caught before the customer received the prescription, ranged from 0.08% to 24% in various studies. Interestingly, the lowest incidence of dispensing errors was found in a study of mail-order pharmacies. The highest rate of errors was found in a study that employed covert patients presenting a prescription for a single medication, either warfarin, carbamazepine, or theophylline, to 100 randomly selected retail pharmacies. These covert patients received the wrong prescription in 24 out of the 100 pharmacies. In results from surveys mailed to pharmacists, 53% admitted making a dispensing error in the last month and 34% thought that at least one dispensing error is made per week. Pharmacy errors occurred at the same rate in supermarket, chain, or independent pharmacies.

To a large extent, many pharmacy errors are made due to the confusion surrounding the names of drugs. There are cognitive (psychological) tests that predict the confusion rates of a proposed new drug name.[6] However, efforts to test new drug names before they are assigned by pharmaceutical companies were rejected as "*too burdensome*" by Big Pharma, that is, too costly. Current FDA guidelines for naming drugs include only the most rudimentary considerations of similarity (similar in spelling or pronunciation to other proprietary names) and do not suggest or mandate cognitive testing of new drug names to see if a new drug would be confused with other drugs.[7] The lack of cognitive testing of drug names for the potential to cause medication errors goes against the FDA's mission and if done for all new drugs, would potentially save thousands of patients from injury or death.

In pharmacies, the main dispensing errors occur by giving a patient the wrong drug or the wrong dose of a prescribed drug.[8] In the latter case, the prescription bottle has the right drug and dose on the label, but the pills in the bottle are a different dose. Most drugs come in multiple dosage forms (10, 20, 40, or 60 mg, for example) and different dose tablets may not be clearly distinguishable. In general, medication errors leading to the wrong dose of the right drug are not as dangerous to a patient as in the first case when the wrong drug is given to a patient. A real-life example of a prescription error leading to the death of an elderly woman is examined next.

Adverse effects of oral diabetes drugs give to a nondiabetic patient

Sulfonylurea drugs are common medicines used to treat Type II diabetes.[9] The medical and pharmacological literature documents the incidence and dangers of sulfonylurea drug-induced hypoglycemia. Hypoglycemia, commonly known as low blood sugar, is usually defined as blood sugar below 70 mg/dL (milligrams per deciliter).[10] Severe hypoglycemia is considered to be blood sugar measurements below 40 mg/dL.

To determine hypoglycemia, the sugar that is measured in the blood is *glucose*. Glucose is the main fuel that the brain requires to properly function.[11] Normal blood glucose levels range from 60 to 100 mg/dL. Glucose levels are dependent on when and what one last ate. When blood glucose falls below about 36 mg/dL, there is not enough glucose left in the brain and it ceases to function correctly. Severe hypoglycemia can cause irreversible brain injury. Patients brought to the ER with hypoglycemia show the following signs and symptoms: confusion, cognitive impairment,

[2] Makary MA, Daniel M (2016) Medical error-the third leading cause of death in the US. BMJ 353:i2139.

[3] Weeks EA (2006) Beyond compensation: using torts to promote public health. J Health Care Law Pol. 10:101-136.

[4] Calculated from the ratio of medical error death and medication error deaths reported in Kohn LT et al. (2000) To err is human: building a safer health system. Institute of Medicine, National Academies Press.

[5] James KL et al. (2009) Incidence, type and causes of dispensing errors: a review of the literature. Int J Pharm Pract. 17:9-30.

[6] Schroeder SR et al. (2017) Cognitive tests predict real-world errors: the relationship between drug name confusion rates in laboratory-based memory and perception tests and corresponding error rates in large pharmacy chains. BMJ Qual Saf. 26:395-407.

[7] FDA (2012) Guidance for Industry: Best practices in developing proprietary names for drug. At: *www.fda.gov/downloads/drugs/guidances/ucm398997.pdf.*

[8] James KL et al. (2009) *Op. cit.*; Aspden P et al. (2007) Preventing medication errors. Institute of Medicine, National Academies Press.

[9] Brenner GM, Stevens CW (2018) *Brenner and Stevens' Pharmacology, 5th Edition*, Chapter 35: Drugs for Diabetes, pp. 404-406. Elsevier, Philadelphia, PA, USA.

[10] Lacherade JC et al. (2009) An overview of hypoglycemia in the critically ill. J. Diabetes Sci Technol. 3:1242-1249.

[11] Bartlett D1 (2005) Confusion, somnolence, seizures, tachycardia? Question drug-induced hypoglycemia. J Emerg Nurs. 31:206-208.

speech difficulty, and blurred vision. Additionally, severe hypoglycemia causes cardiac arrhythmias, seizures, coma, and possible death.[12]

Glipizide is available as a brand name drug called Glucotrol® and also available in many generic formulations. The major adverse effect of glipizide is hypoglycemia, a direct result of its pharmacological action on the insulin-producing cells of the pancreas. The FDA-approved label (full prescribing information) for glipizide includes the following precautions:

All sulfonylurea drugs are capable of producing severe hypoglycemia. Elderly, debilitated or malnourished patients are particularly susceptible to the hypoglycemic action of glucose-lowering drugs. Hypoglycemia may be difficult to recognize in the elderly. Hypoglycemia is more likely to occur when caloric intake is deficient.

[original edited for brevity][13]

Glipizide is a potent, second-generation sulfonylurea. Taking glipizide lowers blood sugar for 12 to 24h.[14] Comparing glipizide/sulfonylurea drugs to other antidiabetic drugs, studies show that more users of glipizide/sulfonylurea drugs experienced hypoglycemia than users of other oral antidiabetic medications.[15] Glipizide and other sulfonylurea drugs accounted for more than 60% of all drug-induced hypoglycemia cases.[16]

There are a number of reports of accidents or errors of unintended ingestion of glipizide and other sulfonylurea drugs leading to severe hypoglycemia and death.[17] Authors note that medication errors due to erroneous dispensing of wrong medications should be considered in cases of unexpected hypoglycemia.[18]

Elderly and critically ill patients are more susceptible to the hypoglycemic effect of glipizide and other sulfonylurea drugs and are more likely to suffer ill effects from hypoglycemia including death.[19] In the elderly patient, drug-induced hypoglycemia is the most common cause of hypoglycemia.[20] Hospitalized patients who are 65 years or older are at increased risk of hypoglycemia caused by sulfonylurea drugs including glipizide, with study authors warning that sulfonylurea drugs should not be used in such elderly patients.[21]

Hypoglycemia due to insulin and sulfonylureas are among the four most common drugs leading to emergency hospitalizations in elderly aged 65 years or older.[22] There are cases in the medical literature of elderly patients experiencing repeated hypoglycemia from a sulfonylurea drug given mistakenly by a pharmacy and the patient dying a few days after a second hypoglycemic episode.[23]

Generic and Brand Name Drugs

Like any other manufactured product,[24] a drug may have more than one name. Typically, drugs have two names, a *generic* name and a *brand* name (also called a *proprietary* or *trade* name). As befitting any major marketing campaign, brand name

---

[12] Mullens DJ, Shubrook JH (2014) Hypoglycaemia in a 94-year-old man without diabetes. BMJ Case Rep. pii: bcr2014204067. http://dx.doi.org/10.1136/bcr-2014-204067.

[13] Glucotrol® Full Prescribing Information, Pfizer, May 2010.

[14] Abraham A et al. (2015) Hypoglycemia secondary to sulfonylurea ingestion in a patient with end stage renal disease: results from a 72-hour fast. Case Rep Endocrinol. 742781. http://dx.doi.org/10.1155/2015/742781.

[15] Bodmer M et al. (2008) Metformin, sulfonylureas, or other antidiabetes drugs and the risk of lactic acidosis or hypoglycemia: a nested case-control analysis. Diabetes Care 31:2086-2091; Bron M et al. (2014) A post hoc analysis of HbA1c, hypoglycemia, and weight change outcomes with alogliptin vs glipizide in older patients with type 2 diabetes. Diabetes Ther. 5:521-534; Arjona Ferreira JC et al. (2013) Efficacy and safety of sitagliptin versus glipizide in patients with type 2 diabetes and moderate-to-severe chronic renal insufficiency. Diabetes Care 36:1067-1073; Nauck MA et al. (2007) Efficacy and safety of the dipeptidyl peptidase-4 inhibitor, sitagliptin, compared with the sulfonylurea, glipizide, in patients with type 2 diabetes inadequately controlled on metformin alone: a randomized, double-blind, non-inferiority trial. Diabetes Obes Metab. 9:194-205.

[16] Seltzer HS (1989) Drug-induced hypoglycemia. A review of 1418 cases. Endocrinol Metab Clin North Am. 18:163-183.

[17] Abraham A et al. (2015) Hypoglycemia secondary to sulfonylurea ingestion in a patient with end stage renal disease: results from a 72-hour fast. Case Rep Endocrinol. 742781. http://dx.doi.org/10.1155/2015/742781; Walfish PG et al. (1975) Sulfonylurea-induced factitious hypoglycemia in a nondiabetic nurse. Can Med Assoc J. 112:71-72; Trenque T et al. (2002) Prevalence of factitious hypoglycaemia associated with sulphonylurea drugs in France in the year 2000. Br J Clin Pharmacol. 54:548; Henry K, Harris CR (2006) Deadly ingestions. Pediatr Clin North Am. 53:293-315.

[18] Huminer D et al. (1989) Inadvertent sulfonylurea-induced hypoglycemia. A dangerous, but preventable condition. Arch Intern Med. 149:1890-1892; Ludman P et al. (1986) Dangerous misuse of sulphonylureas. Br Med J 293:1287-1288.

[19] Lheureux PE et al. (2005) Bench-to-bedside review: Antidotal treatment of sulfonylurea-induced hypoglycaemia with octreotide. Crit Care. 9:543-549.

[20] Arora A (2013) Hypoglycaemia begets hypoglycaemia. BMJ Case Rep. 8, http://dx.doi.org/10.1136/bcr-2013-010156.

[21] Deusenberry CM et al. (2012) Hypoglycemia in hospitalized patients treated with sulfonylureas. Pharmacotherapy 32:613-617.

[22] Klein-Schwartz W et al. (2015) Treatment of sulfonylurea and insulin overdose. Br J Clin Pharmacol. 81:496-504.

[23] ISMP Canada (2007) Unexpected hypoglycemia: consider medication error in the differential diagnosis. ISMP Canada Safety Bulletin, Volume 7, Issue 1.

[24] *Kleenex*™ is a brand name and *facial tissue* is a generic name for the same product. Note there can be many products with the same generic name but only one with a brand name. Same for marketed drugs.

drugs become universally known, like Advil®, OxyContin®, Lipitor®, and Xanax®. Less known are the generic names, like ibuprofen, oxycodone, atorvastatin, and alprazolam, for the above brand name drugs. In the second case of this chapter, a man injured on the job claimed that he is allergic to generic medications. The drug issues that surfaced in this case are presented next.

Generic drugs and generic substitution

The makers of the generic version of the drug do not have to submit clinical data on the safety and efficacy to the FDA but only bioequivalence data.[25] Bioequivalence means that the generic drug dissolves and gets into the bloodstream as fast and as completely as the approved brand name drug. Because the generic manufacturer does not have to recoup the tremendous costs of discovering the new drug, preclinical animal testing, clinical trials, and bringing a new drug to the market, the generic manufacturers charge significantly less for their products compared to the branded drugs. This is evident for OTC (over the counter) drugs as well. While at the Walmart pharmacy or elsewhere, note the difference in price between the branded ibuprofen sold as Advil® and the Walmart labeled generic ibuprofen.

Generic drugs contain the same *active pharmaceutical ingredient* (API) as the branded drug. For example, each tablet of generic ibuprofen (Walmart) contains 200 mg of the drug ibuprofen and so does each ibuprofen tablet marketed as Advil®. What often differs between two *formulations* of the same drug (generic and branded, or between generic and generic) are the other ingredients of the tablet that give it shape, color, and allow for breakdown of the tablet in the gut. However, all these "other ingredients" (known as *excipients*) are themselves approved along with the API by the FDA.[26] Generic drug manufacturers use excipients already in FDA-approved medications to avoid new safety testing.[27] There have been rare cases where a drug allergy was linked to a change in medication and more specifically the "other ingredients" in the pill (see later).

The states have various laws and regulations concerning generic substitution for brand name drugs. About half the states mandate generic substitution carried out by the pharmacist.[28] In Oklahoma, it is mandatory that the pharmacist use generic medications unless the prescribing physician specifically requests that no generic substitutions should be made. Oklahoma law also states that patient consent for filling prescriptions with generic medications is not required. Legislators in states like Oklahoma enjoy lower health care costs by substituting or prescribing generic drugs in place of brand name drugs. States can save millions of dollars by Medicare Part D programs by the implementation of this substitution practices.[29] Overall, generic versions of drugs saved Americans more than $33 billion dollars per year in health care costs.[30] Currently, about 85% of all prescriptions in the United States are filled with generic medications.[31]

Are generic and branded drugs the same?

The FDA approves generic drugs if their pharmacological parameters are consistent with the parameters of the branded drug.[32] The two parameters measured in generic drugs are the rate of absorption (how fast the drug goes from stomach and into the bloodstream) and the bioavailability (how much of the drug gets into the bloodstream over time). If these parameters are close enough to the branded drug's parameters (within about 20%) the generic drug is approved by the FDA. The generic drug is considered *bioequivalent* and a therapeutic equivalent to the branded drug.

A number of clinical studies confirm that generic drugs are similar to branded drugs in terms of pharmacological parameters and clinical effects. A systematic review of health outcomes among patients starting a new medication or continuing an existing medication did not differ for patients taking generic or branded versions of the same drug.[33] A meta-analysis

[25] Kesselheim AS et al. (2015) Modified regulatory pathways to approve generic drugs in the us and a systematic review of their outcomes. Drugs 75:633-650.

[26] Rayavarapu S et al. (2015) Comparative risk assessment of formulation changes in generic drug products: a pharmacology/toxicology perspective. Toxicol Sci. 146:2-10.

[27] Carbon M, Correll CU. Rational use of generic psychotropic drugs. CNS Drugs 27:353-365 (2013).

[28] Sarpatwari A et al. (2016) The case for reforming drug naming: should brand name trademark protections expire upon generic entry? PLoS Med. 2016 Feb 9;13(2):e1001955.

[29] Shrank WH et al. (2010) State generic substitution laws can lower drug outlays under Medicaid. Health Aff (Millwood) 29:1383-1390.

[30] Hoadley JF et al. (2012) Medicare Part D plans, low or zero copays and other features to encourage the use of generic statins work, could save billions. Health Aff (Millwood) 31:2266-2275.

[31] Rayavarapu S et al. (2015) *Op cit.*

[32] Brenner GM, Stevens CW (2018) *Brenner and Stevens' Pharmacology, 5th edition.* Pharmacology textbook for medical and health professional students. Elsevier, Philadelphia.

[33] Gothe H et al. (2015) The impact of generic substitution on health and economic outcomes: a systematic review. Appl Health Econ Health Policy 13 Suppl 1:S21-33.

study of 26 cardiovascular drugs found that in all studies that were reviewed, there were no differences in clinical effects or adverse effects taking generic or branded medications.[34] A clinical study of drugs used to treat osteoporosis found no differences in the use of generic or brand name drugs in preventing bone fractures.[35]

Background on drug hypersensitivity ("drug allergy")

Like many substances than are foreign to the human body, drugs can also cause allergic reactions. True drug allergies are rare and the term "*drug allergy*" is nonspecific, widely misused, and often diagnosed without clinical evidence.[36] Drug allergies are frequently self-reported by patients and poorly documented.[37] Drug allergies are medically known as drug hypersensitivity reactions (DHR). Studies show that about 2%–4% of hospital patients develop a skin rash hypersensitivity reaction to an administered drug.[38] Diagnostic tests for true drug hypersensitivity reactions include skin test, delayed-read intradermal test, patch test, white blood cell proliferation test, and others.[39] Most patients that report a "drug allergy" likely have experienced an adverse effect with the drug, like nausea and vomiting, and not a true and documented immunological drug hypersensitivity reaction.

As previously noted, both brand name drugs and generic drugs contain inactive ingredients called excipients. An excipient is added to the drug tablet to help dissolve the pill, or improve stability, taste, or appearance.[40] There have been rare cases where a drug allergy was linked to a change in medication and more specifically to a particular excipient.[41] These single patient case reports state the rarity of the drug hypersensitivity reaction and each patient was hypersensitive to one excipient. Additionally some generic drugs have the same excipients as the branded drug.

There is only one case in the medical literature that reports on a single patient who believed she was allergic to all generic medicines.[42] This 69-year-old woman was treated by a psychiatrist and was diagnosed as having a somatization disorder (e.g., hypochondria). The patient was further characterized as being a "problem patient." There was no medical evidence that the patient was allergic to all generic medicines.

Drug Interference in Alcohol Testing

In the third case of this chapter, an individual was refused insurance benefits due to alcohol found in a blood sample after administration of a number of hospital medications.

Metabolism of ethanol

The active drug ingredient of all alcoholic beverages is a simple molecule called ethyl alcohol, more commonly known as *ethanol*. Ethanol is one type of alcohol among many[43] and is the alcohol that is measured to yield the blood alcohol concentration (BAC), although more correctly this should be referred to as the blood *ethanol* concentration. Ethanol is metabolized by two enzyme systems in the liver.[44] As shown in Fig. 9.1, ethanol is metabolized in the first system (A) by the enzyme alcohol dehydrogenase (ADH) to give aldehyde, then broken down the enzyme aldehyde dehydrogenase (ALDH) to make acetate. The end product, acetate, is a simple molecule that is then used by the body as a source of fuel.[45]

---

[34] Manzoli L et al. (2016) Generic versus brand-name drugs used in cardiovascular diseases. Eur J Epidemiol. 31:351-368.

[35] Michieli R, Callegaro C (2015) Generic brands in the prevention of fragility fractures. Clin Cases Miner Bone Metab. 12:109-110.

[36] Unsworth DJ, Tsiougkos N (2015) Improving detection and management of drug allergy. Practitioner 259:25-27.

[37] Chiriac AM, Demoly P (2014) Drug allergy diagnosis. Immunol Allergy Clin North Am. 34:461-471.

[38] Roujeau JC et al. (2014) Management of nonimmediate hypersensitivity reactions to drugs. Immunol Allergy Clin North Am. 34:473-487.

[39] Alam R (2014) The complexity of drug hypersensitivity. Foreword. Immunol Allergy Clin North Am. 34:xiii-xiv.

[40] Barbaud A (2014) Place of excipients in systemic drug allergy. Immunol Allergy Clin North Am. 34:671-679.

[41] Hebron BS et al. (2009) Aspirin sensitivity: acetylsalicylate or excipients. Intern Med J. 39:546-549; Mumoli N et al. (2010) Allergic reaction to Croscarmellose sodium used as excipient of a generic drug. QJM 104:709-710; Garrido-Siles M et al. (2015) New cutaneous toxicities with generic docetaxel: are the excipients guilty? Support Care Cancer 23:1917-1923.

[42] Brennan TA, Lee TH (2004) Allergic to generics. Ann Intern Med. 141:126-130 (2004).

[43] Other common alcohols that are encountered in daily life are isopropyl alcohol ("rubbing alcohol"), methanol ("wood alcohol," main ingredient in windshield wiper fluid), and ethylene glycol (active ingredient in antifreeze and coolant solutions).

[44] Brenner GM, Stevens CW (2018) *Brenner and Stevens' Pharmacology, 5th Edition*. Elsevier/Springer, Philadelphia PA, USA.

[45] Acetate is used in the body mainly in the form of acetyl-CoA which enters the citric acid cycle (Kreb's cycle) to produce energy stored in the form of high energy phosphate bonds in adenosine triphosphate (ATP).

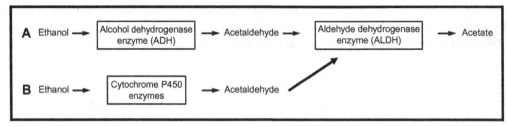

FIG. 9.1   Ethanol metabolic pathways.

In the second system in the liver, the so-called cytochrome P450 enzymes (B) metabolize ethanol into acetaldehyde.[46] This aldehyde is also metabolized by the second enzyme (ALDH) in pathway A to yield acetate. Inhibition or blockade of metabolic pathways in the liver by other drugs prevents the metabolism of ethanol and increases alcohol blood concentrations. This leads to an increase in the measured BAC.

Drugs that interfere with alcohol metabolism

There are two FDA-approved medications that are designed to interfere with ethanol metabolism. The first one is disulfiram (Antabuse®), which inhibits the action of the second enzyme, aldehyde dehydrogenase (ALDH, see Fig. 9.1) which causes toxic levels of acetaldehyde to build up. Disulfiram is an old drug whose inhibition of ethanol metabolism was discovered by serendipity, like the novel actions of so many other drugs.[47] A Danish biochemist in 1945, who had the disturbing habit of testing new drugs on himself, took disulfiram which was being developed as an antiworming drug. The biochemist attended a dinner party and became violently ill after drinking beer.[48] Marketed first in Denmark and Europe, disulfiram was soon available throughout the United States and the world for the treatment of chronic alcoholism. By inhibiting ALDH, the resulting buildup of acetaldehyde in the blood produces upper torso and face flushing, rapid heart rate, and nausea. The *extreme physical discomfort* punishes the alcoholic who continues to drink while taking disulfiram.[49] Disulfiram thereby links negative reinforcement with alcohol use and is an effective deterrent to those who continue taking it. Disulfiram is still marketed today as the brand drug Antabuse® and as generic disulfiram.

The second FDA-approved drug that inhibits alcohol metabolism is fomepizole (Antisol® and generic formulations). Fomepizole inhibits the first enzyme in alcohol metabolism, alcohol dehydrogenase (ADH, see Figure above). It is indicated for the treatment of methanol or ethylene glycol poisoning.[50] Fomepizole prevents ADH from processing methanol or ethylene glycol into toxic metabolites and prevents metabolic acidosis and kidney damage.

Besides drugs that specifically target alcohol metabolic pathways, there are a number of prescription and OTC medications that inhibit alcohol metabolism indirectly and may cause false readings in a BAC determination.[51] These medications include antibiotics, antidepressants, antihistamines, barbiturates, benzodiazepines, muscle relaxants, opioids, and NSAIDs.[52] The strategy for the drug expert is to obtain good medical and pharmacy records and then do the research to find out if the drugs in question alter ethanol metabolism. The three drugs that were administered to the plaintiff in the chapter that interfere with alcohol metabolism are highlighted next. The drugs are etomidate, cefazolin, and acetaminophen.

---

[46] Gilman AG, Goodman LS, Gilman A (1980) *Goodman and Gilman's The Pharmacological Basis of Therapeutics*, Macmillan Publishing Co., New York, NY.

[47] Serendipity plays a major role in drug discovery and in all branches of science. Perhaps my favorite example is the accidental discovery of sildenafil's (Viagra®) uplifting effects during testing mice for antihypertensive effects. Some graduate student probably noticed diminutive but long-lasting erections in the little lab mice but it was not until clinical trials for treating angina that male patients reported an increase in sturdy erections and Pfizer realized they had a blockbuster drug on their hands. See Ban TA (2006) The role of serendipity in drug discovery. Dialogues Clin Neurosci. 8: 335–344.

[48] Kragh H (2008) From disulfiram to Antabuse®: the invention of a drug. Bull. Hist. Chem. 33:82-88.

[49] Bennett AE et al. (1950) Antabuse in the treatment of alcoholism in a private general hospital. Calif Med. 73:141-143.

[50] *Antizol® Prescribing Information*, from the FDA website.

[51] Weathermon R, Crabb DW (1999) Alcohol and medication interactions. Alchol Res. Health 23:40-54.

[52] NSAIDs (pronounced "en-said"; for **n**onsteroidal **a**nti**i**nflammatory **d**rugs) is a good acronym to know as just about everyone occasionally takes an NSAID for headaches or minor aches and pains. Commonly used NSAIDs are ibuprofen (Advil®), acetaminophen (Tylenol®), naproxen (Aleve®), and the ever-present generic aspirin.

Etomidate

Etomidate is an anesthetic drug with a short duration of action used for induction of anesthesia.[53] Etomidate was introduced into clinical practice in 1972 but its use has fallen out of favor due to its side effect of decreasing the production of adrenal corticosteroids. Etomidate remains useful in the emergency room for rapid intubation.[54] Because etomidate does not easily dissolve into solutions for IV administration, etomidate is formulated to contain 35% propylene glycol. Etomidate in this formulation is intended for the induction of general anesthesia by intravenous injection.[55] There are two known mechanisms that etomidate interferes with ethanol metabolism and increases blood ethanol levels. Firstly, the etomidate molecule is metabolized, or broken down to, a carboxylic acid molecule and an ethanol molecule.[56] Therefore administration of etomidate directly increases the amount of ethanol in the blood. Secondly, the propylene glycol, which is a type of alcohol and is added to the etomidate solution at the high concentration of 35%, also inhibits the liver enzymes that metabolize ethanol and other alcohols. Propylene glycol directly competes with alcohol at the alcohol dehydrogenase (ADH) enzyme.[57] Inhibition of ethanol metabolism by propylene glycol additionally increases the blood ethanol concentration.

Cefazolin

Cefazolin is an antibiotic of the class called *cephalosporin* antibiotics and used for prophylaxis (prevention) of surgical infections. Cefazolin is considered a first-generation cephalosporin and available as Cefazolin for Injection given in 1 to 2 g doses 30 to 60 min before the start of surgery.[58] Cephalosporin antibiotics are potent inhibitors of the second enzyme of the ethanol metabolic pathway (A) shown before, namely, aldehyde dehydrogenase (ALDH). The inhibition of ALDH by cephalosporin antibiotics, like cefazolin in this chapter's third case, prevents the complete metabolism of ethanol and produces a buildup of acetaldehyde.[59] Acetaldehyde is also an inhibitor of the first enzyme of ethanol metabolism, alcohol dehydrogenase (ADH).[60] The net result is that cephalosporin antibiotics, like cefazolin, inhibit ethanol metabolism and increase the blood levels of alcohol.

Acetaminophen

Acetaminophen is grouped with the large class of NSAIDs that includes common OTC remedies such as ibuprofen and aspirin. Acetaminophen by itself is available in a number of formulations including the brand name product Tylenol®. Acetaminophen and ethanol exert a well-known drug-drug interaction that is mediated by two distinct mechanisms involving both ethanol metabolic pathways. In the first ethanol metabolic pathway (A), acetaminophen directly inhibits alcohol dehydrogenase (ADH) in a noncompetitive fashion. This inhibition of ethanol metabolism by acetaminophen produces as much as a 31% inhibition of the human alcohol dehydrogenase enzymes.[61] Acetaminophen inhibition in this manner has clinical relevance as it may raise blood alcohol levels and influence the performance of drivers who consume alcohol. In the second metabolic pathway (B), ethanol is metabolized by a certain type of cytochrome P450 enzyme, namely, CYP2E1. This is the same type of P450 enzyme that metabolizes acetaminophen.[62] Competition of acetaminophen and ethanol for the same type of P450 enzyme also decreases the metabolism of ethanol and increases the measurement of blood alcohol content.

[53] Molina DK et al. (2008) Distribution of etomidate in a fatal intoxication. J Anal Toxicol. 32:715-718.

[54] Forman SA (2011) Clinical and molecular pharmacology of etomidate. Anesthesiology 114:695-707.

[55] *Amidate® Full Prescribing Information*, rev. 09/2011, manufactured by Hospira.

[56] Forman SA (2011) *Op. cit.*

[57] Brooks DE, Wallace KL (2002) Acute propylene glycol ingestion. J Toxicol Clin Toxicol. 40:513-516; Zosel A et al. (2010) Severe lactic acidosis after an iatrogenic propylene glycol overdose. Pharmacotherapy 30:219.

[58] *Cefazolin for Injection, USP, Full Prescribing Information*, rev. 01/2012, Braun Medical Inc.

[59] Kline SS et al. (1987) Cefotetan-induced disulfiram-type re-actions and hypoprothrombinemia. Antimicrob Agents Chemother. 31:1328-1331; Uri JV, Parks DB (1983) Disulfiram-like reaction to certain cephalosporins. Ther Drug Monit. 5:219-224; Yamanaka Y et al. (1983) Effects of cephem antibiotics on rat liver aldehyde dehydrogenases. Jpn J Pharmacol. 33:717-723.

[60] Yin SJ et al. (2003) Human class IV alcohol dehydrogenase: kinetic mechanism, functional roles and medical relevance. Chem Biol Interact. 143-144:219-227.

[61] Lee YP et al. (2013) Inhibition of human alcohol and aldehyde dehydrogenases by acetaminophen: Assessment of the effects on first-pass metabolism of ethanol. Alcohol 47:559-565.

[62] Lieber CS et al. (1987) The microsomal ethanol oxidizing system and its interaction with other drugs, carcinogens, and vitamins. Ann N Y Acad Sci. 492:11-24; Slattery JT et al. (1996) The complex interaction between ethanol and acetaminophen. Clin Pharmacol Ther. 60:241-246.

In this chapter's last case, the plaintiff was administered 11 different medications from the time of the accident until the time that blood samples were obtained for toxicological analysis. Three of the 11 drugs interfere with BAC measurement and increase the blood levels of ethanol according to medical and pharmacological studies. The drug expert concluded that known interactions of the administered drugs alter the reliability of the BAC obtained from the blood sample and this interference more likely than not increased the BAC value.

The Drug Expert and Medical Records

Although the first case reports of medical procedures are found in ancient papyrus texts from Egypt *circa* 1600 BCE, the first complete medical records system used in the United States was developed by Dr. Henry Plummer at the Mayo Clinic in 1907.[63] Early medical records consisted of handwritten notes by nurses and physicians. This did not change much until the advent of the digital age and electronic medical records. With the passage of the Patient Protection and Affordable Care Act of 2010 (more commonly known as the Affordable Care Act, or *Obamacare*) use of electronic medical records was mandated, primarily as a cost-cutting measure. The US health care system is the world's largest health care system but also the world's most inefficient operation.[64] Thomson-Reuters, a major think-tank company, estimates that the system wastes from $505 to $850 billion annually. This amount of waste equals about one-third of health care costs. Using electronic medical records instead of paper-based systems is expected to yield annual savings for physicians and hospitals of $9 billion and $25 billion, respectively.

The drug expert is a doctor but is not a physician.[65] The medical records are the domain of physicians, nurses, medical technicians, and hospital specialists. However, the drug expert can search medical records with confidence to find orders for drug administration, current medications, adverse effects of drugs, and results of toxicology tests. An excerpt of the medical records from the prescription error case is provided in Appendix H.

[Narrative continued]
In the first case, the drug expert first requested photographic evidence of the prescription bottle and the remaining pills. Using the online Physicians' Desk Reference, he verified that the pills taken by the decedent, Betty Curtison, were not levofloxacin but instead glipizide 10 mg tablets. The drug expert also suggested that the attorney send one of the tablets in question to a forensic laboratory. While waiting for the results, the drug expert researched the adverse effects of glipizide and literature reports of ensuing fatalities. The drug expert also examined the medical records for the decedent, showing a time course of severe hypoglycemia consistent with inadvertent administration of glipizide. The pharmacy report confirmed that the date of prescription on the pill bottle matched the date of filling the prescription. The report from the forensic laboratory confirmed that glipizide tablets were mistakenly placed in the bottle labeled levofloxacin. After receiving the drug expert report, the team of lawyers for the large-chain pharmacy settled with the attorney representing the estate of Betty Curtison for an undisclosed amount.

For the second case, the drug expert researched the phenomena of "drug allergy" and generic medicines and found no support for allergies or adverse effects restricted to all generic medicine except one case report of a psychiatric patient claiming generic drug allergy like Mr. Joel Orsten. Additionally, by a close examination of Mr. Olsten's pharmacy records, it was clear that half of his ongoing medications were already being prescribed in generic formulations and medical records revealed no history of drug allergies or adverse effects to those generic medications. After the drug expert's report was submitted to the Worker's Compensation Court, Mr. Orsten's case was summarily dismissed and the insurance company continued to pay only for generic medications whenever available.

In the third case, the drug expert researched the effects of each drug administered to Carl Wainwright by the EMT and Medical Center staff. Mr. Wainwright was administered 11 different medications from the time of the accident until the time that blood samples were obtained for toxicological analysis of alcohol. Three drugs were given that increase the blood levels of ethanol; namely etomidate, cefazolin, and acetaminophen. Additionally, according to State Board of Toxicology and Alcohol guidelines, a second test that yielded a BAC that was +/− 0.03 of the first test was not performed to confirm the original BAC. The drug expert testified in court and a settlement with the insurance company was made in Mr. Wainwright's favor.

---

[63] Gillum RF (2013) From papyrus to the electronic tablet: a brief history of the clinical medical record with lessons for the digital age. Am J Med. 126:853-857. As I found out during my Ph.D. studies at the Mayo Clinic in Rochester, Minnesota, ole' Dr. Henry's mansion is still used for fancy affairs and euphemistically named the *"Plummer House."*

[64] Adkinson JM, Chung KC (2014) The patient protection and Affordable Care Act: a primer for hand surgeons. Hand Clin. 30:345-352.

[65] Not that it is a sensitive issue, but I've had to correct an opposing attorney during cross-examination when they called me *"Mr. Stevens"* instead of *"Dr. Stevens"* in court. This is an obvious attempt to undermine the drug expert's credentials. If pressed, I can wax on about how professorial Ph.D. types were called *"Doctor"* (it is, after all, a word derived from the Latin, *docēre*, to teach) at a time when physicians were still called *"Mister"* and still blood-letting their patients in barber shops.

Chapter 10

Through the Looking-Glass: A bank-robbery witness and alleged victim on drugs

Drug Effects on Memory and Perception—Cognitive Effects of Common Drugs

The Public Defender's Office and the Drug Expert

The Drug Expert and Pharmacy Records

[Narrative]

Todd Lewis was a 58 year-old black man who made his living working odd jobs as a handyman. While working on a job in a small, rural town far from home, Mr. Lewis stopped at a bank and tried to cash a check. The bank teller panicked as Mr. Lewis approached her and pushed the emergency alarm. Mr. Lewis did not brandish a firearm or other weapon, nor did he pass a note to the teller. The video surveillance showed that he was not wearing a hood or mask, did not appear to be agitated or threatening nor demanding money from the teller. Upon hearing the alarm, Mr. Lewis fled the bank and sped off in his car. When the local police gave chase, Mr. Lewis swerved his car and struck another car head-on, instantly killing the driver. Mr. Lewis was apprehended and charged with attempted bank robbery and felony murder in the death of the driver. The federal public defender obtained the teller's prescription records and contacted a local drug expert to render an opinion on the effects of drugs on the perception and memory of the eyewitness bank teller.

In a second case, Rob Scott, a 21-year old male, was charged with rape in the first degree and forcible sodomy. The alleged victim, Drew Jacobs, an 18-year senior, accompanied by the principal of the high school, met with the town's Chief of Police. The principal told the Chief of Police that Jacobs relayed information to him that he was sexually assaulted at the mobile home of Mr. Scott three nights ago. Jacobs was interviewed and said that he met Mr. Scott the night of the incident at a convenience store. Mr. Scott purchased two 12-packs of beer and then they went together to a party. Jacobs stated that they left the party and went to Mr. Scott's mobile home. After they arrived, they drank a number of beers and Jacobs admitted that he took some "bars"[1] and smoked marijuana. Jacobs said he passed out and awoke to find Mr. Scott committing oral sodomy, passed out again and then awoke to find Mr. Scott engaging in anal sodomy. The state public defender for Mr. Scott contacted a regional drug expert to investigate the effects of alcohol, Xanax,® and marijuana on the memory and perception of the alleged victim.

Drug Effects on Memory and Perception

The memory function of the brain is often erroneously compared to a video tape recording, faithfully documenting reality as it occurs.[2] But the brain is not a tape recorder. Research has shown that what memory encodes is highly dependent on personal goals and expectations. People remember what they want to remember; memories are biased and based on cultural and personal prejudices. Memory retrieval is not like rewinding a tape and playing it again, but instead is a reconstructed "on the fly" and colored by experience, knowledge, and beliefs.[3]

The reliability of memory should be questioned with all eyewitness testimony. Errors of recall by eyewitnesses are the leading cause of wrongful convictions, with erroneous identification of the perpetrator occurring 30% of the time.[4] Eyewitness misidentification was the main evidence that led to wrongful convictions in 70% of DNA-based exonerations nationwide.[5]

---

[1] *Bar* is the slang term for alprazolam (Xanax®), which comes as a rectangular-shaped tablet, scored into four sections or "bars." Note that alprazolam is a benzodiazepine drug like diazepam (Valium®), midazolam (Versed®), and lorazepam (Ativan®); also note that most benzodiazepine drugs end with the prefixes "olam" or "epam."

[2] Simons DJ, Chabris CF (2011) What people believe about how memory works: a representative survey of the U.S. population. PLoS One 6:e22757.

[3] Simons DJ, Chabris CF (2011) *Ibid.*

[4] Wise RA et al. (2014) An examination of the causes and solutions to eyewitness error. Front Psychiatry 5:102.

[5] *www.innocenceproject.org/causes/eyewitness-misidentification/.*

The Drug Expert. https://doi.org/10.1016/B978-0-12-800048-9.00010-9

There are no studies on the effects of drugs on eyewitness testimony, except for the effect of alcohol (see later). However, there is much research on the effects of drugs on the brain and memory. The function of the brain and memory, and its alteration by drugs, is an underlying state to eyewitness testimony. For prescription drugs, the brain effects of a marketed drug, if any, are usually known from clinical trials data and the FDA label. For OTC and illegal drugs, adverse brain effects may not be as well known and researched.

Drug effects on the brainstate

The state of the brain, or *brainstate*,[6] is a concept explained best by example. Trekking around Nepal, one can visit a Buddhist monastery with rows of monks chanting with eyes closed and sitting cross-legged on the floor. It is easy to understand an idea of the brainstate in the monks; they are in a *meditative state*. The brainstate arises from the composite action of all substances that affect brain cells, including neurotransmitters, nutrients, and drugs. And in the case of the chanting monks, their brain is likely full of endorphins and dopamine floating around.

Psychologists and pharmacologists discovered long ago that memory and learning works best when the brainstates at the time of acquisition match the brainstate at the time of recall.[7]

This phenomenon is called *state-dependent learning* or a *state-dependent effect*. For example, persons with bipolar (manic depressive disorder) had better memories of events that occurred and recalled later in the same brainstate (manic-manic) than when in opposite states (manic-depressive).[8] State-dependent effects on memory are also found when the brainstate includes intoxication from alcohol, chlorpromazine, and pentobarbital. This is important when arguments are made in court on the veracity of eyewitnesses who may have been intoxicated, such as incidents arising during or after a house party or a binge at the bar. They may have been drunk at the time of the incident but (hopefully) not in the courtroom when giving testimony.

Substances of abuse or any type of drug effect on the brain is not only germane to the intent and behavior of the alleged perpetrator of a crime. Drug effects are also pertinent to victims and witnesses.[9] Among victims of drug-facilitated sexual assault, the pharmacological effect of a "date-rape drug" includes amnesia, sedation, and confusion.[10] These victims of drug-facilitated sexual assault will therefore have inadequate recall of the rape event and the perpetrator. About 20% of all rapes coming into the hospital ER show evidence of drug-facilitation. Victims are the most important eyewitnesses in cases of alleged date-rape facilitated by drugs and will need the support of expert testimony by pharmacologists to inform the court of drug effects on victim/eyewitness accounts.

Cognitive Effects of Common Drugs

In this chapter's first case, an elderly woman teller who served as the only eyewitness was taking five common prescription medications: duloxetine, tramadol, oxycodone, clonazepam, and pregabalin. These drugs are introduced and their known effects on the brain detailed next.

Duloxetine

Duloxetine (Cymbalta®) is a newer antidepressant approved for use in the treatment of major depressive disorder, generalized anxiety disorder, neuropathic pain, fibromyalgia, and musculoskeletal pain.[11] Duloxetine is a prescription-only medicine but is not associated with drug or substance abuse. Antidepressants work by increasing the amount of brain neurotransmitters, specifically norepinephrine and/or serotonin. Depression is thought to be a lack of these neurotransmitters in the brain; the antidepressants correct this underlying deficit that manifest as depression. These same mechanisms of increasing the levels of brain neurotransmitters are also thought to provide therapeutic benefit in generalized anxiety disorder, neuropathic pain, fibromyalgia, and in patients with musculoskeletal pain.

---

[6] I am aware that this is a neologism. It will be spread all over Google™ by the time you read this.

[7] Bower GH et al. (1978) Emotional mood as a context for learning and recall. J. Verbal Learn. Behav. 17:573–585.

[8] Bower GH et al. (1978) *Ibid.*

[9] Mack AH (2015) Chapter 52 Forensic Addiction Psychiatry. In: *Textbook of Substance Abuse Treatment, 5th Ed.*, edited by Galanter, M et al., The American Psychiatric Publishing Company.

[10] Common date-rape drugs include *gamma*-hydroxybutyric acid (GHB), a drug used to treat narcolepsy, and flunitrazepam, a potent benzodiazepine illegal in the United States but sold unregulated elsewhere, like Mexico, under the brand name of Rohypnol® (called "*roofies*").

[11] *Cymbalta® Prescribing Information.*

Duloxetine prescribing information includes "black box" warnings of suicidal thoughts and behaviors. Black box warnings are the highest level of FDA warning and are presented at the beginning of the prescribing information document. As evident in the prescribing information, it is clear that duloxetine can adversely affect cognitive function with the following reported characteristics: anxiety, agitation, irritation, irritability, hostility, aggressiveness, impulsivity, unusual changes in behavior, disturbance in attention, disorientation/confusional state, aggression and anger, and hallucinations. Additional reports of cognitive adverse effects of antidepressants and duloxetine in the medical/pharmacological literature include cognitive toxicity of antidepressants in treating anxiety.[12] Greater than 30% of patients treated for depression had adverse cognitive effects of apathy, inattentiveness, forgetfulness, word-finding difficulty, and mental slowing.[13] Antidepressants reduced attentional performance in adults with anxiety.[14] There were also two case reports of a depressed patient and elderly patient having visual hallucinations during duloxetine treatment.[15] Besides duloxetine, other commonly used antidepressants include fluoxetine (Prozac®), citalopram (Celexa®), escitalopram (Lexapro®), and sertraline (Zooloft®).

Tramadol

Tramadol is a centrally acting synthetic opioid analgesic marketed in the United States since 1995 under the trade name Ultram®. Opioid analgesics are the class of drugs used for moderate to severe pain and besides tramadol, include drugs like morphine, oxycodone, and hydrocodone. Tramadol has a unique dual mechanism of action, it acts at opioid receptors on pain neurons in the brain and spinal cord (see *oxycodone* later) and it acts like an antidepressant by inhibition of norepinephrine and serotonin reuptake. Tramadol is indicated for the management of moderate to moderately severe pain in adults.[16] It is available by prescription only in tablet formulation at a single dosage of 50 mg. Due to its substance abuse liability, tramadol is a Schedule IV Controlled Substance.[17]

The prescribing information of tramadol highlights a number of cognitive adverse effects that occur with tramadol use including impairment of the mental abilities, nervousness, anxiety, euphoria, emotional lability, amnesia, cognitive dysfunction, delirium, difficulty in concentration, and hallucinations. Additional reports of cognitive adverse effects of opioids and specifically tramadol in the medical/pharmacological literature include direct neurotoxic effects and death of brain neurons in rats with chronic administration of morphine or tramadol,[18] tramadol-induced seizures,[19] and case reports of nightmares and visual hallucinations, auditory hallucinations, delirium, and mania with tramadol use.[20]

Oxycodone

Oxycodone (OxyContin®) is a strong opioid analgesic ("painkiller") drug in the same class as morphine, or heroin for that matter.[21] Oxycodone is indicated for the treatment of moderate to severe pain.[22] It is available in different oral forms

---

[12] Hindmarch I (2009) Cognitive toxicity of pharmacotherapeutic agents used in social anxiety disorder. Int J Clin Pract 63:1085–1094.

[13] Fava M et al. (2006) A cross-sectional study of the prevalence of cognitive and physical symptoms during long-term antidepressant treatment. J Clin Psychiatry 67:1754–1759.

[14] Lenze EJ et al. (2013) Escitalopram reduces attentional performance in anxious older adults with high-expression genetic variants at serotonin 2A and 1B receptors. Int J Neuropsychopharmacol 16:279–288.

[15] Rolma G et al. (2013) Combined duloxetine and benzodiazepine-induced visual hallucinations in prodromal dementia with Lewy bodies. General Hospital Psychiatry 35: 678e7–678e9; Tomita T et al. (2013) Visual hallucinations during duloxtine treatment in a patient with major depressive disorder. Clin Neuropharmacol 36:175–176.

[16] *Ultram® Prescribing Information.*

[17] Scheduling of controlled substances is done by their propensity of drug abuse and legit medical use with Schedule I drugs being highly addictive with no medical use and Schedules II-V progressively less so. See Chapter 11 for further details.

[18] Atici S et al. (2004) Opioid neurotoxicity: comparison of morphine and tramadol in an experimental rat model. Intern J Neuroscience 114:1001–1011.

[19] Farajidana H, Hassanian-Moghaddam H, Zamani N, Sanaei-Zadeh H (2012) Tramadol-induced seizures and trauma. Eur Rev Med Pharmacol Sci 16:S34-S37.

[20] Devulder J et al. (1996) Nightmares and hallucinations after long-term intake of tramadol combined with antidepressants. Acta Clin Belg 51:184–186; Ghosh S et al. (2013) Acute delirium due to parenteral tramadol. Case Reports in Emergency Medicine ID 492685:1–2; Gonzalez-Pinto A et al. (2001) Mania and tramadol-fluoxetine combination. Am J Psychiatry 158:964–965; Keeley PW et al. (2000) Hear my song: auditory hallucinations with tramadol hydrochloride. BMJ 321:1608; Watts BV, Grady TA (1997) Tramadol-induced mania. Am J Psychiatry 154:1624.

[21] Heroin is simply a morphine molecule with two acetyl groups stuck on, thus heroin's generic name is *diacetylmorphine*. Bayer marketed Heroin® as a cough-suppressant in 1898; it was freely available OTC at the corner drugstore in every American town and city until 1924. *See*: Sneader W (1998) The discovery of heroin. Lancet 352:1697–1699. Heroin (like Kleenex, registered trademark symbol no longer needed) has been considered for use in hospice or chronic pain patients; its onset of action is faster than morphine and it is more water soluble so larger doses could be administered. Because it is metabolized to morphine after administration, heroin has the same analgesic potency at opioid receptors as morphine.

[22] *OxyContin Prescribing Information.*

including formulations for around-the-clock treatment and others for more immediate pain control. The OxyContin® formulation is an opioid analgesic for the management of pain when a continuous, around-the-clock opioid analgesic is needed. Like morphine, oxycodone and a number of other opioid analgesics work by binding to specific protein targets (opioid receptors) on pain neurons of the CNS (central nervous system, i.e., brain and spinal cord). When opioid analgesics bind to the opioid receptor, the activity of pain neurons decreases, producing analgesia. Because of their potential for abuse, oxycodone and other opioid analgesics are classified as Schedule II Controlled Substances under the federal act of the same name.[23]

Oxycodone is an opioid analgesic that has quickly become one of the most commonly prescribed opioids for chronic pain in the United States and Canada mainly due to the aggressive marketing[24] of its controlled-release formulation called OxyContin®. Subjective and psychomotor assessment studies of oxycodone and morphine show that at equal doses, oxycodone produced stronger effects and greater cognitive dysfunction (in terms of psychomotor impairment) than morphine in healthy young volunteers.[25] Single low doses of oxycodone produced a slight but significant cognitive dysfunction characterized by decreased function of working memory in healthy young adults.[26] Oxycodone showed a dose-related cognitive and psychomotor impairment in nondrug abusing health volunteers.[27] In comparing two formulations of oxymorphone and oxycodone, the controlled-release oxycodone produced more cognitive and psychomotor impairment than extended-release oxymorphone at equal analgesic doses.[28]

Neurocognitive adverse effects are a major concern in elderly patients because even a minor decrement in functioning can have catastrophic consequences for frail older adults, including accidents, falls, impaired judgment, delirium, and a loss of independence.[29] For this reason, the American Geriatrics Society recommends that patients on opioid therapy be regularly monitored for cognitive adverse effects.[30] Additionally, the decreased metabolic capacity of elderly patients results in higher blood plasma concentrations of opioids, especially oxycodone.[31] Besides oxycodone (OxyContin®), other commonly used opioid analgesics are hydrocodone (in generic and Lortab®, Vicodin®, Norco®, and other formulations), fentanyl patches (Duragesic®), and meperidine (Demerol®).

Clonazepam

Clonazepam is a benzodiazepine drug better known by its trade name Klonopin®. Like other benzodiazepines, clonazepam is a sedative-hypnotic drug under the general class of CNS depressants. Unlike most other benzodiazepines, clonazepam is approved for treatment of seizure disorders (epilepsy) as well as a type of anxiety disorder called panic disorder (with *panic attacks*).[32] Due to substance abuse liability, clonazepam is classified under the Controlled Substances Act of 1970 as a Schedule IV drug. Clonazepam works by enhancing the effect of the inhibitory neurotransmitter, GABA, in the brain to produce a calming effect in persons with anxiety. It does this by binding to the GABA receptor and increasing the effect of naturally occurring GABA. This in turn decreases the activity of neurons in the brain. The decrease in neuronal activity leads to clonazepam's classification as a CNS depressant and its sedative effects. Adverse or side effects of clonazepam on brain function are common; clonazepam is a benzodiazepine.

Benzodiazepines, as CNS depressants, carry strong warnings of interfering with cognitive functions and mental alertness and noted to impair judgment and thinking. Psychiatric symptoms such as anxiety, aggressive reactions, and illusions, are noted in the warnings. Other literature on the cognitive adverse effects of clonazepam include reports showing that clonazepam affected memory and attention in healthy volunteers,[33] psychomotor performance in healthy volunteers,[34] and

---

[23] See Chapter 11 *I Want a New Drug* for background on the Controlled Substances Act.

[24] Lexchin J, Kohler JC (2011) The danger of imperfect regulation: OxyContin® use in the United States and Canada. Int J Risk Saf Med. 23:233–40.

[25] Zacny JP, Gutierrez S. (2003) Characterizing the subjective, psychomotor, and physiological effects of oral oxycodone in non-drug-abusing volunteers. Psychopharmacology (Berl). 170:242–54.

[26] Friswell J et al. (2008) Acute effects of opioids on memory functions of healthy men and women. Psychopharmacology (Berl). 198:243–50.

[27] Zacny JP, Gutierrez S. (2003) *Op. cit.*

[28] Schoedel KA et al. (2010) Reduced cognitive and psychomotor impairment with extended-release oxymorphone versus controlled-release oxycodone. Pain Physician. 13:561–73.

[29] Cherrier MM et al. (2009) Comparative cognitive and subjective side effects of immediate-release oxycodone in healthy middle-aged and older adults. J Pain. 10:1038–50.

[30] American Geriatrics Society (2002) The management of persistent pain in older persons. J Am Geriatr Soc. 50:S205–224.

[31] Liukas A et al. (2008) Plasma concentrations of oral oxycodone are greatly increased in the elderly. Clin Pharmacol Ther 84:462–467.

[32] *Klonopin® Prescribing Information.*

[33] Dowd SM et al. (2002) The behavioral and cognitive effects of two benzodiazepines associated with drug-facilitated sexual assault. J Forensic Sci 47:1101–1107.

[34] dos Santos FM et al. (2009) Pharmacokinetic/pharmacodynamic modeling of psychomotor impairment induced by oral clonazepam in healthy volunteers. The Drug Monitor 31:566–574.

cognitive impairment in anxiety patients.[35] There are case reports demonstrating clonazepam-induced mania,[36] behavioral disinhibition, suicide ideation, self-mutilation,[37] and psychosis.[38] Besides clonazepam, other benzodiazepine antianxiety medications include alprazolam (Xanax®), diazepam (Valium®), and lorazepam (Ativan®).

Pregabalin

Pregabalin is a newer drug approved by the FDA in 2004 and given the brand name of Lyrica®. It is approved for the treatment of fibromyalgia, partial onset seizures (epilepsy), postherpetic neuralgia, and neuropathic pain.[39] The mechanism of action of pregabalin is not entirely known but it binds to and reduces the activity of calcium channels on neurons in the CNS. Due to abuse liability, pregabalin is a Schedule V Controlled Substance.

Pregabalin Prescribing Information (for Lyrica®) displays the following warnings of ophthalmological adverse effects such as blurred vision, diplopia ("double vision"), disturbance in attention, memory impairment, confusional states, anxiety, hallucinations, and disorientation. Pregabalin use was associated in clinical trials with neurocognitive disturbances such as confusion, disturbed attention, abnormal thinking, euphoric mood, and ophthalmological problems (blurred vision).[40] Cognitive adverse effects of pregabalin include deterioration of verbal and episodic memory, and abnormal thinking.[41] In healthy volunteers, pregabalin at conventional doses induced mild cognitive adverse effects and neurotoxicity.[42] Case reports also show that pregabalin use is associated with delirium,[43] confused state, stupor,[44] acute psychosis,[45] delirium, psychosis, visual hallucinations,[46] and self-harm behavior.[47]

In this chapter's second case, the alleged victim of forced oral and anal sodomy admitted to taking alprazolam (Xanax®), drinking beer, and smoking marijuana. The effects on memory and perception when under the influence of these three drugs are detailed next.

Alprazolam

Alprazolam is a benzodiazepine drug better known by its prescription trade name of Xanax®.[48] Benzodiazepines are very common drugs and alprazolam (Xanax®) is one of the most commonly prescribed benzodiazepine drug, along with diazepam (Valium®) and lorazepam (Ativan®). Alprazolam is FDA approved for the treatment of anxiety, and also indicated for the treatment of panic disorder, with or without agoraphobia ("fear of the marketplace"). Alprazolam is a leading antianxiety medicine (sedative), with millions of Americans taking Xanax® on a daily basis. Alprazolam works the same way as clonazepam detailed before. Like clonazepam, alprazolam (Xanax®) is a strong CNS depressant drug. Because of its widespread abuse, alprazolam and other benzodiazepines are Schedule IV controlled substances.

As early as 1982, neuropsychiatric adverse effects were noted with the use of benzodiazepines like alprazolam.[49] Adverse effects noted in this study included delirium, hallucinations, confusion, and memory impairment. A larger study documented the side effects of anger or violence, impulsivity, self-harming, depression, and manic behaviors after taking alprazolam and other benzodiazepines.[50] Sexual fantasies were also reported to be associated with benzodiazepine use, often leading to unfounded allegations of sexual abuse by persons taking benzodiazepines.[51] One of the best-studied adverse

[35] Hindmarch I (2009) Cognitive toxicity of pharmacotherapeutic agents used in social anxiety disorder. Int J Clin Pract 63:1085–1094.

[36] Ikeda M et al. (1998) Clonazepam-induced maniacal reaction in a patient with bipolar disorder. Internat Clin Psychopharm. 13:189–190.

[37] Kandemir H et al. (2008) Behavioral disinhibition, suicidal ideation, and self-mutilation related to clonazepam. J Child Adol Psychopharm. 18:409–410.

[38] White MC et al. (1982) Psychosis associated with clonazepam therapy for blepharospasm. J Nerv Mental Dis. 170:117–119.

[39] *Lyrica® Prescribing Information.*

[40] Hauser W et al. (2010) Comparative efficacy and harms of duloxetine, milnacipran, and pregabalin in fibromyalgia syndrome. J. Pain 11:505–521.

[41] Eddy CM et al. (2011) The cognitive impact of antiepileptic drugs. Ther Adv Neural Disord. 4:385–407.

[42] Salinsky M et al. (2010) Cognitive effects of pregabalin in healthy volunteers. Neurology 74:755–761.

[43] Hickey C, Thomas B (2011) Delirium secondary to pregabalin. General Hospital Psychiatry 34:436e1–436e2.

[44] Lee S (2012) Pregabalin intoxication-induced encephalopathy with triphasic waves. Epilep Behav. 25:170–173.

[45] Olaizola I et al. (2006) Pregabalin-associated acute psychosis and epileptiform EEG-changes. Seizure 15:208–210.

[46] Pedroso JL et al. (2012) Delirium, psychosis, and visual hallucinations induced by pregabalin. Arq Neurosiquiatr 70:960–966.

[47] Tandon VR et al. (2013) Pregabalin-induced self-harm behavior. Indian Journal of Pharmacology 45:638–639.

[48] Brenner GM, Stevens CW (2018) *Brenner and Stevens' Pharmacology, 5th edition.* Elsevier, Philadelphia, PA, USA.

[49] Ong BY et al. (1982) Lorazepam and diazepam as adjuncts to epidural anaesthesia for caesarean section. Can Anaesth Soc J 29:31–34.

[50] Cole JO, Kando JC (1993) Adverse behavioral events reported in patients taking alprazolam and other benzodiazepines. J Clin Psychiatry 54 Suppl:49–61.

[51] Brahams D (1989) Benzodiazepine sedation and allegations of sexual assault. Lancet 1:1339–1340; Brahams D (1990) Benzodiazepines and sexual fantasies. Lancet 335:157.

cognitive effects of the benzodiazepines is their inhibition of memory formation.[52] Numerous clinical studies show that alprazolam and other benzodiazepines prevent recall of memories while on the drug, called anterograde amnesia.[53] Among the types of memories affected by benzodiazepines, episodic memory is particularly affected.[54] Episodic memory is the ability to recall events that one experiences, like a story of what happened.

Marijuana

Marijuana is the most abused illegal drug in the United States. A profile of marijuana including the action of its main active ingredient, THC, was given earlier in the book in Chapter 6 *Hairs of the Innocent*.[55] Adverse effects of marijuana on the brain include reduction in performance on tests of memory, reaction time, attention, tracking, and motor function.[56] The impairment of memory by the use of marijuana was shown by human volunteer experiments in clinical studies where controlled doses of marijuana were smoked.[57] Like alprazolam before, one of the most consistent findings is that marijuana use causes a decrement in episodic memory and recall.[58] Marijuana targets (cannabinoid receptors) are found in high concentrations in the brain regions responsible for working and episodic memory function.[59] One of those brain regions, called the hippocampus, is actually smaller in chronic marijuana users and the decrease in the hippocampus correlates with the decrement in episodic memory.[60] Marijuana users show a lack of inhibitory control and decreased episodic memory which is associated with risky sexual behavior in young adult users.[61] Significantly, marijuana users show an increased susceptibility to false memories.[62]

Alcohol (ethanol)

Alcohol was introduced in Chapter 7 *Firewater* and only its effects on memory will be added here. A major effect of alcohol on cognitive function has to do with memory formation and recall. Numerous individuals have described a period of "blackout" after heavy drinking of alcohol that is characterized by complete or partial memory loss (amnesia) during the time alcohol was being consumed and alcohol intoxication occurred. Alcohol primarily interferes with the ability of the brain to form new memories and leaves intact previously established memories.[63] Detectable impairments of memory occur after just one or two drinks. At the molecular level, alcohol inhibits the formation of long-term potentiation between brain synapses, which results in a detrimental effect on memory.[64] Increasing the dose of alcohol increases the degree of memory impairment, leading from fragmentary blackouts to complete blackouts. During amnesic events, persons using alcohol are capable of being involved in dramatic and emotional events that they cannot later recall.[65] Significantly, persons with fragmentary blackouts can become somewhat aware of events that occurred only after being reminded about them.[66]

[52] Beracochea D (2006) Anterograde and retrograde effects of benzodiazepines on memory. Sci. World Journal 6:1460–1465; Savić MM et al. (2005) Memory effects of benzodiazepines: memory stages and types versus binding-site subtypes. Neural Plast. 12:289–298.

[53] Roth T et al. (1984) Benzodiazepines and memory. Br J Clin Pharmacol. 18 Suppl 1:45S–49S; Langlois S et al. (1987) Midazolam: kinetics and effects on memory, sensorium, and haemodynamics. Br J Clin Pharmacol. 23:273–278; Bareggi SR et al. (1998) Impairment of memory and plasma flunitrazepam levels. Psychopharm. (Berl). 140:157–163; Carter LP et al. (2013) Acute cognitive effects of high doses of dextromethorphan relative to triazolam in humans. Drug Alcohol Depend. 128:206–213; Hall-Porter JM et al. (2014) The effect of two benzodiazepine receptor agonist hypnotics on sleep-dependent memory consolidation. J Clin Sleep Med. 10:27–34.

[54] Milgrom P et al. (1994) The efficacy and memory effects of oral triazolam premedication in highly anxious dental patients. Anesth Prog. 41:70–76.

[55] See also chapter 16 *Reefer Madness* for more information in marijuana intoxication and driving.

[56] Kramer JL (2015) Medical marijuana for cancer. CA Cancer J Clin. 65:109–122.

[57] Heishman SJ et al. (1997) Comparative effects of alcohol and marijuana on mood, memory, and performance. Pharmacol Biochem Behav. 58:93–101; Viñals X et al. (2015) Cognitive Impairment Induced by Delta9-tetrahydrocannabinol Occurs through Heteromers between Cannabinoid CB1 and Serotonin 5-HT2A Receptors. PLoS Biol. 13:e1002194.

[58] Crane NA et al. (2013) Effects of cannabis on neurocognitive functioning: recent advances, neurodevelopmental influences, and sex differences. Neuropsychol Rev. 23:117–137.

[59] Ilan AB et al. (2004) Effects of marijuana on neurophysiological signals of working and episodic memory. Psychopharm. (Berl). 176:214–222.

[60] Smith MJ et al. (2015) Cannabis-related episodic memory deficits and hippocampal morphological differences in healthy individuals and schizophrenia subjects. Hippocampus 25:1042–1051.

[61] Schuster RM et al. (2012) The influence of inhibitory control and episodic memory on the risky sexual behavior of young adult cannabis users. J Int Neuropsychol Soc. 18:827–833.

[62] Riba J et al. (2015) Telling true from false: cannabis users show increased susceptibility to false memories. Mol Psychiatry 20:772–777.

[63] White, AM (2003) What happened? Alcohol, memory blackouts, and the brain. Alcohol Res Health 27:186–196.

[64] Lücke C et al. (2014) Deleterious effects of a low amount of ethanol on LTP-like plasticity in human cortex. Neuropsychopharm. 39:1508–1518.

[65] Goodwin DW (1995) Alcohol amnesia. Addiction 90:315–7.

[66] Goodwin DW et al. (1969) Alcoholic "blackouts": a review and clinical study of 100 alcoholics. Am J Psych. 126:191–198.

Skillful investigators may elicit better recall during blackout periods from alcoholic perpetrators by prompting them during questioning.

Interactions among drugs used by the witness and alleged victim

A general pharmacological principle is that adverse effects are magnified when two drugs have the same adverse effects. For example, alcohol and benzodiazepines are two drugs that each have CNS depressant effects that cause impairment; taking these two drugs together causes even greater impairment than the total of either drug alone. Adding more drugs increases the likelihood for more adverse effects. In the case of the bank teller, there were five drugs on board that are classified as CNS-acting drugs. Each one of these five prescription medicines has strong warnings in their FDA-approved Prescribing Information against concurrent use of other CNS depressant or psychoactive drugs.

In the second case alprazolam, marijuana, and alcohol were taken by the alleged victim. There are few studies examining the combination drug effects on memory. It is common to use marijuana and alcohol together as shown by its high rate of occurrence from epidemiological studies in drivers suspected of driving under the influence of drugs.[67] As both marijuana and alprazolam exert detrimental effects on memory, the pharmacological effect of both together are likely to be at least additive.[68] The combined effects of alcohol and marijuana have mostly been examined in the context of driving impairment. In laboratory tests of performance, a greater decrease in psychomotor tests was observed with the coadministration of alcohol and marijuana.[69] Performance in a driving simulator was more impaired when marijuana and alcohol were coadministered.[70] With regards to memory function, one study did show that combined alcohol and marijuana use did lead to greater memory deficits than when used alone.[71] The use of alcohol and alprazolam produces a greater degree of brain dysfunction than either drug alone. Alprazolam and all the other benzodiazepines contain strong warning of this drug-drug interaction in their FDA-approved label.

Another aspect of drug effects on testimony is the special case of statements by the alleged perpetrator, that is, when a suspect makes a confession. We will see in Chapter 14 *The Truth Shall Not Set You Free*, that drug-induced confessions have a long and sordid history in American justice. While drugs are no longer used overtly by law enforcement agencies for extracting a confession, interrogation of witnesses and suspects while intoxicated is prevalent.[72]

What is the effect of drugs on eyewitness testimony? As mentioned before, there is not a significant body of research papers examining drugs and eyewitness testimony.[73] The exception is alcohol, whose brain effects after consumption increased eyewitness suggestibility to misinformation.[74] Short of an instantaneous drug test for all known drugs and their metabolites, there is no way of knowing when and which member of the public is under the influence of legal or illegal drugs and may be providing testimony from recall of events while under drug influence. Both prosecutors and defense attorneys should be aware of possible drug effects and consult with their friendly neighborhood drug expert when needed.

The Public Defender's Office and the Drug Expert

Anyone charged with a crime and arrested under a felony warrant is entitled to an attorney. Whether the defendant's attorney is hired and paid for by hard-working, professional parents,[75] or reimbursed from public funds, the ability of the defendant to pay for his attorney should not prevent him from adequate representation before the court. Because it is obvious that persons with lower socioeconomic status are more likely to enter the justice system, the amount of public funds for indigent defense is quite large. Historically, federal district judges would appoint defendant's counsel and depend on the

---

[67] Augsburger M et al. (2005) Concentration of drugs in blood of suspected impaired drivers. Forensic Sci Int. 153:11–15.

[68] *Additive* pharmacological effects example: one painkiller gives 10% pain relief and another one 40% relief; taking both together gives 50% pain relief. Pharmacological *potentiation* or *synergy* occurs when the total effect of both painkillers taken together is greater than 50%, like say 85% pain relief.

[69] Perez-Reyes M et al. (1988) Interaction between marihuana and ethanol: effects on psychomotor performance. Alcohol Clin Exp Res. 12:268–276.

[70] Downey LA et al. (2012) The effects of cannabis and alcohol on simulated driving: Influences of dose and experience. Accid Anal Prev. 50:879–886.

[71] Mahmood OM et al. (2010) Learning and memory performances in adolescent users of alcohol and marijuana: interactive effects. J Stud Alcohol Drugs 71:885–894.

[72] Palmer FT et al. (2013) Intoxicated witnesses and suspects: an archival analysis of their involvement in criminal case processing. Law Human Behav. 37:54–59.

[73] At least not in the usual places I look, like *PubMed* and others. An enterprising law student or attorney might want to do legal search and let me know if you find anything.

[74] Gawrylowicz J (2017) Alcohol-induced retrograde facilitation renders witnesses of crime less suggestible to misinformation. Psychopharmacology (Berl). 234:1267–1275.

[75] Don't ask.

attorney to provide *pro bono* services for those accused who could not afford to hire a lawyer. Providing services for free became untenable as the number of indigent defendants grew and attorneys rightly bemoaned the lack of billable hours. The passage of the *Criminal Justice Act* (CJA) in 1964 established a system for appointing and paying lawyers by funds appropriated from the U.S. Treasury. At that time, the law stated that public defenders were compensated at a rate of $15 per hour for court time and $10 per hour for out of court time, with a maximum of $500 per case.[76] Amendments to the CJA in 1970 established federal defender organizations as counterparts to the prosecutors in US Attorneys' offices. There are now federal defender offices attached to each of the 94 district courts.

States must also provide counsel to indigent defendants which costs about $2.3 billion per year.[77] The annual cost of the federal public defender program adds an additional $1 billion.[78] The court appointment of a paid attorney does not apply in all criminal cases, but reserved for serious felony crimes. Also, a court-paid attorney is not available for either plaintiff nor defendant in civil litigation.

The Supreme Court consistently upheld that the government is required to provide effective counsel to persons accused of a crime but who cannot afford to hire a defense attorney. The right of free counsel for indigent defendants in federal cases is guaranteed in the Sixth Amendment of the US Constitution. The Supreme Court ruled that state governments must also provide this right to counsel under the due process clause of the Fourteenth Amendment, in *Gideon v. Wainwright*, 1963. The Sixth Amendment gives defendants the right to counsel in federal prosecutions, but it was not until the decision in *Gideon v. Wainwright* that the right to counsel was applied to state prosecutions for felony offenses.[79] Like the federal system, the right to free counsel does not always apply to state nonfelony cases.

Today there is an outcry from public defenders across the country that state and federal budget cuts are decimating staff and services, leading to ineffective counsel.[80] With the cuts to the public defenders program, courts have to rely more on court-appointed private lawyers (*CJA panel attorneys*, for example) to represent indigent clients. These lawyers are paid from the same budget as the public defenders, but they cost more since they are paid by the hour, and they tend to be less experienced and less effective. According to recent studies, indigent defendants who had court-appointed private lawyers were more often found guilty and spent more time in prison than similar defendants represented by federal public defenders.[81]

The right to hire and the reimbursement of drug experts

The CJA also established the right of indigent or otherwise cash-strapped defendants to hire investigators, expert witness, or other services necessary for adequate representation. Upon request and prior approval of the federal judge, an expert may be reimbursed up to $2400. If time does not allow, or if the public defender has not taken the step of getting prior authorization for expert services from the judge, the reimbursement for an expert without prior court approval is limited to $800.[82] State federal defender programs may be less limited in the amount paid to an expert witness.

Depending on the case, the drug expert may find that a portion of the time spent on the case will be *pro bono* with partial reimbursement for services rendered even with prior approval. Those drug experts that work full-time for publicly funded universities or medical school should view "*lost*" income as payback to the community or the state that pays the full-time salary of the drug expert. *Payback for paycheck,* as it were. Other drug experts, either the "*hired-gun*" types who do not hold a full-time job as a Pharmacologist or Toxicologist, or those experts employed by private or business institutions, may not take the case due to fiduciary concerns. The material advantage of taking on a federal or state public defender case for any drug expert is the potential future cases that might come through word-of-mouth referrals.

Similar to the federal defender organizations, many states and counties have their own public defender systems. Some states organize all public defenders at the state level, called simply state public defender systems. Oklahoma's state public

---

[76] It is now increased to $132 per hour for noncapital cases, with a case maximum of $10,300 for felony defense and $2900 for defense of a misdemeanor offense.

[77] Herberman E, Kyckelhahn T (2015) Government Indigent Defense Expenditures, FY 2008–2012 – Updated. U.S. Department of Justice, Office of Justice Programs, Bureau of Justice Statistics.

[78] The Judiciary FY 2017 Congressional Budget Summary (2016) Prepared by the Administrative Office of the U.S. Courts, Washington, DC. Available at: *www.uscourts.gov/sites/default/files/fy_2017_federal_judiciary_congressional_budget_summary_0.pdf*.

[79] Rapping JA (2014) Reclaiming our rightful place: reviving the hero image of the public defender. Iowa Law Rev. 99:1893–1904.

[80] Marcus P (2016) The United States Supreme Court (mostly) gives up its review role with ineffective assistance of counsel cases. Minnesota Law Rev. 100:1745–1768.

[81] Joy PA, McMunigal KC (2012) Does the lawyer make a difference? Public defender v. appointed counsel. Criminal Justice, Spring issue, pp. 46–48, 63.

[82] This has happened. For more details and exceptions, see the code at *www.law.cornell.edu/uscode/text/18/3006A*.

defense system goes under the mellifluous acronym of *OIDS*, standing for the *Oklahoma Indigent Defense System*. Other states have county-level organization, while a few operate with a hybrid of state and county-wide organizations. Funding may come from state appropriations or a combination of state and local (county) revenues. There is a more of a paperwork burden working with the state or federal public defender systems. In both federal and state systems, the drug expert may need to first register as an official vendor, and the application process may be tedious and slow. Each case may involve submission of forms for approval of the drug expert's fees before work on the case begins and other forms for the reimbursement for amount due after the case ends.

Finally, as elaborated in Chapter 7 *Firewater*, the Federal Rules of Evidence *Rule 706, Court-Appointed Expert Witnesses,* details the process whereby a judge may appoint a drug expert, an impartial court-appointed expert witness. Although rarely used, in this case the expert is paid from court funds.

The Drug Expert and Pharmacy Records

The pharmacy records are essential to many cases investigated by the drug expert. The pharmacy records consist of a list of the time, type, dosage, and quantity of a prescription drug picked up from a retail pharmacy. The format of the records varies slightly from pharmacy to pharmacy but they are all suboptimal for easy comprehension. The pharmacy records supplied by Walmart pharmacies may be the worst, with column headers and data looping around and interfering with the next row of data. The record entries end up splattered across the pages like a *Jackson Pollock* painting. The drug expert will find it necessary to extract the needed data and reformat into a timeline or calendar format for inclusion in the litigation report. Examples of the pharmacy records and the data from pharmacy records converted to an easier to read format for inclusion in the litigation report are given in Appendix I.

In any event, pharmacy records give some important data on the person's use of a prescribed drug. If pharmacy records show that a monthly supply of a medication is filled and picked up once every 3–4 months, it is likely that the person does not regularly take that drug. If the prescription is picked up like clockwork, once a month without fail for the last six months, then it is likely that the person is taking the drug as prescribed. If a 30-day supply is consistently refilled earlier than a month (or is resupplied due to "loss" of the pills) and creeps forward in time month by month, then it is likely that the person is abusing the drug and not taking the drug as prescribed.

[Narrative continued]
In the first case, Todd Lewis was charged with two counts in the federal trial court; attempted bank robbery and killing a person while attempting to avoid apprehension. The drug expert researched the brain effects of prescription medications taken by the bank teller, wrote a litigation report to support testimony, and testified in federal court. The jury was not overly persuaded and Mr. Lewis was sentenced to the maximum sentence of 20 years in prison for attempted bank robbery. The second charge of killing a person while attempting to avoid apprehension was dropped.

In the second case, Mr. Scott was accused of oral and anal sodomy, and represented by a state public defender. The drug expert researched the effects of the drugs used by the alleged victim, wrote a litigation report, but did not give a deposition or testify in court. At the first hearing, the district court dismissed the charges after receiving the drug expert's report which called into question the reliability of the alleged victim's memory and recall. Additional evidence suggested that the incident described by the alleged victim was consensual.

Chapter 11

I Want a New Drug: Fake marijuana, designer stimulants, and hallucinogens

Designer Drugs in the Age of Synthetics—The Controlled Substances Act

Scheduling of Controlled Substances—Federal Drug Sentencing Guidelines

The Business of Being a Drug Expert

[Narrative]
Kamal Nepali immigrated to the USA to escape the poverty of his native country. With the help of family and friends, Mr. Nepali purchased a gas-station/convenience store in a small Midwestern town. After numerous customers asked him if he carried any "K2" or "Spice," Mr. Nepali calls his distributor and orders a gross of these "herbal incense" products. Undercover federal agents purchased packets of K2 at the convenience store, had the contents analyzed at the DEA lab, and convicted Mr. Nepali under the Controlled Substances Analogue Act for selling XLR-11, a synthetic cannabinoid. The US Sentencing Memorandum quantifies his offense by using the total weight of all packages of leafy material sold to determine the amount of the illegal drug. However, XLR-11 is sprayed on innocuous and legal plant leaves with a trace concentration of only 0.6% in the K2 packets. Mr. Nepali's criminal defense attorney calls a local drug expert to determine the type and the amount of the synthetic substance Mr. Nepali sold.

In a separate case, 24-year old Dan Blazer is arrested under the Controlled Substances Act for possession and distribution of BZP (benzylpiperazine), a synthetic amphetamine-like drug used at raves. Like most designer drugs, BZP is not listed as a specific agent in the Federal Drug Sentencing tables for the determination of offense level. Both methamphetamine ("meth") and MDMA ("Ecstasy") are chemical analogs to BZP but have different pharmacological effects and different patterns of abuse. A determination is made by the DEA that BDZ is most similar to methamphetamine and not MDMA, leading to severe sentencing terms under the Federal Drug Sentencing Guidelines. Mr. Blazer's defense attorney contacts a drug expert to research the pharmacology of BZP with respect its similarity to methamphetamine or MDMA.

Designer Drugs in the Age of Synthetics

As if there weren't enough mind-altering substances found in nature to be taken, there is now a tsunami of synthetic drugs available for abuse in America. These newer synthetic drugs are called *designer drugs,* a term first used in the early 1980s to describe compounds which were made in small home laboratories using freely available over-the-counter (OTC) drugs and chemical precursors.[1] Initially, designer drugs were not illegal because they were structurally different from substances listed as illegal under the *Controlled Substances Act of 1970* (see later).

Nearly every synthetic chemical process can be duplicated in a clandestine laboratory; from making meth using Sudafed® precursors with match tips in an empty 2-L pop bottle to the more sophisticated methods of multistep laboratory synthesis of LSD (*acid*). There are now designer drugs for nearly every drug of abuse class, including opioids, amphetamines, MDMA (*Ecstasy, X*), and cannabinoids. This chapter's cases are based on real-life issues with the designer drugs, XLR-11 (*5-fluoro-UR-144*, a synthetic cannabinoid), and BZP (*benzylpiperazine*, a synthetic stimulant) profiled next.

---

[1] German CL et al. (2014) Bath salts and synthetic cathinones: an emerging designer drug phenomenon. Life Sci. 97:2–8.

Synthetic marijuana (THC)-like drugs

There are more than 100 designer drugs made to mimic the action of the active ingredient of marijuana, THC.[2] These synthetic cannabinoids are sold as "*incense*" or "*plant food*" at convenience stores and truck stops. The most popular brands are known as *Spice* and *K2*.[3] The typical package consists of a dollop of marijuana-looking dried leaves that were sprayed with a solution containing a synthetic cannabinoid or two. As noted in Chapter 6 *Hairs of the Innocent*, the psychoactive active ingredient in marijuana is *delta*-tetrahydrocannabinol (THC). THC produces its effects by binding and activating a cannabinoid receptor. Synthetic cannabinoids share the same pharmacological mechanism of action with THC but are much more potent. Synthetic cannabinoids have acute adverse effects not shared by natural marijuana, like severe agitation, seizures, and psychosis.[4] Synthetic cannabinoid overdose admissions to emergency rooms have sky-rocketed in the last decade and there is evidence that synthetic cannabinoids destroy kidney function.[5]

XLR-11 is one of the synthetic cannabinoids that is sprayed onto unregulated plant substances and sold in packets as *Spice* or *K2*.[6] These unregulated plant substances include various species such as the leaves and flowers of the licorice plant, the Mongolian milkvetch plant, or the Great mullein plant.[7] It is not illegal to possess or sell these unregulated plant species. Studies show that the amount of synthetic cannabinoids in *Spice* or *K2* products ranges from 0.1% to 1.0% by weight (equal to 0.1%–1.0% purity).[8] From limited studies using cell cultures that express cannabinoid receptors, XLR-11 acted like a cannabinoid agonist. XLR-11 bound to and activated cannabinoid receptors just like THC. However, XLR-11 produced cannabinoid effects in the rat with a potency of 4–17 times greater than THC, the natural cannabinoid in marijuana.[9]

Synthetic CNS stimulant/hallucinogenic drugs

The profiles of amphetamine and methamphetamine were given in Chapter 5 *Wrong Place at the Wrong Time*. The synthesis of methamphetamine (*making meth*) is well known from the ubiquity of meth labs around the country, fueled by the easy access to meth recipes on the internet and readily available ingredients.[10] Methamphetamine is also a legal prescription medication, used to treat narcolepsy and obesity. Amphetamine shares the same pharmacological effects as methamphetamine but is not synthesized in clandestine labs. Amphetamine abuse is characterized by diversion of prescription medications for ADHD, like the amphetamines in Adderall®.

Many designer drugs were originally synthesized for research purposes by medicinal chemists employed at academic research institutions or the pharmaceutical industry. The resulting publications describing the method of synthesis and pharmacological effects of these designer drugs were used to synthesize these research drugs for the black market. For example, the methamphetamine derivative, MDMA (*Ecstasy*), was first developed and patented by Merck in 1912, but was not discovered as a street drug until 1970 and was not widely abused until the 1980s.[11]

MDMA, called *Ecstasy* or simply *X*, is chemically known as 3,4-*methylened*ioxy-*meth*amphetamine, the origin of its initialism *MDMA*. MDMA use soared during the last two decades of the 20th century, with abuse propelled by communal use during dance parties known as *raves*.[12] Besides CNS stimulation, MDMA produces a unique *pro-social* pharmacological

[2] Dasgupta A, Wahed A (2014) Chapter 17 – Challenges in drugs of abuse testing: magic mushrooms, peyote cactus, and designer drugs. In: *Clinical Chemistry, Immunology and Laboratory Quality Control*, pp. 307–316, Elsevier, Philadelphia, PA, USA.

[3] The marketing of synthetic cannabinoids is designed for the junior high to high school crowd with all sorts of snazzy names and flavors. Drug dealers often market to the young, as in the Joe Camel ad campaign for cigarettes. China remains the source of most synthetic cannabinoids sold in the United States. See Schwarz A (2015) Arrest underscores China's role in the making and spread of a lethal drug, New York Times, May 28.

[4] Harris CR, Brown A (2013) Synthetic cannabinoid intoxication: a case series and review. J Emerg Med. 44:360–366.

[5] Vardakou I et al. (2010) Spice drugs as a new trend: mode of action, identification and legislation. Toxicol Lett. 197:157–162; Seely KA et al. (2012) Spice drugs are more than harmless herbal blends: a review of the pharmacology and toxicology of synthetic cannabinoids. Prog Neuropsychopharmacol Biol Psychiatry 39:234–243; Spaderna M et al. (2013) Spicing things up: synthetic cannabinoids. Psychopharmacology (Berl). 228:525–540.

[6] Seely KA et al. (2013) Forensic investigation of K2, Spice, and "bath salt" commercial preparations: a three-year study of new designer drug products containing synthetic cannabinoid, stimulant, and hallucinogenic compounds. Forensic Sci Int. 233:416–422.

[7] Uchiyama N et al. (2010) Chemical analysis of synthetic cannabinoids as designer drugs in herbal products. Forensic Sci Int. 198:31–38.

[8] Zuba D et al. (2011) Comparison of "herbal highs" composition. Anal Bioanal Chem. 400:119–126.

[9] Wiley JL (2013) Cannabinoids in disguise: Δ^9-tetrahydrocannabinol-like effects of tetramethylcyclopropyl ketone indoles. Neuropharmacology 75:145–154.

[10] A case for internet censorship? There are more Google™ hits after entering "making methamphetamine" (2,590,000 hits) than "making apple pie" (2,330,000 hits).

[11] German CL et al. (2014) *Op. cit.*

[12] Bahora M et al. (2009) Understanding recreational ecstasy use in the United States: a qualitative inquiry. Int J Drug Policy 20:62–69.

effect. This results in users reporting an increased desire to socialize with greater empathy and closeness to others.[13] MDMA also produces acute toxicity including cardiovascular toxicity, nephrotoxicity (toxicity of the kidneys), and uncontrolled hyperthermia. The acute toxic effects of MDMA cause fatalities in many users.

The mechanism of action for MDMA and methamphetamine is similar in that they both affect dopamine and serotonin neurotransmitter systems, increasing their concentration in the brain. However, MDMA primarily inhibits serotonin reuptake and stimulates serotonin release, while methamphetamine mostly inhibits dopamine reuptake and stimulates dopamine release.[14] While dopamine is known for its role in drug reward and addiction, serotonin is famous for its action in producing hallucinations.[15] For this reason, MDMA is classified as a hallucinogen and methamphetamine as a stimulant, although there is some overlap in pharmacological effects.

There are recent clinical studies reporting the use of MDMA as part of psychotherapy.[16] The treatment for psychiatric disorders is best accomplished using a combination of pharmacology and psychotherapy. Psychiatrists do this by prescribing an FDA-approved drug during cognitive or behavioral therapy.[17] However, MDMA is not an FDA-approved drug. MDMA is a schedule I controlled substance and clinical trials on the safety and efficacy of MDMA have not been done. Additionally, MDMA produces neurotoxicity in animal models as noted by destruction of serotonin-containing neurons.[18]

Benzylpiperazine (BZP) is a common chemical used in the manufacture of industrial chemicals and other drugs. BZP was designed as a legal alternative to Ecstasy (MDMA), branded with the street names of *Legal X* or *Legal E*. BZP was originally synthesized in 1944 by pharmaceutical manufacturers to test as an antiparasitic or antidepressant drug. BZP was not a good antiparasitic or antidepressant drug and never developed further.[19] Like MDMA, BZP is used during electronic dance parties (*raves*) and like MDMA, can cause life-threatening toxicity.[20] In an attempt to curb growing abuse, BZP was listed as a Schedule I controlled substance by DEA in 2004.

The Controlled Substances Act

After the heyday of hopped-up hippies and prescription pill-poppers in the 1960s, the Nixon administration and Congress responded to the growing drug abuse problem by introducing massive legislation to regulate legal and illegal drugs. The omnibus bill that became law was called the *Comprehensive Drug Abuse Prevention and Control Act* of 1970. The stated purpose of this act was *"to amend the Public Health Service Act and other laws to provide increased research, into, and prevention of, drug abuse and drug dependence; to provide for treatment and rehabilitation of drug abusers and drug dependent persons; and to strengthen existing law enforcement authority in the field of drug abuse."*[21] The *Comprehensive Drug Abuse Prevention and Control Act* of 1970 also funded the expansion of the Bureau of Narcotics and Dangerous Drugs (BNDD) in the Justice Department, increasing the Bureau mission and budget, and emerging as the renamed *Drug Enforcement Administration* (DEA) in 1973.[22] A section of this omnibus bill contains the *Controlled Substances Act* or CSA.

---

[13] Wardle MC, de Wit H (2014) MDMA alters emotional processing and facilitates positive social interaction. Psychopharmacology (Berl). 231:4219–4229. Indeed, MDMA produces spontaneous ejaculation in male rats: Bilsky EJ et al (1991) MDMA produces a conditioned place preference and elicits ejaculation in mare rats: a modulatory role for the endogenous opioids. Pharm. Biochem. Behav. 40:443–447.

[14] Stough C et al. (2011) The acute effects of 3,4-methylenedioxymethamphetamine and d-methamphetamine on human cognitive functioning. Psychopharmacology (Berl). 220:799–807.

[15] For example, LSD is a serotonergic receptor agonist and an extremely potent hallucinogen.

[16] MDMA has been used in posttraumatic stress disorder (PTSD) patients and in autistic adults. See Mithoefer MC et al. (2011) The safety and efficacy of {+/−}3,4-methylenedioxymethamphetamine-assisted psychotherapy in subjects with chronic, treatment-resistant posttraumatic stress disorder: the first randomized controlled pilot study. J Psychopharmacol. 25:439–452; Danforth AL et al. (2016) MDMA-assisted therapy: A new treatment model for social anxiety in autistic adults. Prog Neuropsychopharmacol Biol Psychiatry 64:237–249. See also Chapter 18 *The Devil Made Me Do it* section on Psychedelic Drugs used in Psychiatry.

[17] For example, the anxious acrophobic who takes the benzodiazepine alprazolam (*Xanax*®) while undergoing exposure therapy by riding a glass-sided elevator with a therapist.

[18] Verrico CD et al. (2007) MDMA (Ecstasy) and human dopamine, norepinephrine, and serotonin transporters: implications for MDMA-induced neurotoxicity and treatment. Psychopharmacology (Berl) 189:489–503. Since depressive disorders are associated with decreased serotonin in the brain and MDMA is toxic to serotonergic neurons, today's *ravers* abusing MDMA may be tomorrow's depressives and suicides.

[19] Campbell H et al. (1973) Comparison of the effects of dexamphetamine and 1-benzylpiperazine in former addicts. Eur J Clin Pharmacol. 6:170–176; DEA (2007) Drugs and chemicals of concern: N-Benzylpiperazine. Office of Diversion Control, Drug Enforcement Administration, Dept. of Justice, USA.

[20] Gee P et al. (2010 Multiorgan failure from 1-benzylpiperazine ingestion--legal high or lethal high? Clin Toxicol (Phila). 48:230–233.

[21] Comprehensive Drug Abuse Prevention and Control Act of 1970, Pub. L. No. 91-513, 84 Stat. 1236 (Oct. 27, 1970).

[22] Spillane JF, McAllister WB (2003) Keeping the lid on: a century of drug regulation and control. Drug Alcohol Depend. 70:S5–12.

The CSA establishes US drug policy regulating the manufacture, importation, possession, use, and distribution of certain substances, called *controlled substances*. Both legal (e.g., morphine) and illegal drugs (heroin) are denoted as controlled substances. The CSA details a mechanism for emerging drugs of abuse to be controlled (added to the list or *scheduled*) or removed from the controlled substances list (*de-scheduled*). In general, the proceedings to add, delete, or change the schedule of a drug may be started by the DEA, the Department of Health and Human Services (HHS), or by petition from any interested party, like the manufacturer of a drug or a medical society or pharmacy association.[23] Substances are considered *scheduled* when they are listed in 21 USC § 812. Up-to-date and revised schedules are published in the Code of Federal Regulations, Part 1308 of Title 21, Food and Drugs. The current federal list of *Schedules of Controlled Substances* is available on the DEA site.[24]

Controlled Substances Analogue Enforcement Act

In the last few decades, Congress passed a number of new regulations to address the scourge of designer drugs hitting the streets. The *Analogue Enforcement Act of 1986* was enacted as *Subtitle E of the Anti-Drug Abuse Act of 1986* to include designer drugs (the analogues) as controlled substances. Under this law, a controlled substance *analogue* is defined as a substance if:

(i) *the chemical structure of which is substantially similar to the chemical structure of a controlled substance in schedule I or II;*

(ii) *which has a stimulant, depressant, or hallucinogenic effect on the central nervous system that is substantially similar to or greater than the stimulant, depressant, or hallucinogenic effect on the central nervous system of a controlled substance in schedule I or II; or*

(iii) *with respect to a particular person, which such person represents or intends to have a stimulant, depressant, or hallucinogenic effect on the central nervous system that is substantially similar to or greater than the stimulant, depressant, or hallucinogenic effect on the central nervous system of a controlled substance in schedule I or II.*[25]

The *Analogue Enforcement Act* swiftly classified designer drugs that differed only slightly from a Schedule I or II controlled substance as *controlled substances analogues* which inherited the scheduling of the related listed drug. This act provides a stopgap measure when new designer drugs are first seized by the DEA in that they can be quickly determined to be controlled substances analogues, therefore illegal, and criminals can be prosecuted. Eventually, the DEA moves to schedule the new analogue drugs so that they are listed and become controlled substances. For example, when synthetic cannabinoids were first introduced in the late 1980s, they were already illegal under the *Analogue Enforcement Act*. After synthetic cannabinoids were identified, they were placed into Schedule I listing of the CSA by DEA action. Now synthetic cannabinoids are illegal to manufacture, possess, and distribute directly under the CSA.

Scheduling of Controlled Substances

The scheduling of controlled substances has wide-reaching ramifications affecting the federal and state mandatory minimum sentencing guidelines used for criminal punishment (see later). In general, possession or trafficking of Schedule I drugs elicit more draconian prison sentences than Schedule V drugs. The mandatory minimum drug sentencing guidelines set by the United States Sentencing Commission for federal courts and similar drug sentencing laws in the states led to the unbridled growth of incarcerated persons. Nonviolent drug offenses carry mandatory life sentences for some defendants who had prior drug-related convictions, even though they were caught with relatively minor quantities of certain Schedule I or II controlled substances.[26]

The CSA mandates the scheduling of licit and illicit drugs (controlled substances) according to their addictive potential, safety, and medical use.[27] There are five schedules, labeled in Roman numerals from I to V, with Schedule I drugs have high abuse potential and no approved medical use like heroin, LSD, and marijuana.[28] Schedule II drugs have relatively less

---

[23] Controlled Substances Act, from the DEA website at: *www.dea.gov/druginfo/csa.shtml.*

[24] *www.deadiversion.usdoj.gov/schedules/#list.*

[25] 21 U.S.C. §802(32)(A).

[26] See the Families Against Mandatory Minimums (FAMM) website at *famm.org.* Crack cocaine is notorious for demanding severe mandatory minimum sentences compared to powder cocaine, with an initial 100-1 and later an 18-1 sentencing ratio compared to cocaine powder. See upcoming text for further details.

[27] Spillan JF (2004) Debating the Controlled Substances Act. Drug Alcohol Depend. 76:17–29.

[28] We will get to the special case of marijuana scheduling in Chapter 16 *Reefer Madness.*

TABLE 11.1 Scheduling of controlled substances

Controlled substances			
Schedule	Symbol	Characteristics	Examples
I (C I)	C	High abuse potential. May lead to severe dependence. NO ACCEPTED MEDICAL USE.	Heroin Marijuana Peyote
II (C II)	C	High abuse potential. May lead to severe dependence.	Cocaine Morphine Codeine Methadone Amphetamine
III (C III)	C	Abuse potential less than Schedules I and II. May lead to moderate dependence.	Drugs that are combinations of opiate and nonnarcotic drugs, such as hydrocodone and acetaminophen (VICODIN)
IV (C IV)	C	Moderate abuse potential. May lead to limited dependence.	Alprazolam (XANAX) Zolpidem (AMBIEN) Phenobarbital (LUMINAL) Modafinil (PROVIGIL)
V (C V)	C	Small abuse potential. May lead to limited dependence.	Cough medications with codeine, certain antidiarrheals.

(From Brenner, G. M., & Stevens, C. W. (2018). Brenner and Stevens' pharmacology (5th ed.). Philadelphia, PA: Elsevier.)

abuse potential and medical use; morphine and oxycodone come to mind. Likewise down to the lowest level of Schedule V drugs.[29] Table 11.1 illustrates the Schedules of Controlled Substances and example drugs for each schedule.[30]

Congress established 8 criteria that determine the particular Schedule for a drug in question.[31] The statutes list these criteria for scheduling a controlled substance as follows:

(1) Its actual or relative potential for abuse.
(2) Scientific evidence of its pharmacological effect, if known.
(3) The state of current scientific knowledge regarding the drug or other substance.
(4) Its history and current pattern of abuse.
(5) The scope, duration, and significance of abuse.
(6) What, it any, risk there is to the public health.
(7) Its psychic or physiological dependence liability.
(8) Whether the substance is an immediate precursor of a substance already controlled under this title

The scheduling of drugs according to these criteria of abuse likelihood, safety, and medical utility also correlates with the severity of drug sentences for the unlawful possession, distribution, and manufacture of controlled substances. As per usual, State legislatures passed their own *Controlled Substances Acts*, following the scheduling model and controlled substances list of the federal CSA. For the most part, the State's Controlled Substances lists are consistent with the Federal

---

[29] Courtwright DT (2004) The Controlled Substances Act: how a "big tent" reform became a punitive drug law. Drug Alcohol Depend. 76:9–15.

[30] Adapted from Table 4.2 in Brenner GM, Stevens CW (2018) Brenner and Stevens' Pharmacology, 5th Edition. Elsevier, Philadelphia, PA, USA.

[31] According to Congress. While drugs in Schedules II–V are similar to each other in structure or function, the cast of characters that make up Schedule I drugs vary greatly in actual abuse patterns, frequency of use, and harm to user and society. For example, the Schedule I drugs LSD, mescaline, peyote, MDMA (ecstasy), heroin, and marijuana have very different pharmacological actions and impact on the individual and society.

listing.[32] As we see in Chapter 16 *Reefer Madness* in the context of medical marijuana, the scheduling of a controlled substance is key to whether this drug can be marketed and used clinically as medicine, or if the weedy drug is forever banished to passing between unknown hands in dark alleys.

The CSA also enacted minimum mandatory drug sentencing for select drugs that were of concern in 1970 for two levels of drug amounts. For example, possession with intent to distribute 1 kg or more of a mixture or substance containing a detectable amount of heroin carries a mandatory prison sentence of 10 years to life.[33] A drug offense based on 100 g of heroin (or a detectable amount of heroin within a substance weighing 100 g) carries a mandatory sentence of not less than 5 years and not more than 40 years. However, for drugs not specifically listed in the CSA and for amounts lower than either threshold stated in the CSA, drug sentencing was not consistent among the federal courts. A disparity of sentencing for other federal crimes was noted as well. This led to the *Sentencing Reform Act (SRA) of 1984* which established Federal Sentencing Guidelines including an elaborate scheme for drug offense sentencing, as seen next.

Federal Drug Sentencing Guidelines

The United States Sentencing Commission (USSC) was created with the passage of *Sentencing Reform Act of 1984* under the Reagan Administration.[34] Congress charged the USSC with enacting guidelines and sentencing policies for the federal courts. The specific purposes of the Guidelines promulgated by the Commission are to:

(1) incorporate the underlying purposes of sentencing (i.e., deterrence); (2) provide certainty and fairness in meeting the purposes of sentencing by avoiding unwanted sentencing disparity among offenders with similar characteristics who are convicted of similar conduct, while permitting sufficient judicial flexibility to consider relevant aggravating and mitigating factors; and (3) reflect, to the extent practicable, advancement in the knowledge of human behavior as it relates to the criminal justice process.[35]

As early as 1991, prison officials reported problems with the new sentencing guidelines.[36] This prescient paper, authored by the Federal Bureau of Prisons, warned over two decades ago that the new sentencing guidelines will lead to a *burgeoning inmate population*. In their study, the average sentence imposed for a drug offense more than doubled from 23 months to 58 months with the new federal guidelines. In just three years since the drug sentencing guidelines were promulgated, the number of federal inmates incarcerated for drug offenses doubled from 14,556 inmates in 1988 to 27,908 in 1991. At the beginning of 2018, there were 183,493 federal inmates, with 49.1% of them classified as drug offenders.[37] Of the drug offenders, 72.3% of them were convicted of a drug offense carrying a mandatory minimum sentence. In 1976 federal prisons cost the public about $184 million to run and maintain for a year; in 2016 federal prisons cost over $6.75 billion a year. Mandatory minimum sentencing of nonviolent drug offenders is a major cause of the current over-incarceration of Americans and a tremendous drain on public monies and services.[38]

We saw in the previous chapter that drug intoxication is a poor defense for most crimes. However, Congress directed the USSC to draft the sentencing guidelines with the issue of drug dependence as a factor to be considered in mitigating the sentencing of criminals.[39] Seemingly deaf to the will of Congress, the USSC went out of its way to make sure that the issue of drug dependence was specifically *excluded*. As stated "*drug dependence or alcohol abuse is not a reason for imposing a*

---

[32] A few interesting differences may be seen. For example, Oklahoma legislature scheduled the muscle relaxant carisoprodol (Soma®) as a controlled substance before the feds did. This was due to high levels of abuse of this drug in the state. See "Soma – Fast Facts" produced by the National Drug Intelligence Center which was a component of the DOJ back in 2004: *www.justice.gov/archive/ndic/pubs10/10913/10913p.pdf.*

[33] Title 21 Controlled Substances Act, USC, SUBCHAPTER I—CONTROL AND ENFORCEMENT, Part D—Offenses and Penalties, §841. Prohibited acts A.

[34] Kannenberg CC (2008) From Booker to Gall: The evolution of the reasonableness doctrine as applied to white-collar criminals and sentencing variances. J Corp Law 34: 349–358.

[35] Available on the USSC website at: *www.ussc.gov.*

[36] Luttrell MH (1991) The impact of the Sentencing Reform Act on prison management. Fed. Probation 55:54–57.

[37] Doyle C (2018) Mandatory Minimum Sentencing of Federal Drug Offenses in Short. Congressional Research Service, *www.crs.gov.*

[38] Not to mention the impact on families, communities, and society. The United States has 5% of world's population but incarcerates 25% of the world's prisoners. See Cassidy RM (2014) (Ad)ministering justice: a prosecutor's ethical duty to support sentencing reform. Loyola Univ Chicago Law J. 45:101–145.

[39] 28 U.S. Code § 994 - Duties of the Commission, *(d) The Commission in establishing categories of defendants for use in the guidelines and policy statements governing the imposition of sentences of probation, a fine, or imprisonment, governing the imposition of other authorized sanctions, governing the size of a fine or the length of a term of probation, imprisonment, or supervised release, and governing the conditions of probation, supervised release, or imprisonment, shall consider whether the following matters, among others, with respect to a defendant, have any relevance to the nature, extent, place of service, or other incidents of an appropriate sentence, and shall take them into account only to the extent that they do have relevance— (1) age; (2) education; (3) vocational skills; (4) mental and emotional condition to the extent that such condition mitigates the defendant's culpability or to the extent that such condition is otherwise plainly relevant; (5) physical condition, **including drug dependence**; and others.* [bold added]

sentence below the guidelines."[40] The USSC Guidelines also made sure that in validating sentencing departures for nonviolent crimes in those with diminished capacity, drug use was specifically excluded. To wit, departures are not warranted if "*resulting from the voluntary use of drugs or other intoxicants.*"[41] The idea promulgated by the USSC is that someone with a drug dependence or drug addiction *voluntarily* uses drugs. All medical and pharmacological studies show that this view of drug dependence is extremely anachronistic in light of the brain changes and chronic disease state imposed by chronic drug use. There is no such thing as pure voluntary drug use in a person with drug dependence or drug addiction; it is a compulsion like a morning cup of coffee to the rest of us but infinitely greater.

Drug offender sentencing guidelines

The USSC sets sentencing levels for all criminal offenses, but it is the *USSC Sentencing Guidelines Chapter 2, Part D—Offenses Involving Drugs and Narco-Terrorism* that is of most interest to the drug expert. In general, the USSC determines drug offender sentences by consideration of the following six qualifiers: (1) chemical structure, (2) pharmacological effects, (3) legislative and scheduling history, (4) potential for addiction and abuse, (5) the patterns of abuse and harms associated with their abuse, and (6) the patterns of trafficking and harms associated with their trafficking.[42] In this way, possession and trafficking of drugs that are more addicting and more harmful to users, and drugs that exert a greater cost to society, are punished more severely. To account for these differences in harmfulness of drugs, the USSC decided to compare all controlled substances to marijuana.[43] Elaborate *Drug Equivalency Tables* were created correlating 1 g of drug to an equivalent amount of marijuana in grams.[44] Using marijuana equivalents are as base unit remained in the guidelines until 2018, when the "*of marijuana*" was removed and marijuana equivalents were given the new term of "*Converted Drug Weight*" (see excerpt of table in Fig. 11.1).

The rational and justification behind the marijuana equivalents or new converted drug weights (CDW) in the renamed but unchanged drug conversion tables are not readily apparent nor explained by the USSC.[45] There does not seem to be any comprehensible relationship between single gram amounts of the drugs on the left of the table and the CDW values on the

(D) Drug ~~Equivalency~~ Conversion Tables.—	
COCAINE AND OTHER SCHEDULE I AND II STIMULANTS (AND THEIR IMMEDIATE PRECURSORS)*	CONVERTED DRUG WEIGHT
1 gm of Cocaine =	200 gm ~~of marihuann~~
1 gm of N-Ethylamphetamine =	80 gm ~~of marihuann~~
1 gm of Fenethylline =	40 gm ~~of marihuann~~
1 gm of Amphetamine =	2 kg ~~of marihuann~~
1 gm of Amphetamine (Actual) =	20 kg ~~of marihuann~~
1 gm of Methamphetamine =	2 kg ~~of marihuann~~
1 gm of Methamphetamine (Actual) =	20 kg ~~of marihuann~~
1 gm of "Ice" =	20 kg ~~of marihuann~~
1 gm of Khat =	.01 gm ~~of marihuann~~
1 gm of 4-Methylaminorex ("Euphoria") =	100 gm ~~of marihuann~~
1 gm of Methylphenidate (Ritalin) =	100 gm ~~of marihuann~~
1 gm of Phenmetrazine =	80 gm ~~of marihuann~~
1 gm Phenylacetone/P_2P (when possessed for the purpose of manufacturing methamphetamine) =	416 gm ~~of marihuann~~
1 gm Phenylacetone/P_2P (in any other case) =	75 gm ~~of marihuann~~
1 gm Cocaine Base ("Crack") =	3,571 gm ~~of marihuann~~
1 gm of Aminorex =	100 gm ~~of marihuann~~
1 gm of N-N-Dimethylamphetamine =	40 gm ~~of marihuann~~
1 gm of N-Benzylpiperazine =	100 gm ~~of marihuann~~

FIG. 11.1 Editing changes for the new Drug Conversion Tables in the USSC Sentencing Guidelines. (*From* Amendments to the USSC Sentencing Guidelines, *April 30, 2018.*)

---

[40] U.S.S.G. § 5H1.4, p.s.

[41] U.S.S.G. § 5K2.13, p.s.

[42] USSC Request for Public Comment: Drugs from the August 17, 2017 meeting. Available at the USSC website: *www.ussc.gov/sites/default/files/pdf/amendment-process/reader-friendly-amendments/20170817_prelim_IFC.pdf.*

[43] In the USSC guidelines and other federal documents, marijuana is spelled archaically (still) as marihuana.

[44] Drug Conversion Tables are found in USSC §2D1.1 page 158 of the latest version (2018) of the guidelines.

[45] I am still in correspondence with the USSC over this matter. Unfortunately, the USSC is exempt from FOIA and other Sunshine Act regulations.

```
• At least 10 G but less than 20 G of Heroin;                              Level 14
• At least 50 G but less than 100 G of Cocaine;
• At least 2.8 G but less than 5.6 G of Cocaine Base;
• At least 10 G but less than 20 G of PCP, or
        at least 1 G but less than 2 G of PCP (actual);
• At least 5 G but less than 10 G of Methamphetamine, or
        at least 500 MG but less than 1 G of Methamphetamine (actual), or
        at least 500 MG but less than 1 G of "Ice";
• At least 5 G but less than 10 G of Amphetamine, or
        at least 500 MG but less than 1 G of Amphetamine (actual);
• At least 100 MG but less than 200 MG of LSD;
• At least 4 G but less than 8 G of Fentanyl (N-phenyl-N-[1-(2-phenylethyl)-4-piperidinyl]
        Propanamide);
• At least 1 G but less than 2 G of Fentanyl Analogue;
• At least 10 KG but less than 20 KG of Marihuana;
• At least 2 KG but less than 5 KG of Hashish;
• At least 200 G but less than 500 G of Hashish Oil;
• At least 10,000 but less than 20,000 units of Ketamine;
• At least 10,000 but less than 20,000 units of Schedule I or II Depressants;
• At least 10,000 but less than 20,000 units of Schedule III substances (except Ketamine);
• At least 625 but less than 1,250 units of Flunitrazepam;
• At least 10 KG but less than 20 KG of Converted Drug Weight.
```

FIG. 11.2   USSC Drug Quantity Table, excerpt for Offense Level 14 showing PCP (actual), methamphetamine (actual) and amphetamine (actual). *(See text for further details. USSC Sentencing Guidelines, November 2018.)*

right. There are certainly no pharmacological principles at play discernable by this drug expert. For example, how does 1 g of cocaine (powder) equal to 200 g of marijuana or CDW (see first row of table)? And why does 1 g of crack cocaine equal 3571 g of marijuana or CDW?[46] Indeed the USSC includes a statement that *precludes* a basis in pharmacology stating: "*Because of the statutory equivalences, the ratios in the Drug Conversion Tables do not necessarily reflect dosages based on pharmacological equivalents.*"[47]

Besides the irrational assignment of drug equivalency using the drug conversion tables, the USSC distinguishes between a "drug" and a "drug (actual)" for some controlled substances.[48] For example, in the 4th row of the previous table, 1 g of amphetamine is equal to 2 kg of marijuana or CDW. In the 5th row, 1 g of amphetamine (actual) is equal to 20 kg of marijuana or CDW. Actual weights are used also for methamphetamine and PCP, but not most other drugs in the table. Once the amount of controlled substance or actual amount of controlled substance is determined, prosecutors look at the Drug Quantity Table in the USSC sentencing guidelines to determine the offense level for that amount of drug. The offense levels run from 38 (highest) to 6 (lowest) depending on the amount and type of controlled substance. The chart for offense level 14 is shown as follows (Fig. 11.2).

USSC explains what the "drug (actual)" listing means. *"The terms "PCP (actual)," "Amphetamine (actual)," and "Methamphetamine (actual)" refer to the weight of the controlled substance, itself, contained in the mixture or substance. For example, a mixture weighing 10 g containing PCP at 50% purity contains 5 g of PCP (actual). In the case of a mixture or substance containing PCP, amphetamine, or methamphetamine, use the offense level determined by the entire weight of the mixture or substance, or the offense level determined by the weight of the PCP (actual), amphetamine (actual), or methamphetamine (actual), whichever is greater."*[49] The addition of the "actual" amount of a controlled substance to be used as a basis of drug sentencing is a step in the right direction, although the USSC still maintains the opposite that the amount of the controlled substance used for sentencing is the total amount of a mixture that the controlled substance may only be a small part of. It is illogical and irrational for the USSC to maintain both methods of determining controlled substances amounts in the guidelines. Commonsense application of the *USSC Sentencing Guidelines* would demand that the amount of the controlled substance used for sentencing be limited to the actual quantity of the controlled substance or analogue and not

---

[46] This ratio of about 18 between powder cocaine and crack cocaine (3571/200=17.86) is somewhat understandable as the *Fair Sentencing Act of 2010* reduced the sentencing ratio of the two forms of cocaine from 100 to 18. The previous 100-fold sentencing ratio was roundly accepted to be racially biased to crack cocaine users versus powder cocaine users. The *First Step Act* passed in December 2018 made the 18-fold sentencing ratio retroactive to inmates sentenced prior to the *Fair Sentencing Act*.

[47] Note after USSC §2D1.1 Sec 8.B in the 2018 guidelines.

[48] Thanks to Tara Valouch, Director of Forensic Laboratory for the Tulsa Police Department, for ongoing discussions about this issue and other enlightening discussion on forensic drug analysis.

[49] Notes to Drug Quantity Table in USSC §2D1.1, 2018 sentencing guidelines.

include the quantity of nonregulated carrier plant substance, cutting agents, or other fillers.[50] In any event, the seized controlled substance is first changed to equivalent amount of marijuana or CDW using the Drug Conversion Table (Fig. 11.1), then the base level of offense found by using the Drug Quantity Table (Fig. 11.2). The final step is using the offense level to determine the prison sentence by using the Sentencing Table (not shown, in the USSC guidelines).

The *Sentencing Reform Act of 1984* created mandatory minimum sentences for drug offenses, essentially altering the judge's role from a sentencing expert to a mechanistic tabulator of drug amounts and offense levels.[51] The USSC guidelines determined the sentence range and judges could only sentence within that narrow range. Prison populations swelled under the drug sentencing guidelines and mandatory sentencing continued until 2005 with the *United States v. Booker* opinion by SCOTUS. *Booker* was found guilty by a jury of possessing 92 g of crack cocaine which translated into a guideline of maximum of 10 years. However, the federal district judge sentenced *Booker* to 30 years on additional facts presented at the sentencing hearing. Booker rightly maintained that sentencing guidelines violated the Sixth Amendment because the judge was able to base his sentence on additional facts in the absence of a jury. On appeal by the government to SCOTUS, the Justices ruled 5–4 in favor of *Booker* and their remedy was to simply change the language in the *Sentencing Reform Act* from "mandatory" sentencing to "advisory" guidelines. The case was remanded back to the district court and *Booker* received the same 30-year sentence now that the judge wasn't under mandatory sentencing. Although the ability of the trial judge to deviate downward as well as upward from the sentencing guidelines exists after *Booker*, data from the USSC shows that average sentences for drug offenses increased after *Booker*.[52]

The Business of Being a Drug Expert

A scientist working as a litigation consultant, if successful, will be pleasantly surprised at the business aspects of this challenging moonlighting career. First of all, remuneration for services rendered can be substantial, reaching more than six figures a year in hard-working drug experts. The drug expert or pharmacologist charging a modest $150 to $300 per hour for research or writing litigation reports, and $300 to $500 per hour for deposition or trial testimony will be amazed at the total invoice when the case is closed. The average one-drug case may run about $5000 with more complicated cases earning the drug expert $8000 or more when out-of-town trial testimony is also given. The windfall in extra income[53] will be useful in home improvement projects, international travel adventures, the constant payments and "loans" to offspring, or a substantial contribution to retirement accounts.[54]

Record-keeping is essential in tracking extra income that won't show up on your university or medical school's W-2 form in late January. As previously stated, it is recommended that a spreadsheet be maintained with each row listing in separate columns the hiring attorney with firm address and contact information, date when the letter of engagement was signed, a brief description of case, title of litigation report, date of deposition, date of court testimony, date invoice sent, date invoice paid, and the amount received in last column. This Master List of Cases is extremely useful when preparing the last four years of testimony document for federal courts and to prepare a separate document with an annual listing. This latter document might be titled *Table of Invoices Paid for Year 2019* or such and show the total annual income for tax purposes. This ongoing yearly document also can have a place to indicate whether a 1099-MISC form was received from the law firm or insurance company.[55] Such organization will be appreciated at tax time.

Consulting income can be reported as regular income or through a business set up as a limited partnership, limited liability corporation (LLC), or various other means. This may provide some tax advantages that outweighs the cost (an attorney may be needed) of creating such an entity in highly successful drug experts. Of course, such tax advice is specific to each expert's financial situation and desires.[56]

---

[50] There is no undue burden for the Government to determine the purity of seized samples from which the actual amount of controlled substances can be determined. The level of purity of seized samples is reported for all drug classes on the DEA website and quantifying the actual controlled substance amount is the only method that can reliably lead to fair sentencing for all offenders.

[51] Bilsborrow JJ (2007) Sentencing acquitted conduct to the post-*Booker* dustbin. William Mary Law Rev. 49:289–334.

[52] USSC (2012) Report on the Continuing Impact of *United States v. Booker* on Federal Sentencing.

[53] *Extra income* used as the assumption throughout the book is that the drug expert has a main, full-time Pharmacologist job.

[54] The expert will need to make quarterly tax payments to both the feds and in most states as taxes are not taken out when the drug expert is paid. If not, the expert will be hit with a huge tax bill come the following April. Additionally, many law firms will be contacting the expert in December to obtain a copy of their W-9 form to process their payments for tax purposes.

[55] Many times the check will be sent directly from an insurance company to the drug expert without reference to the attorney or case. Some will be kind enough to include a copy of the invoice with the check but in a few cases the drug expert needs to figure out who the payment is from by matching invoices recently sent.

[56] The author does not imply any knowledge of tax or business law so *caveat emptor* hereby applies to the reader.

[Narrative continued]

The drug expert for Mr. Nepali confirmed that the active ingredient in Spice and K2 products he sold was XLR-11 which is a synthetic cannabinoid drug. However, the drug expert argued that the appropriate sentencing correlate would be a direct comparison of seized leafy material to the same amount of marijuana, not equating the whole packet weight directly to the same amount in kilograms of THC, the active ingredient in marijuana. The sentence for Mr. Nepali was reduced in accordance to the drug expert's findings.

In the second case, Dan Blazer was arrested under the Controlled Substances Analog (CSA) Act for selling benzylpiperazine (BZP), a designer drug used at raves and other get-togethers. Like most designer drugs, BZP is not listed in the Drug Quantity Table of the USSC Sentencing Guidelines. Because BZP is an unlisted drug, a determination of the closest analog of BZP on the controlled substances list needs to be made under the Controlled Substances Analog Act. Both methamphetamine and MDMA ("Ecstasy") are chemical analogs but have different pharmacological effects when taken. Under the USSC Sentencing Guidelines, possession and distribution of methamphetamine yield more severe sentences than possession and distribution of MDMA. The DEA maintained that BZP was an analogue of methamphetamine. Although preclinical and clinical studies were occasionally contradictory, the most basic pharmacological parameter of the mechanism of drug action, that of its binding properties, proved that BZP was most similar to MDMA and not methamphetamine. The drug expert argued this conclusion in federal court and waxed eloquently on the true nature of a drug. Sentencing was given according to the USSC Guideline tables for MDMA which resulted in a prison sentence reduced by 12 months.

Chapter 12

Where There's a Will, There's a Way: Cancer chemotherapy and probate

Anticancer Drugs and *Chemobrain*—Chronic Alcoholism and Neurotoxicity

Making a Will and Drug Use—Drug-Induced Diminished Capacity

Estimation of BAC From Alcohol Consumed

[Narrative]
Mrs. Alberta Robinson was a wealthy widow after the death of her husband, the CEO of Robinson Oil Company in Tulsa, Oklahoma. There were millions of dollars in the estate and Mrs. Robinson's natural heirs, a daughter and a son, were expected to each receive a large inheritance per stirpes.[1] After Mrs. Robinson died, they were shocked when their mother's young male caretaker was awarded one-third of the estate in a will that was changed two weeks before her death. In this civil suit, the plaintiffs argued that a last-minute change in the will by her mother was made because of the undue influence of the mother's caretaker. Additionally, the daughter and son challenged the will on grounds of testamentary capacity as their mother was a chronic alcoholic and underwent multiple rounds of chemotherapy that affected her brain function. The estate attorney hired by the parties contesting the will sought the services of a drug expert to determine the adverse effects, if any, of chronic alcohol use and anti-cancer drugs on the brain and mental function of the mother at the time the will was executed.

Anticancer Drugs and *Chemobrain*

The most common treatment after a cancer diagnosis is the use of chemotherapeutic agents (anticancer drugs) alongside or after surgery and radiation.[2] While the use of anticancer drugs is beneficial in a number of different types of cancers, the adverse effects of their use include peripheral and central neurotoxicity, the latter leading to a decrease in cognitive (mental) function. Neurotoxicity after anticancer drugs is noted in a large number of medical studies and there are numerous papers documenting cognitive decline in cancer patients. Cognitive dysfunction is manifest by severe memory deficit, attention deficit, and other problems, and occurs in up to 70% of cancer patients.[3] Moreover, only about half of affected patients show long-term improvement of this cognitive dysfunction.[4] The acute effects of chemotherapy causing cognitive dysfunction within weeks of receiving chemotherapy are common.[5] These acute adverse cognitive effects are so common that a term has circulated among cancer patients and their doctors naming it "*chemobrain*" or "*chemofog*".[6] Indeed, it is

---

[1] A legal term meaning equal share of the estate, from the Latin for "*by branch*," as in each branch of the offspring.

[2] Hutchinson AD et al. (2012) Objective and subjective cognitive impairment following chemotherapy for cancer: a systematic review. Cancer Treat Rev. 38:926–934.

[3] Ahles TA et al. (2002) Neuropsychologic impact of standard-dose systemic chemotherapy in long-term survivors of breast cancer and lymphoma. J Clin Oncol 20:485–493; Wefel JS et al. (2004) The cognitive sequelae of standard-dose adjuvant chemotherapy in women with breast carcinoma: results of a prospective, randomized, longitudinal trial. Cancer 100:2292–2299.

[4] Wefel JS et al. (2004) The cognitive sequelae of standard-dose adjuvant chemotherapy in women with breast carcinoma: results of a prospective, randomized, longitudinal trial. Cancer 100:2292–2299; Wefel JS, Schagen SB (2012) Chemotherapy-related cognitive dysfunction. Curr Neurol Neurosci Rep. 12:267–275.

[5] Ahles TA, Saykin AJ (2007) Candidate mechanisms for chemotherapy-induced cognitive changes. Nat Rev Cancer 7:192–201.

[6] Mehnert A et al. (2007) The association between neuropsychological impairment, self-perceived cognitive deficits, fatigue and health related quality of life in breast cancer survivors following standard adjuvant versus high-dose chemotherapy. Patient Educ Couns. 66:108–118.

The Drug Expert. https://doi.org/10.1016/B978-0-12-800048-9.00012-2

usually the neurotoxic adverse effects of chemotherapeutic agents that limits the dose of anticancer drugs or causes cessation of treatment.[7]

Functional brain imaging studies in cancer survivors who received chemotherapy for five to ten years show deficits in brain activity that correlate to their present cognitive dysfunction.[8] Although not generally appreciated by the oncology community or their cancer patients, cancer and the chemotherapeutic treatment of cancer is now considered a strong risk factor for long-term cognitive deficits and dementia.[9]

Neurotoxicity and cognitive dysfunction due to fluorouracil treatment (5-FU)

Fluorouracil (5-FU) is a common anticancer drug indicated for the treatment of colon, rectum, breast, stomach, and pancreatic cancers.[10] 5-FU works by inhibiting the synthesis of DNA in carcinoma (tumor) cells. Tumor cells take up 5-FU to a greater extent than normal cells and 5-FU has a greater effect on the tumor cells because they are undergoing more rapid growth (cell division) than normal cells.

Neurotoxic effects of fluorouracil after treatment of cancer patients were noted as early as 1964.[11] Some of the first studies noted that administration of fluorouracil caused central neurotoxicity in the form of cerebellar ataxia, a syndrome characterized by failure of muscular coordination and jerky movement.[12] Later it was shown that a single dose of fluorouracil produced somnolence and confusion which developed within four to 6 weeks and was slow to recover.[13] The administration of fluorouracil alone or in combination with other chemotherapeutic agents produced both acute and late phase cognitive dysfunction in breast cancer patients.[14] In this study, cognitive dysfunction was found most disrupted in the domains of memory and executive function. Executive function is a central control system that manages other cognitive processes including planning, initiating appropriate behavior and inhibiting inappropriate behavior, and attention to relevant information. Executive function is carried out by the front part of the brain in an area called the prefrontal cortex.[15]

Fluorouracil-induced central neurotoxicity has been reported to cause confusion, cognitive disturbances, and seizures due to *leukoencephalopathy* in cancer patients.[16] Leukoencephalopathy is a pathological state of the brain characterized by degeneration of the white matter tracts of the brain, leading to severe cognitive dysfunction. Fluorouracil treatment was shown to cause leukoencephalopathy in breast cancer patients,[17] esophageal cancer patients,[18] and in colorectal cancer patients.[19]

Preclinical studies show that fluorouracil treatment causes brain cell death and depresses neuronal cell proliferation in the brain.[20] Fluorouracil causes both acute brain damage and delayed damage due to demyelination pathology.[21] Fluorouracil chemotherapy interrupts spatial working memory and learning in animal models.[22]

[7] Sioka C, Kyritsis AP (2009) Central and peripheral nervous system toxicity of common chemotherapeutic agents. Cancer Chemother Pharmacol. 63:761–767.

[8] Dietrich J et al. (2008) Clinical patterns and biological correlates of cognitive dysfunction associated with cancer therapy. Oncologist 13:1285–1295.

[9] Heflin LH et al. (2005) Cancer as a risk factor for long-term cognitive deficits and dementia. J Natl Cancer Inst. 97:854–856; Roe CM et al. (2005) Alzheimer disease and cancer. Neurology 64:895–898; Vardy J, Tannock I. (2007) Cognitive function after chemotherapy in adults with solid tumours. Crit Rev Oncol Hematol. 63:183-202; Wefel JS, Meyers CA (2005) Cancer as a risk factor for dementia: A house built on shifting sand. J Natl Cancer Inst. 97:788–789.

[10] *Fluorouracil Prescribing Information*, from Sagent Pharmaceuticals, Schaumburg, IL, USA.

[11] Moertel CG et al. (1964) Cerebellar ataxia associated with fluorinated pyrimidine therapy. Cancer Chemother Rep. 41:15–18.

[12] Greenwald ES. (1976) Letter: Organic mental changes with fluorouracil therapy. JAMA. 235:248-249; Weiss HD et al. (1974) Neurotoxicity of commonly used antineoplastic agents. N Engl J Med. 291:75–81.

[13] Bagley CM (1975) Single intravenous doses of 5-fluorouracil: A phase I study. Proc Am Assn Cancer Res. 16:12.

[14] Wefel JS et al. (2010) Acute and late onset cognitive dysfunction associated with chemotherapy in women with breast cancer. Cancer. 116:3348–3356.

[15] Ahles TA et al. (2002) Neuropsychologic impact of standard-dose systemic chemotherapy in long-term survivors of breast cancer and lymphoma. J Clin Oncol 20:485–493.

[16] Cheung WY et al. (2008) The confused cancer patient: a case of 5-fluorouracil-induced encephalopathy. Curr Oncol. 15:234-236; Pirzada NA et al. (2000) Fluorouracil-induced neurotoxicity. Ann Pharmacother. 34:35-38; Yeh KH, Cheng AL (1997) High-dose 5-fluorouracil infusional therapy is associated with hyper-ammonaemia, lactic acidosis and encephalopathy. Br J Cancer 75:464–465.

[17] Choi S-M et al. (2001) 5-Fluorouracil-induced leukoencephalopathy in patients with breast cancer. J Korean Med Sci. 16:328–34.

[18] Akitake R et al. (2011) Early detection of 5-FU-induced acute leukoencephalopathy on diffusion-weighted MRI. Jpn J Clin Oncol 41:121–124.

[19] Kim Y-A et al. (2006) Intermediate dose 5-fluorouracil-induced encephalopathy. Jpn J Clin Oncol. 36:55–59.

[20] Wigmore PM et al. (2010) Effects of 5-FU. Adv Exp Med Biol. 678:157–64.

[21] Han R et al. (2008) Systemic 5-fluorouracil treatment causes a syndrome of delayed myelin destruction in the central nervous system. J Biol. 7:12.

[22] Foley JJ et al. (2008) Effects of chemotherapeutic agents 5-fluorouracil and methotrexate alone and combined in a mouse model of learning and memory. Psychopharma-cology (Berl). 199:527–538; Mustafa S et al. (2008) 5-Fluorouracil chemotherapy affects spatial working memory and new-born neurons in the adult rat hippocampus. Eur J Neurosci. 28:323–330; Winocur G et al. (2006) The effects of the anti-cancer drugs, methotrexate and 5-fluorouracil, on cognitive function in mice. Pharmacol Biochem Behav. 85:66–75.

Neurotoxicity and cognitive dysfunction due to oxaliplatin

Oxaliplatin (Eloxatin®) is a platinum-based anticancer drug used with 5-FU in the treatment of colorectal cancer.[23] Oxaliplatin has a well-known neurotoxic effect at treatment doses that is described as peripheral neurotoxicity or peripheral neuropathy.[24] Oxaliplatin produces both acute and chronic peripheral nerve damage.[25] This chemotherapeutic neurotoxicity is characterized by a symmetrical distal sensory neuropathy ("stocking-glove" pattern) that is gradual in onset and worsens with repeated cycles of treatment.[26]

In preclinical studies, oxaliplatin alone impairs learning and memory in animal models.[27] This cognitive impairment of oxaliplatin is greater when given with fluorouracil.[28] The pattern of the cognitive deficits observed is consistent with brain damage in the regions associated with memory and executive function. In pancreatic cancer patients, one large study showed that all the quality of life measures improved except cognitive function with the addition of oxaliplatin to a fluorouracil-based treatment.[29] As pointed out by preclinical studies and a recent review, the common mechanism of producing cognitive dysfunction by all cytotoxic chemotherapeutic agents including oxaliplatin is the destruction of newly forming brain cells and the glial cells that support them.[30]

Neurotoxicity and cognitive dysfunction due to bevacizumab

Unlike fluorouracil and oxaliplatin, bevacizumab (Avastin®) is not a cytotoxic ("cell-killing") anticancer drug but rather inhibits the formation of new blood vessels to support the tumor. Bevacizumab is indicated for treatment of metastatic colorectal cancer.[31] In clinical trials, the most significant adverse effect of bevacizumab was life threatening and fatal bleeding, primarily from the lungs.[32] Monoclonal antibody drugs, like bevacizumab, can enter the brain capillaries where they can exert their beneficial and neurotoxic effects.[33]

Like 5-FU, neurotoxicity and cognitive dysfunction due to leukoencephalopathy with bevacizumab treatment of cancer patients is documented in the medical literature. In a patient treated for colorectal cancer, bevacizumab was considered the causative agent for *reversible posterior leukoencephalopathy syndrome* (RPLS) which was diagnosed by radiographic imaging.[34] This patient developed global aphasia (severe impairment of both comprehension and expression of language, and mutism), bouts of confusion, and agitation. In a patient being treated for renal carcinoma, bevacizumab was shown to cause reversible posterior leukoencephalopathy syndrome (RPLS) and experienced seizures and cortical blindness.[35] An additional patient with rectal cancer treated with bevacizumab developed reversible posterior leukoencephalopathy syndrome (RPLS) that led to loss of vision and confusion.[36] In response to these clinical cases, Genentech, the manufacturers

[23] *Eloxatin® Prescribing Information*, Sanofi-Aventis, USA.

[24] Cersosimo RJ (2005) Oxaliplatin-associated neuropathy: a review. Ann Pharmacother. 39:128–135; Hartmann JT, Lipp HP (2003) Toxicity of platinum compounds. Expert Opin Pharmacother. 4:889–901; Markman M (2003) Toxicities of the platinum antineoplastic agents. Expert Opin Drug Saf. 2:597–607; Ocean AJ, Vahdat LT (2004) Chemotherapy-induced peripheral neuropathy: pathogenesis and emerging therapies. Support Care Cancer 12:619–625; Pasetto LM et al. (2006) Oxaliplatin related neurotoxicity: how and why? Crit Rev Oncol Hematol. 59:159–168.

[25] Argyriou AA et al. (2008) A review on oxaliplatin-induced peripheral nerve damage. Cancer Treat Rev. 34:368–377.

[26] Kidwell KM et al. (2012) Long-term neurotoxicity effects of oxaliplatin added to fluorouracil and leucovorin as adjuvant therapy for colon cancer: results from National Surgical Adjuvant Breast and Bowel Project trials C-07 and LTS-01. Cancer 118:5614–5622; Raymond E et al. (1998) Oxaliplatin: A review of preclinical and clinical studies. Ann Oncology 9:1053–1071.

[27] Fardell JE et al. (2012) Cognitive impairments caused by oxaliplatin and 5-fluorouracil chemotherapy are ameliorated by physical activity. Psychopharmacology (Berl). 220:183–193; Sharpe MJ et al. (2012) The chemotherapy agent oxaliplatin impairs the renewal of fear to an extinguished conditioned stimulus in rats. Behav Brain Res. 227:295–299.

[28] Fardell JE et al. (2012) *Ibid.*

[29] Conroy T et al. (2005) Irinotecan plus oxaliplatin and leucovorin-modulated fluorouracil in advanced pancreatic cancer—a *Groupe Tumeurs Digestives of the Fédération Nationale des Centres de Lutte Contre le Cancer* Study. J Clin Oncol. 23:1228–1236.

[30] Dietrich J et al. (2006) CNS progenitor cells and oligodendrocytes are targets of chemotherapeutic agents *in vitro* and *in vivo*. J Biol. 5:22; Dietrich J et al. (2008) Clinical patterns and biological correlates of cognitive dysfunction associated with cancer therapy. Oncologist 13:1285–1295.

[31] *Avastin® Prescribing Information*, Genentech, South San Francisco, CA, USA.

[32] Ferrara N et al. (2005) Bevacizumab (Avastin®), a humanized anti-VEGF monoclonal antibody for cancer therapy. Biochem Biophys Res Comm. 333:328–335.

[33] Paris-Robidas S et al. (2011) *In vivo* labeling of brain capillary endothelial cells after intravenous injection of monoclonal antibodies targeting the transferrin receptor. Mol Pharmacol. 80:32–39.

[34] Allen JA et al. (2006) Reversible posterior leukoencephalopathy syndrome after bevacizumab/FOLFIRI regimen for metastatic colon cancer. Arch Neurol. 63:1475–1478.

[35] Glusker P et al. (2006) Reversible posterior leukoencephalopathy syndrome and bevacizumab. N Engl J Med. 354:980–981.

[36] Ozcan C, Wong SJ, Hari P (2006) Reversible posterior leukoencephalopathy syndrome and bevacizumab. N Engl J Med. 354:981–982.

of bevacizumab (Avastin®), stated in a letter published in the New England Journal of Medicine that they would change the prescription label for bevacizumab.[37] The revised FDA label for bevacizumab now clearly states the risk of *reversible posterior leukoencephalopathy syndrome* (RPLS) with bevacizumab treatment.

Chronic Alcoholism and Neurotoxicity

To reiterate, alcohol is an insidious drug that is exceedingly more dangerous than commonly known. Alcohol's active drug is ethanol; the term alcohol is actually generic and refers to a class of chemicals called alcohols which includes ethanol, methanol (wood alcohol), and isopropyl alcohol (rubbing alcohol). However, as is the case in most writings, this book uses ethanol or alcohol interchangeably.

Alcohol is a drug that, while socially acceptable in moderation, is abused to a greater degree and exacts more detrimental costs on society than any other legal or illegal drug in the United States. In monetary terms, the total cost to society of excessive alcohol consumption was $249 billion in 2010 or about $2.05 per drink.[38] Alcohol consumption is a leading cause of premature death in the United States, with excessive drinking accounting for 1 in 10 deaths among working-age adults.[39] The widespread availability and cultural acceptance of alcohol masks the fact that alcohol is a neurotoxic drug with devastating effects on brain function and behavior. Alcoholism, now termed alcohol dependence, is a chronic medical disease and classified in psychiatric listings alongside other mental disorders such as schizophrenia and depression.

Alcohol's active ingredient is ethanol, a simple molecule that freely distributes throughout the body water, soaking every organ and crossing into the brain with impunity. The brain is literally "pickled" in a solution of alcohol in a chronic alcoholic and physical changes such as an enlargement of the spaces of the brain and decreases in brain density are observed.[40] At the cellular level, brain neurons atrophy and inflammation of the brain occurs.

Alcohol increases impulsivity due to decreased brain inhibition. Impulsivity is defined as *a predisposition toward rapid, unplanned reactions to internal or external stimuli with diminished regard to the negative consequences of these reactions to the impulsive individual or others*.[41] Much research has focused on the detrimental effects of alcohol use and alcohol-related behaviors by showing that alcohol increases impulsivity.[42] This increase in impulsivity has been shown by human experiments in the laboratory setting with alcohol use.[43] The degree of impulsivity was correlated with the amount of alcohol used.

Much of the effects of alcohol on brain function have concentrated on the area of the brain known as the prefrontal cortex. This part of the brain is responsible for *executive function* which has been defined as *higher-order mental abilities, such as attention, planning, organization, abstract reasoning, self-monitoring, and the ability to use external feedback to modulate future behavior*.[44] Using brain imaging, it was shown that chronic alcohol use was more detrimental to the prefrontal cortex than chronic cocaine use.[45] Acute alcohol consumption was also shown to disrupt executive function in the prefrontal cortex.[46]

Making a Will and Drug Use

Making a will and testament ensures that the inheritance of one's property and assets is distributed as desired upon death. In most cases, the will is carried out, as written, upon death. However, the contesting of wills in America occurs in 3 out of 10 probate proceedings.[47] The grounds for most cases in contesting a will are *undue influence*, followed next by *testamentary capacity* and *fraud*.

---

[37] Barron H (2006) Response to: Reversible posterior leukoencephalopathy syndrome and bevacizumab. N Engl J Med. 354:982.

[38] Sacks JJ et al. (2015) 2010 National and state costs of excessive alcohol consumption. Am J Prev Med. 49:e73–79.

[39] Stahre M et al. (2014) Contribution of excessive alcohol consumption to deaths and years of potential life lost in the United States. Prev Chronic Dis. 11:E109.

[40] Oscar-Berman M, Marinkovic K (2003) Alcoholism and the brain: an overview. Alcohol Res Health 27:125–133.

[41] Moeller FG et al. (2001) Psychiatric aspects of impulsivity. Am J Psychiatry 158:1783–1793; Potenza MN, de Wit H (2010) Control yourself: alcohol and impulsivity. Alcohol Clin Exp Res. 34:1303–1305.

[42] Lejuez CW et al. (2010) Behavioral and biological indicators of impulsivity in the development of alcohol use, problems, and disorders. Alcohol Clin Exp Res. 34:1334–1345.

[43] Mitchell JM et al. (2005) Impulsive responding in alcoholics. Alcohol Clin Exp Res. 29:2158–2169.

[44] Foster J et al. (1994) The cognitive neuropsychology of attention: A frontal lobe perspective. Cog Neuropsych. 11:133–147.

[45] Goldstein RZ et al. (2004) Severity of neuropsychological impairment in cocaine and alcohol addiction: association with metabolism in the prefrontal cortex. Neuropsychologia 42:1447–1458.

[46] Hoaken PN et al. (1998) Executive cognitive functions as mediators of alcohol-related aggression. Alcohol Alcohol. 33:47–54.

[47] With over a million will contests per year, even a 3% rate yields a large number of cases. Ryznar M, Devaux A (2013) *Au Revoir*, will contests: comparative lessons for preventing will contests. Nev. Law J. 14:1–24.

Testamentary capacity not only applies to making a will but also to the process or creation of other legally binding documents.[48] Such documents include deeds, contracts, powers of attorney, estate planning, wills, and testamentary gifts. The client making the will (the testator) must be of *sound mind* when making the will.[49] Contesting the will thrusts the witnesses that signed the will into the spotlight; they have direct eyewitness accounts of the testator's state of mind and behavior at the time of the will. Additional evidence of testamentary capacity, or lack thereof, comes from various medical experts (drug experts, for example), personal physicians, psychologists, and other forensic evidence that will be needed to buttress or refute statements from attesting witnesses. The drug expert or other lay or expert witness cannot testify whether the testator had the *legal capacity to execute a will* as that is a legal conclusion rather than a statement of fact.[50] The drug expert is not a lawyer and cannot make such an ultimate legal conclusion. The drug expert can, however, make statements of facts from studies showing that anticancer drugs cause brain dysfunction and chronic alcoholism causes neurotoxicity. Careful direct examination by the hiring attorney can bring out expert testimony that all but determines a legal conclusion in the minds(s) of the trier-of-fact.

The attorney should make sure that the client is not visibly under the influence of drugs or alcohol when executing a will. Obviously a client who reeks of alcohol should be ushered out with the thin promise of another appointment in a few days. Similarly, the aging, pony-tailed stoner reeking of marijuana will be an easy tell, and politely shown the door. Other cultural stereotypes are an opioid or heroin addict with unfocused eyes and incoherent chatter, and an agitated cocaine user or crack-head who is extremely hyper and rapidly talking with bad teeth. However, the acutely intoxicated clients are rare compared to the millions of clients who may cross the office threshold with drug-diminished capacity, and lack of testamentary capacity, from the chronic use of prescription and nonprescription drugs.[51]

First of all, testamentary capacity is predicated on the client knowing what a will is; that it is a set of instructions on how property should be disposed of after death. Secondly, the testator should generally be aware of assets that are to be disposed or dispersed of after death, such as property, bank accounts, and so on, as well as their personal items. Thirdly, the testator should show recognition of the natural heirs, such as a spouse or offspring, in deciding how to apportion the estate.[52]

Most states in the United States place the burden to prove testamentary incapacity on the person challenging or contesting the will. Usually that means the will is upheld as valid, if the question of testamentary capacity is too close to call. Likewise, the critical threshold for incapacity in executing a will in most states is a *preponderance of the evidence* (i.e., 51% or more likely) but some states set the threshold higher in that the challenger to the will must prove by *clear and convincing evidence* (75% or higher confidence) that the testator lacked mental capacity.[53] The bottom line is that contesting a will due to drug-induced lack of capacity or undue influence should include the testimony of a drug expert based on solid evidence of drug use by the testator in order to be successful.

Interestingly, the attorney does not have a legal obligation to assess his will-maker client for *testamentary capacity* or *undue influence* from drugs.[54] Drugs may even be involved in will contests due to *fraud*, insofar as drug use is rampant and those attempting fraud may also be influenced by drug use and addiction problems. Legal scholars have long recognized the impact of drugs on testamentary capacity.[55] As few people outside the medical profession understand and appreciate the impact of medications on mental impairment, medication as a threat to testamentary capacity is recognized as a "*latent legal problem*."[56] Flash-forward to the present society in which many of its citizens are under nearly constant drug influence and the legal issue of testamentary capacity does not appear so latent.

The previous sections of this chapter highlight the real-life example of cognitive dysfunction induced by anticancer drugs and chronic alcoholism. Trial testimony of the adverse effects of these drugs, along with supporting medical records, was strong evidence that a will was altered when the testator (person making the will) was more likely than not incapable of independently initiating or altering valid estate or will documents.

Although the day is not here yet, one can imagine someday that an attorney[57] might greet a client with a plastic cup for urine drug testing in their hand. Medical and pharmacy records would also be provided by the client. Or passing a

---

[48] Quinn MJ et al. (2010) Undue influence: definitions and applications. Final Report to the *Borchard Foundation Center on Law and Aging*. California Administrative Office of the Courts. At: *www.courts.ca.gov/documents/UndueInfluence.*

[49] Frolik LA, Radford MF (2006) "Sufficient" capacity: the contrasting capacity requirements for different documents. NAELA J. 2:303–323.

[50] Frolik LA, Radford MF (2006) *Ibid.*

[51] Illegal drugs and especially alcohol, too.

[52] Ferner RE (1997) Drugs and testamentary capacity. J Clin Forensic Med. 4:185–187.

[53] Vars FE (2013) Uncertain testamentary capacity. J Forensic Leg Med. 20:1098.

[54] Champine P (2006) Expertise and instinct in the assessment of testamentary capacity. Villanova Law Rev. 51:26–94.

[55] Sharpe DJ (1957) Medication as a threat to testamentary capacity. N. Carolina Law Rev.35:380–399.

[56] Sharpe DJ (1957) *Ibid.*

[57] More likely the receptionist, legal assistant, or even the newest attorney to join the firm, would have this task.

mini-mental status exam will be required, as suggested by some scholars.[58] Only then may the attorney guarantee that the client is of *sound mind* for executing a will.

Drug-Induced Diminished Capacity

Stepping back from isolated chapter case of the impact of drugs on testamentary capacity, we next examine the impact of drugs on *diminished capacity* in a more general way. Diminished capacity is defined as the inability to form a *mental intent* in committing a crime.[59] The inability to form a mental intent, called *mens rea* in legalese, is the basis for a diminished capacity defense in various jurisdictions. Some states limit the defense to specific intent crimes, such as robbery assault and battery states, whereas other states recognize it in crimes with varying degrees of intensity, as in manslaughter versus murder. Other states only allow diminished capacity defense within the context of insanity hearings. A successful diminished capacity defense usually results in a lesser conviction and not in acquittal of the crime.

Drugs and their intoxicating ways can produce diminished capacity in the commission of crime with acute drug use most assuredly, chronic drug use more insidiously. The over-intoxicated drunk who punches a friend and gets arrested for assault may not have formed the proper mental intent for the crime, and has no memory of event due to alcohol blackout. *Mens rea*, or mental intent or ideation, is only one essential element of a crime. The second element is *actus rea*, or the "*acting out*" of the crime, the actual physical action that resulted in a crime being committed.[60] Drug use can also alter the *actus rea* element of the crime, for example, a case of involuntary intoxication due to a prescription error in an impaired driver resulting in a pedestrian death. The driver was unaware of the dangers of driving due to the prescription error; the pharmacy gave him a sedative-hypnotic drug instead of his usual diabetes medication, for example. Both the *mens rea* and *actus rea* elements of the crime have to be proven beyond a reasonable doubt for the prosecution to be successful.

The use of a diminished capacity defense due to drug intoxication is not uniformly allowed among all the states. In Montana, a young man was camping and drinking liquor with two friends. He was found the next day severely passed out in the rear seat of a car, severely intoxicated with alcohol (0.36% BAC). His two friends were both dead with gunshot wounds in the front seat. The trial court found him guilty of *deliberate homicide*, defined by Montana law as "*purposely*" or "*knowingly*" causing another's death. The young man argued that "*extreme intoxication had rendered him physically incapable of committing the murders and accounted for his inability to recall the events of the night in question.*"[61] After giving the jury instruction that the defendant's claim of intoxication could not be used "*in determining the existence of a mental state which is an element of the offense,*" the jury found him guilty. The decision was reversed by the Supreme Court of Montana, under the Due Process Clause, to have the jury consider all relevant evidence, and that evidence of his voluntary intoxication was "*clearly relevant*" to the issue whether he acted knowingly. However, in yet another 5–4 decision, the Supreme Court of the United States (SCOTUS) agreed with the trial court in *Montana v. Egelhoff 1996* based on long-standing common law tradition. SCOTUS stated that to let a jury hear "*evidence of a defendant's voluntary intoxication where relevant to mens rea has gained considerable acceptance since the 19th century, it is of too recent vintage*"[61] to be uniformly accepted by the Court.

To this pharmacologist and part-time drug expert, SCOTUS did not get it right in the *Montana v. Egelhoff 1996* case. Egelhoff is not as culpable of deliberate murder in his extreme intoxicated state as the spurned ex-husband who plans for months to murder his ex-wife and does so in cold blood. The state cannot simply ignore modern drug intoxication and addiction research and the medical model of drug addiction. A state law explicitly providing jury instructions that drug effects do not matter in a case like this, or in any other case, does not address the impact of drugs in our drug-using society. To rely on common-law tradition and talk about changes in the 19th century as being too recent belies the ultraconservative majority opinion written by the late Justice Scalia.[62] Like it or not, we live in the 21st century. Drugs have an undeniable effect on the brain, and the brain controls behavior. An educated analysis tells one that it is extremely difficult for a person to stop taking addictive drugs, that our society does not offer adequate health care to treat drug addiction, and that the penal system does a crummy job of treating drug addicts. Ignorance of these simple facts keeps our justice system most unfair to those who need to be treated most fairly. Habitual drug abusers are not doing drugs for kicks, they are sick.

We saw in the previous chapter that the Federal Sentencing Guidelines consider drug use and drug addiction during a crime but concluded that a downward departure cannot usually be predicated on drug use or addiction. Specifically, they

---

[58] Zehr MD (2012) The assessment of capacity civil settings. J. Missouri Bar, Mar-Apr issue, pp. 98–102.

[59] Gifis SH (2005) Barron's Law Dictionary, 5th Edition, Barron's Educational Series, Hauppauge, NY, USA.

[60] Shiner RA (1990) Intoxication and responsibility. Int. J. Law Psych. 13:9–35.

[61] *Montana v. Egelhoff*, 518 U.S. 37 (1996).

[62] A point made by a true legal scholar in Allen RJ (1997) *Montana v. Egelhoff*--Reflections on the limits of legislative imagination and judicial authority. J. Crim. Law Crimonol. 87:633–691.

excluded diminished capacity due to voluntary drug use or intoxication as a consideration for downward departure in sentencing. There are exceptions to the intoxication defense in the case of involuntary intoxication, discussed in the context of drug-induced confessions in an upcoming chapter.[63]

Estimation of BAC From Alcohol Consumed

In the life of the drug expert, and for the sake of the hiring attorney, it is often necessary to estimate the blood alcohol concentration (BAC) at a time during or after consuming alcoholic beverages. The ability to do this depends on reliable data on the time of consumption, the number of drinks, and the type of alcoholic drinks consumed. Depending on the case, the time of consumption, type, and number of drinks can be obtained from the restaurant or bar receipt.[64] The weight and gender of the person consuming alcohol is also needed, but usually medical or autopsy records will be available to get that data, or even obtained from a driver's license if that is the only source available.

There are published charts that correlate number of standard alcoholic drinks to resulting BAC by weight and gender of the drinker. A number of BAC charts pop-up after a Google™ search. However, the use of BAC charts provided by the American Prosecutors Research Institute (APRI) is a nice touch and hard for the prosecution to refute when used by the defense attorney.[65] BAC charts are a simple way to estimate BAC levels after a number of drinks. Drinks are standardized such that one drink equals a 12-oz beer, 1-oz of 100 proof distilled spirits, or 5 oz of wine. The first column of the chart runs from top to bottom with different body weights and the remainder of columns run from 1 to 12 drinks. The BAC is estimated by first finding the row of the person of interest's body weight, then moving right until you are in the column of the proper number of drinks. There is a separate chart for males and females (see Appendix J). These charts show, for example, that a 160 lb. male needs 4 drinks to reach a BAC over the legal driving limit of 0.08% whereas a 160 lb. female reaches 0.08% after 3 drinks.[66]

A BAC can also be more precisely calculated using the Widmark formula, the eponymous method from a pioneering Swedish scientist studying alcohol metabolism in the 1930s.[67] The BAC is equal to the amount of alcohol divided by the body weight of the drinker and a Widmark factor that depends if the drinker is male or female. This calculation gives the maximum BAC after drinking a known amount of alcohol.

Calculation of BAC after drinking alcohol is called anterograde ("*going forward*") calculation of BAC. It is useful in cases when the time and amount of alcoholic drinking is known and an incident occurred at a specific time afterwards. Calculation of BAC at the time of an incident (e.g., motor vehicle accident) earlier than the time of obtaining a BAC from a blood sample is called retrograde calculation of BAC. The usefulness and method for retrograde calculation of BAC are saved for a later chapter.

[Narrative continued]

The drug expert studied medical and pharmacy records of the testator, Mrs. Robinson. A timeline of prescription drug doses and clinic chemotherapy administration was made. Research on the brain effects of the three specific anti-cancer drugs taken by Mrs. Robinson to treat her advanced colon cancer gave evidence of drug-induced diminished capacity. Additional information on the type and amount of alcohol consumed by Mrs. Robinson in the years prior to and during the time of the recent will amendment was obtained by eyewitness reports of a housemaid and from liquor store receipts. Research on the alcohol-induced neurotoxicity and brain dysfunction from chronic consumption of hard liquor supported another cause of drug-diminished capacity. An examination of the BAC likely reached by Mrs. Robinson from the daily intake of alcohol was done by making an anterograde calculation of BAC from her body weight and the amount of alcohol consumed, using standard alcohol charts. This method conservatively estimated that Mrs. Robinson reached daily levels of 0.18% BAC from her consumption of whiskey and beer. The drug expert testified before the Judge that the anti-cancer drugs and chronic alcoholism more likely than not caused cognitive dysfunction and lack of clear-headed thinking at the time she amended the will. Based on this evidence, and other testimony from her personal physician and family members, the Court decided that the last-minute amended will was invalid and the previous will executed ten years earlier remained in force. The natural heirs of Mrs. Robinson received equal shares of their mother's estate with no allocation to the young caretaker.

---

[63] See Chapter 14 *The Truth Shall Not Set You Free*.

[64] See Chapter 17 *A Visit to the Dram Shop* to see an example of bar receipts used to determine how many drinks were served.

[65] See Appendix J for the Alcohol Chart for Males from: American Prosecutors Research Institute (2003) Alcohol toxicology for prosecutors: targeting hardcore impaired drivers. APRI, Alexandria, VA, USA. Available at: *www.ndaa.org/pdf/toxicology_final.pdf*.

[66] While it is true that the women have increased BAC with the same amount of alcohol as men, the opposite appears to be true in rats and other laboratory animals.

[67] Posey D, Mozayani A (2007) The estimation of blood alcohol concentration: Widmark revisited. Forensic Sci Med Pathol. 3:33–39.

Chapter 13

Speed Kills: Two cases of methamphetamine abuse and homicide

Drug Addiction in a Nutshell

Methamphetamine-Induced Violence, Aggression, and Psychosis

Phases of Criminal Trials—Admissibility of Scientific Expert Testimony

Daubert Challenge to Drug Expert Testimony

[Narrative]
Brian Diener was charged with first-degree murder in the shooting death of an individual known to be a habitual user of methamphetamine. According to Mr. Diener, the decedent asked to come over to his house because it was raining out. Mr. Diener testified that the decedent began to talk about gangs and locked himself in the bathroom for over 30 min. Mr. Diener could hear him talking on the phone. When the decedent exited the toilet, he was agitated and carrying a knife. Mr. Diener testified that he was afraid for his life and shot him twice with a legally-registered handgun. His defense attorney argues that Mr. Diener was acting in self-defense and hires a local drug expert to investigate methamphetamine use and aggression.

In a second case, Corey Chester was addicted to methamphetamine and sold meth to other users to support his habit. He met a buyer in a seedy motel room, next to the interstate running through the city. On a tip from an informant, police officers showed up at the motel to investigate. Upon officers announcing their presence, Mr. Chester fired a round from a pistol through the door, injuring the shoulder of one of the officers. As the police drew their weapons and entered, Mr. Chester grabbed a female hostage and escaped on foot towards the highway. He fired a warning shot to keep the police at bay. The police returned gunfire, killing the hostage and critically wounding Mr. Chester. Miraculously, Mr. Chester survived and was facing the death penalty for the aggravating factors of using a firearm with drug trafficking charges, wounding a police officer, kidnapping a hostage, and death of a hostage. Blood samples obtained from Mr. Chester at the hospital were positive for very high levels of methamphetamine. His Public Defender contacted a drug expert to assess the effects of methamphetamine on behavior after acute and chronic use.

Drug Addiction in a Nutshell

As discussed previously, the brain operates by the activity of neurons. Crank up the neuronal activity and the brain gets activated, stimulated, and motivated. Slow the activity of the neurons and the brain gets depressed, regressed, and suppressed. The level of neuronal activity is closely regulated in most people, sometimes a little up and a little down but no major swings.[1] This regulation ultimately comes from the amount of neurotransmitters in the brain, which are either inhibitory or excitatory. Too much dopamine acting on excitatory pathways, for example, and one may start hearing voices. Too little serotonin and one may start becoming depressed and think about killing themselves.

Mechanism of drug addiction

The *nucleus accumbens* is a brain structure that is about the size of an almond and is embedded in the front part of the brain—like behind the forehead region and straight back about 4 in.[2] Most importantly, the nucleus accumbens has dopamine fibers impinging on it from areas farther back in the midbrain. The nucleus accumbens is the most important place in

---

[1] Major swings in brain activity are seen as manic-depressive disease, *a.k.a.* bipolar disorder.
[2] Maybe farther in for those with a greater percent of Neanderthal genes, which range from 1% to 4% in all non-African populations. See Wall JD et al. (2013) Higher levels of Neanderthal ancestry in East Asians than in Europeans. Genetics 194:199–209.

The Drug Expert. https://doi.org/10.1016/B978-0-12-800048-9.00013-4

the brain for producing drug addiction. All addicting drugs and behavior become such only because they produce release of dopamine into the nucleus accumbens. Due to the work of many stalwart scientists in the field of addiction, research over the last couples of decades has linked the nucleus accumbens to the reinforcing effects of nearly all abused drugs,[3] but also behaviors that can become addictive including eating, sexual activity, and gambling.[4]

Neurotransmitters are the brain's own set of drugs; conversely, psychoactive drugs act like neurotransmitters when they reach the brain. Drugs acting on the brain often hit the same drug receptors in the brain as neurotransmitters. Drugs that stimulate the brain, called *CNS stimulants*, are among the most abused substances. CNS stimulants produce a large amount of dopamine release in the nucleus accumbens.[5] Other drugs, called CNS depressants, are also abused for the feeling that comes with the lowering of brain activity, and also cause release of dopamine at the nucleus accumbens.

Methamphetamine and Violence, Aggression, and Psychosis

Physically, the brain is not the most handsome internal organ.[6] It is a gray gooey mass with the consistency of day-old Jello.™ The brain is crammed into a bony bowl and folded in upon itself, creating lumpy folds and ridges. From the outside, it doesn't appear that one part of the brain is different than any other, but we now know that each small part of the brain is specific for a particular function. The Latin-named *hippocampus* region of the brain is famous for memory, the occipital lobe in the back of the brain processes vision, and there is a small area of the left temporal (underneath the temple) lobe that enables speech.

The frontal lobe of humans is the part of the brain that lies directly beneath the scalp of the forehead. This area of the brain controls *executive function*, which is the ability to plan, organize, and control behavior. CNS stimulants, such as amphetamines and methamphetamine are associated with a number of adverse effects on the brain. As noted before, amphetamine and methamphetamine are potent stimulators of the brain's sympathetic arousal system and overuse of the arousal system produces changes in brain function. Addiction (preferably called drug dependence) to methamphetamine occurs due to the rewarding aspects produced by the arousal neurotransmitters, especially dopamine.[7] Besides users of cannabis (marijuana and related forms), there are more methamphetamine abusers in the United States than users of any other illegal substance.[8]

Methamphetamine use increases impulsive behavior, hostility, and aggression

The widespread acceptance of methamphetamine use leading to impulsive behavior, hostility, and aggression is shown in the inclusion of such warnings in the legal prescription formulations of methamphetamine and similar drugs. Methamphetamine (trade name Desoxyn®) is prescribed legally to treat obesity and narcolepsy. The FDA-mandated Patient Medication Guide for Desoxyn® warns against new or worse behavior and thought problems, new or worse bipolar illness, and new or worse aggressive behavior or hostility at the front of the guide. These same warnings of aggression are included in the full prescribing information of other amphetamine and amphetamine-like drugs such as amphetamine salts (Adderall®), methylphenidate (Ritalin®), amphetamine (Dexedrine®), atomoxetine (Strattera®), and dexmethylphenidate (Focalin® XR).

The clinical and pharmacological literature supports a strong link between methamphetamine use and impulsive behavior, hostility, and aggression. Methamphetamine users exhibit risky decision-making and impulsive behavior, as shown in clinical tests of delayed versus immediate rewards and impulsive choices, and in their self-report of impulsive behaviors.[9] Due to poor impulse control, 43% of methamphetamine users self-report a loss of control over their behavior with outbursts of anger and rage.[10] In clinical studies, 35%–57% of methamphetamine users demonstrated aggressive behavior while under the influence of methamphetamine.

---

[3] LSD and other types of hallucinogenic drugs are not associated with release of dopamine and explain why few people become addicted to hallucinogens. Even in their hippie heyday, hallucinogens were mainly a weekend drug tried, but seldom overly repeated.

[4] Much of this research was funded by the National Institutes of Health (NIH, a Dept. of Health and Human Services component) at NIDA, the National Institute on Drug Abuse.

[5] See Becker JB et al. (2016) Sex differences in addiction. Dialogues Clin Neurosci. 18:395–402.

[6] Best organ award may go to the firm and interestingly shaped kidney or perhaps the strong and nearly round muscle we call the heart.

[7] Ciccarone D (2011) Stimulant abuse: pharmacology, cocaine, methamphetamine, treatment, attempts at pharmacotherapy. Prim Care 38:41–58.

[8] Cruickshank CC, Dyer KR (2009) A review of the clinical pharmacology of methamphetamine. Addiction 104:1085–1099.

[9] Scott JC et al. (2007) Neurocognitive effects of methamphetamine: a critical review and meta-analysis. Neuropsychol Rev. 17:275–297.

[10] Lapworth K et al. (2009) Impulsivity and positive psychotic symptoms influence hostility in methamphetamine users. Addict Behav. 34:380–385.

Methamphetamine use is associated with violence in both perpetrators and the victims

Methamphetamine use is associated with impulsive, aggressive, antisocial, and homicidal behavior in many studies.[11] Methamphetamine use is linked to both the perpetrators and victims of interpersonal violence.[12] In a study of trauma patients, those who tested positive for methamphetamine were more likely to suffer from violent trauma, such as gunshot wounds, stabbing, or assault than those patients who tested negative for methamphetamine.[13] Methamphetamine-positive patients are also significantly more prone to have attempted suicide, be a victim of interpersonal violence, and have an altercation with police. Upon presentation to the trauma center, methamphetamine users were significantly more agitated, violent, and aggressive than other trauma patients with nonmethamphetamine related intoxication.

A direct comparison of methamphetamine users and heroin addicts showed that regular methamphetamine use was associated with more violent acts than heroin use.[14] Methamphetamine is more likely to induce aggression and violence with higher methamphetamine doses.[15] This study found that violent behaviors occurred with methamphetamine use independent of the violence caused by methamphetamine-induced psychosis. There are at least two ways methamphetamine causes aggression and violence, by the pharmacological and neurotoxic effect of methamphetamine itself, and by the psychotic state that methamphetamine use produces.

Methamphetamine is more closely linked to violent behavior than any other abused drug in the United States.[16] Methamphetamines produce an aroused "fight or flee" state in the brain and therefore methamphetamine use is associated with episodes of sudden, violent behavior.[17] Relative to other drugs of abuse, methamphetamine is highly neurotoxic. Studies in the next section show the brain damage that occurs with methamphetamine use.

Methamphetamine use causes changes in brain structure and function

Methamphetamine use changes the physical structure of the brain in ways that are linked to deficits in brain function.[18] There are changes in the parts of the brain that control executive function and negatively impact the ability to control behaviors and impulsiveness.[19] The areas of the brain that control inhibition of impulsive behaviors were smaller and less connected in methamphetamine users than healthy controls. Neurochemical analysis in postmortem brains of chronic methamphetamine users shows decreased markers of arousal neurotransmitters and other biochemical changes.[20] Changes to the parts of the brain that control emotion and fear are dysfunctional in methamphetamine users, which lead to aggression, paranoia, and violence routinely observed in methamphetamine users.

Researchers believe that the much of the hostility and aggression exhibited by methamphetamine users comes from the psychotic symptoms that they experience which makes their perception of the environment as a hostile and threatening place.[21] The impact of psychosis produced by amphetamine and methamphetamine use is detailed next.

Amphetamine and methamphetamine psychosis

Much like the FDA-mandated warnings for aggressive behavior following the use of prescription methamphetamine and other amphetamines detailed before, there are FDA warnings for psychotic behavior also in the full prescribing information of all amphetamine-like prescription drugs. The earliest studies of methamphetamine-induced psychosis in an experimental

[11] Harro J (2015) Neuropsychiatric adverse effects of amphetamine and methamphetamine. Int Rev Neurobiol. 120:179–204.

[12] Baskin-Sommers A, Sommers I (2006) The co-occurrence of substance use and high-risk behaviors. J Adolesc Health. 38:609–611.

[13] Bunting PJ et al. (2007) Comparison of crystalline methamphetamine ("ice") users and other patients with toxicology-related problems presenting to a hospital emergency department. Med J Aust. 187:564–566; Swanson SM et al. (2007) The scourge of methamphetamine: impact on a level I trauma center. J Trauma 63:531–537; Vearrier D et al. (2012) Methamphetamine: history, pathophysiology, adverse health effects, current trends, and hazards associated with the clandestine manufacture of methamphetamine. Dis Mon. 58:38–89.

[14] Darke S et al. (2010) Comparative rates of violent crime among regular methamphetamine and opioid users: offending and victimization. Addiction 105:916–919.

[15] McKetin R et al. (2014) Does methamphetamine use increase violent behaviour? Evidence from a prospective longitudinal study. Addiction 109:798–806.

[16] Baicy K, London ED (2007) Corticolimbic dysregulation and chronic methamphetamine abuse. Addiction 102 Suppl 1:5–15.

[17] Boles SM, Miotto K (2003) Substance abuse and violence: a review of the literature. Aggress. Viol. Beh. 8:155–174.

[18] Baicy K, London ED (2007) Corticolimbic dysregulation and chronic methamphetamine abuse. Addiction 102 Suppl 1:5–15; Cattie JE et al. (2012) Elevated neurobehavioral symptoms are associated with everyday functioning problems in chronic methamphetamine users. J Neuropsychiatry Clin Neurosci. 24:331–339; Scott JC et al. (2007) Neurocognitive effects of methamphetamine: a critical review and meta-analysis. Neuropsychol Rev. 17:275–297.

[19] Ersche KD et al. (2012) Abnormal brain structure implicated in stimulant drug addiction. Science 335:601–604.

[20] Baicy K, London ED (2007) Corticolimbic dysregulation and chronic methamphetamine abuse. Addiction 102 Suppl 1:5–15.

[21] Lapworth K et al. (2009) Impulsivity and positive psychotic symptoms influence hostility in methamphetamine users. Addict Behav. 34:380–385.

setting occurred in the 1970s; such studies would not be approved today. In one study, healthy volunteers took repeated oral doses of 5–10 mg dextroamphetamine until paranoid delusions were observed. All volunteers became psychotic within an oral methamphetamine dose range of 55–75 mg of methamphetamine (*reviewed in*[22]). In follow-up studies more recently, consensus shows that psychosis can be induced with acute administration of methamphetamine, with characteristics of paranoia and delusional thinking.[23] Also there are reports of psychosis produced by normal therapeutic doses of methamphetamine or amphetamines used clinically in the treatment of ADHD.[24]

Chronic methamphetamine use causes a transient psychotic state (psychosis) which is often accompanied by aggression, violent behavior, and homicide.[25] The clinical presentation of methamphetamine psychosis is often indistinguishable to acute paranoid schizophrenia. However, studies have shown that methamphetamine-induced psychosis does not just occur in persons predisposed to schizophrenia.[26] Clinical studies of methamphetamine users report that 29% to 45% of users had a methamphetamine-induced psychosis.[27] Indeed, methamphetamine abusers show similar degrees of psychosis as persons suffering from schizophrenia.[28]

Phases of Criminal Trials

In most cases, the drug expert will not end up testifying at a trial. After the drug expert's litigation report is submitted, many cases will settle or plea bargain to avoid a trial. Reviewing the author's experience, statistics at the time of this writing show that the drug expert may be deposed in about 20% of cases and provide trial testimony in about 30% of cases.[29]

The drug expert might want to have a general working knowledge of the procedures and phases of trial for civil and criminal cases. If nothing else, knowledge of court proceedings helps the expert understand the big picture of the case and the timeline of potential testimony. The following information will allow the drug expert to ask intelligent questions during the first contact (usually by phone) with a potential client attorney.

Stages of a criminal case[30]

Criminal prosecution develops in stages, starting with an arrest and finishing at some point before, during, or after a trial proceeding. Most criminal cases end with the offender accepting a plea bargain offered by the State or district attorney. A plea bargain allows the defendant to plead guilty before a trial and often to lesser criminal offenses in exchange for a more lenient sentence or the dismissal of other charges.

Most criminals begin their prosecution with an arrest by a police officer. The police officer may arrest someone if they observe a person committing a crime, if they have probable cause that a crime has been committed, or in carrying out an arrest warrant on that person. After booking the person at the police station, the suspect is incarcerated. If the offense is minor (a misdemeanor, for example) the offender may be given a citation with instructions to appear in court at a later date. Bail may be granted to the suspect, which if paid directly or through a bail bondsman can allow the suspect to be released from jail.

The arraignment is the first time the suspect appears in court in front of a judge. At this time, there is no jury present and the judge reads the charges filed against the defendant who answers charges by pleading guilty, not guilty, or no contest.[31] The judge will also set the docket or schedule for future court proceedings.

Depending on the seriousness of the crime and the jurisdiction, the defendant may attend a preliminary hearing to establish the existence of probable cause or the case will go to a grand jury. If an indictment is sought, the case will go before a

---

[22] Berman SM et al. (2009) Potential adverse effects of amphetamine treatment on brain and behavior: a review. Mol Psychiatry 14:123–142.

[23] Glasner-Edwards S, Mooney LJ (2014) Methamphetamine psychosis: epidemiology and management. CNS Drugs 28:1115–1126.

[24] Berman SM et al. (2009) *Op cit.*; Bramness JG et al. (2012) Amphetamine-induced psychosis—a separate diagnostic entity or primary psychosis triggered in the vulnerable? BMC Psychiatry 12:221.

[25] McKetin R et al. (2008) Hostility among methamphetamine users experiencing psychotic symptoms. Am J Addict. 17:235–240.

[26] Bramness JG et al. (2012) Amphetamine-induced psychosis—a separate diagnostic entity or primary psychosis triggered in the vulnerable? BMC Psychiatry 12:221.

[27] Grant KM et al. (2007) Methamphetamine use in rural Midwesterners. Am J Addict. 16:79–84.

[28] Chen CK et al. (2015) Persistence of psychotic symptoms as an indicator of cognitive impairment in methamphetamine users. Drug Alcohol Depend. 148:158–164.

[29] Total cases to date: 85; depositions given in 16 cases; trial testimony in 25 cases; some cases both deposition and trial testimony given.

[30] Much of this section from the *Justia* website at: *www.justia.com/criminal/procedure/stages-criminal-case/.*

[31] Pleading "no contest" known as *nolo contendere,* means the defendant does not admit guilt for the charged crimes, but leaves it to the court to determine the punishment.

grand jury. In federal cases, charges must be established by indictment with a grand jury. States may use preliminary hearings or grand juries to establish probable cause. Either way, failure to convince the judge or grand jury of probable cause will allow the defendant to go free.

In a preliminary hearing, both sides and their attorneys engage in an adversarial process with witness examination, cross-examinations, and a judge making the final determination of probable cause. In a grand jury proceeding, only the prosecutor makes the case and the defendant and defense attorneys are not present. A grand jury may also request further investigation and call their own witnesses. The final decision is made by the grand jury.

A number of pretrial motions may be made by either party. A *Daubert* motion is often filed against an expert witness during this phase of the trial to prevent the expert from testifying. Admissibility of scientific evidence and Daubert motions are discussed in the next two sections.

At the actual trial, the judge (in a bench trial) or the jury (in a jury trial) will find the defendant guilty or not guilty. The State or prosecutor must prove the defendant's guilt beyond a reasonable doubt.[32] In general, the defendant has a right to a jury trial, but may want a bench trial if the crime is especially heinous with graphic pictures. The judge or jury listens to opening and closing statements, and examination and cross-examinations of witnesses before coming to a decision. In most cases, if a jury does not reach a unanimous verdict, the judge may declare a mistrial or dismiss the case, or start the process over by empaneling a new jury.

If the defendant is found guilty, a sentencing phase begins. This may be a separate trial date, as mandated for capital punishment cases,[33] or after the guilt-phase part of the same trial. A judge or jury determines the suitable sentence by specific factors involved in the crime. These factors include the nature and impact of the crime, criminal history, personal circumstances, and remorsefulness of the defendant.

After conviction and sentencing, the defendant may appeal the decision to a higher court, appealing all the way to the highest court of the land, SCOTUS, in some (rare) cases. If an appeals court finds an error in the legal handling of the case or in the sentencing, the appeals court may reverse the finding or send (remand) the case back to the trial court for a do-over.

Admissibility of Scientific Expert Testimony

Expert testimony is only as good as the science of the times. Testimony in the early days of American justice included so-called experts in the Salem witch trials, often relying on spectral evidence in which dreams of the accuser consorting with the devil retold by the accusers were admitted as reliable evidence.[34] However, by the late 18th century expert witnesses began appearing in courts and providing scientific testimony with some degree of reliability based on a nascent understanding of the scientific method. Many experts declined to testify when the question at hand was not answerable with the scientific knowledge available at the time. Early courts requested experts to sit on the jury to help decide the case at hand, circumventing the need for adversarial experts and the outrageous expense of trying a case.[35]

A drug expert is a type of scientific expert witness. In general, the admissibility of testimony from an expert witness relies on the expert qualifications on a particular subject or area of expertise, that the expert's opinion will actually assist the fact finder (judge or jury), and that there be a reliable foundation for the opinion.[36] However, the admissibility of expert testimony is an issue that the courts have struggled with since the introduction of fingerprint matching testimony into the courts in 1902.[37] Since 1923, the decision of the U.S. Court of Appeals for the D.C. Circuit in *Frye v. U.S.* governed the admissibility of expert testimony for nearly 70 years. It set the *general acceptance* standard of the admissibility of expert testimony.[38] The *Frye* standard requires the court to determine whether the scientific method and findings of the expert are generally accepted by the scientific community to which it belongs.

In 1975 Congress enacted laws establishing the Federal Rules of Evidence (FRE). As discussed in Chapter 4 *The Power of the Poppy*, FRE Rule 702 governed expert testimony and allowed expert testimony provided their opinions were based on "*scientific, technical, or other specialized knowledge*" and supported by the expert's "*knowledge, skill, experience, training,*

---

[32] This standard of proof is lower for civil cases, in the realm of "more likely than not."

[33] SCOTUS mandated a separate sentencing trial for capital cases so that aggravating and mitigating issues could be considered when the death penalty is sought. The drug expert may be a part of the sentencing trial. See Chapters 7 and 20 for example cases.

[34] DeCoux EL (2007) The admission of unreliable expert testimony offered by the prosecution: What's wrong with *Daubert* and how to make it right. Utah L. Rev. 131:1–31.

[35] Not a bad idea, eh?

[36] Smithburn JE (2004) The trial court's gatekeeper role under *Frye, Daubert* and *Kumho*: a special look at children's cases. J Child Family Advoc. 4:3–34.

[37] Haack S (2015) The expert witness: lessons from the U.S. experience. Humana.Mente J Philosophical Stud. 28:39–70.

[38] DeCoux EL (2007) *Op. cit.*

or education."[39] From 1975 to 1993 there existed two different standards for the admissibility of scientific testimony; the *Frye* standard based on case law and the statutory law promulgated by Congress in the FRE 702 Rule. The resulting inconsistency in judicial decisions and among the appeals court led to the landmark decision by the Supreme Court of the United States (SCOTUS) that further defined the admissibility of scientific and expert testimony in the early 1990s.[40] The decision in *Daubert v. Merrell Dow Pharmaceuticals Inc.* in 1993 established first that FRE Rule 702 supersedes the *Frye* general acceptance standard. Before *Daubert* it was up to the trier-of-fact (e.g., the jury) to determine the reliability and credibility of the scientific expert witness; after *Daubert* the trial court judge took on the obligatory role of *gatekeeper* for the admission of scientific testimony.

The Court set up a two-pronged test for scientific testimony. Scientific testimony had to be both reliable and relevant. Specific nonexhaustive criteria were given by the Court to help the trial judge. Testimony should be testable, able to be proved right or wrong. This should eliminate the hare-brained testimony of fringe "scientists," espousing Huber's *junk science*. Only science can be tested and if the ideas behind a particular testimony are not testable, it is a belief and not a science. The Court also stated that scientific testimony that is not supported by peer review should be stopped at the gate. Peer review means that primary papers and reviews are published in reputable scientific and medical journals after detailed examination by others in the same scientific discipline, that is, the *Frye* general acceptance standard. Here SCOTUS basically updated the 1923 *Frye* general acceptance finding in more modern terms of peer review. Scientific testimony should also be based on methods that have known or potential error rates and standard measures of reliability. In the second prong of the *Daubert* test, scientific testimony should be relevant. This means the testimony must fit the facts of the case at hand and will assist the trier-of-fact.

Interestingly, the Court did not rule directly in *Daubert v. Merrill-Dow Pharmaceuticals Inc.* but remanded the case back to the circuit court. The Ninth Circuit reconsidered the scientific testimony against Benedictine® using the factors spelled out in *Daubert* and again excluded the testimony from the plaintiff's scientists and granted summary judgment for the defendant.[41]

There were two major outcomes after *Daubert*. The first was the new role it heaved upon the trial court judge as gatekeeper who must screen for reliability and relevance of proffered scientific expertise. Trial judges previously had the power to dismiss inappropriate expert testimony, but now the trial judge was obligated to screen each and every bit of scientific testimony. This encouraged defendants to seek pretrial rulings on the admissibility of expert testimony by filing a *motion in limine* asking for a *Daubert* hearing.[42] If the *Daubert* hearing was favorable, defendants could file a motion for summary judgment if the excluded were essential to the plaintiff's case.[43] This resulted in a tremendous increase in the use of *Daubert* motions by defendants. Second, judges could no longer allow a scientific expert witness with excellent credentials and qualifications to validate their own scientific expertise. Whether the trial judge liked the sciences or avoided any class in science throughout their life, they now had to deal with science and the scientific method.

Daubert Challenge to Drug Expert Testimony

There is a wealth of research on the impact of the *Daubert* ruling on the justice system. One clear finding is the increased filing of a *motion in limine* to block the admission of scientific testimony (*Daubert motion*). The end result is fewer cases going to trial and an overwhelmingly percentage (90%) of *Daubert* motions in which the defendant prevails, at least in civil tort cases.[44] According to a survey of judges, the most frequent reasons for excluding testimony were because it was not relevant (47%), because the expert witness was not qualified (42%), or because the expert's testimony would not assist the trier-of-fact (40%).[45]

Daubert comes into play early in the timeline of proceedings leading to a trial. After the initial filings are made that start the legal proceeding, experts for both sides (if not just one *unilateral* expert) submit litigation reports that provide the basis

[39] See Chapter 4 *Power of the Poppy*, section *Federal Rules of Evidence and the Drug Expert* for the complete text of FRE Rule 702.

[40] Bernstein B (2013) The misbegotten judicial resistance to the *Daubert* revolution. Notre Dame Law Rev. 89:27–70.

[41] Berger MA (2001) Upsetting the balance between adverse interests: The impact of the Supreme Court's trilogy on expert testimony in toxic tort litigation. Law Contemp. Prob. 64:289–326.

[42] A *Daubert* hearing may ensue after filing of a *Daubert* motion.

[43] Berger MA (2001) *Op. cit.*

[44] Cranor CF (2005) The science veil over tort law policy: how should scientific evidence be utilized in toxic tort law? Law Phil. 24:139–210.

[45] Krafka C et al. (2002) Judge and attorney experiences, practices, and concerns regarding expert testimony in federal civil trials. Psych. Public Pol. Law 8:309–332.

of their testimony.[46] After discovery, which may include depositions of both experts by opposing attorneys, one side or the other (or both) may file a *Daubert* motion to have the opposing expert excluded from testifying.

In a pretrial hearing before the judge (no jury) the judge listens to the attorneys and experts, and decides, based on *Daubert* criteria, whether the expert may testify. If a scientific expert with testimony critical to the case is not admitted, *"the litigant (typically the plaintiff) may be unable to establish needed factual premises, in which case the judge can dismiss the attempted legal action by means of a summary judgment because there is no material issue of fact for the jury to decide (the issue of the legal sufficiency of a party's evidence compared with the evidence offered by the other party)."*[47]

The drug expert, like any scientific expert witness, relies on the known facts of the drug issue at hand, garnered from hours of research and the gathered results of peer-reviewed studies in the medical and pharmacological literature. For this reason, the drug expert should be safe from exclusion of testimony after a *Daubert* motion.[48] However, clinical studies yield group data with methodological and statistical reliability, resulting in average (mean) values in control and treatment groups. The legal process is concerned with an individual before the court, and the job of the drug expert is to transfer the group data to the particular individual with a specific drug issue. The basic challenge for trial court judges is determining how scientific knowledge derived from studying group data applies to the individual cases before them.[49] The equitable transfer of group data to an individual's situation is at the heart of relevancy, a key consideration for the admissibility of scientific testimony.

If the *Daubert* motion fails, then the drug expert will continue in the litigation process and testify at the trial. If the judge does not allow the expert's testimony, the drug expert submits the final invoice to the hiring attorney and perhaps rather sheepishly part ways. Failing a *Daubert* challenge is a serious mark on the expert's record. This is one reason in particular why the selection of drug cases is important; the drug issue at hand must be researchable and there must be published evidence to answer the specific drug question. During cross-examination, the drug expert will likely be asked about any previous *Daubert* challenges by the opposing attorney, especially if the opposing attorney is aware of one.[50] An excerpt of a *Daubert* motion against a drug expert is shown in Appendix K.

[Narrative continued]

In the courtroom, Brian Diener insisted that he was in fear for his life. The drug expert testified that the extremely high levels of methamphetamine in the decedent's post-mortem blood samples, along with the ME's report listing syringes among personal effects, suggested that the decedent very recently injected methamphetamine. This is consistent with the longer than usual time the decedent remained in the bathroom before the incident. The drug expert also offered evidence-based testimony on the acute and chronic effects of methamphetamine use on the control of impulses and aggression. A jury found the drug expert's testimony credible and acquitted Mr. Diener of homicide.

In the second case, the chronic meth user shot a hostage and the prosecutor sought the death penalty. Testifying at the sentencing hearing, the drug expert testified to the extensive research studies of methamphetamine and effects on brain function. In particular, the impact of meth use on impulsivity, decision-making, aggression and psychosis was researched and reported to the court. The jury was instructed on aggravating and mitigating factors in the case of the death penalty and returned a sentence of life without parole.

---

[46] In Federal civil courts, Rule 26(a)(2)[a] mandates submission of a written litigation report by all testifying experts. This may also be the case in state courts, but either way, a drug expert should not even think about testifying at trial without at least a preliminary report to summarize and refer to when needed. I've never gone to the witness box without a copy of my report handed to me by my client-attorney during direct examination and/or carried with me in a manila folder.[b]

[a]See Chapter 5 *Wrong Place at the Wrong Time*, section *Rules of Discovery for the Drug Expert*.

[b]Carrying a manila folder with you to the stand looks professional and impresses upon the courtroom your seriousness. Besides the litigation report, the folder may contain actual hardcopies of key references from the report or other records discovered since the submission of the litigation report.

[47] Cranor CF (2005) *Op. cit.*

[48] In the event that a *Daubert* motion is filed, the drug expert should receive a copy and be prepared to assist in the response filing.

[49] Faigman DL et al. (2014) Group to individual (G2i) inference in scientific expert testimony. Univ. Chicago Law Rev. 81:417–480.

[50] Of course, the drug expert must reveal the outcome of any *Daubert* challenges to the court if asked. However, the drug expert can use this opportunity to emphasize that *Daubert* motions have never been successful if this is indeed the case, fortifying the expert's position and credibility in the court.

Chapter 14

The *Truth Shall* Not *Set You Free*: A drug-induced confession

A Short History of Drug-Induced Confessions

Drug-Induced Confessions and the Drug Expert

Disruption of Thinking and Memory Due to Drugs—Involuntary Drug Intoxication

The Pharmacist Versus the Pharmacologist Drug Expert

[Narrative]

Austin Braden lived in a dilapidated apartment building on the bad side of town. His business was making and selling metham-phetamine, using a meth lab set-up in his kitchen. During a recent meth-making run, he purportedly fell asleep and the kitchen caught on fire. The fire and smoke spread to the adjoining apartments, severely injuring an elderly woman. Austin was rescued by the fire department and transferred to a burn center with third-degree burns. Two days after the incident, a police detective and the fire chief interrogated Austin about the fire as he lay bedridden in the hospital burn unit. In the hours before the interrogation, Austin received six different drugs that are known to affect the brain. There was no attorney for Austin present during the bedside interrogation. After lengthy questioning, Austin admitted that the fire started when he was making meth and he was subsequently charged with methamphetamine possession and manufacturing and other charges related to injuries of the elderly neighbor. Austin's defense attorney obtained recordings of the police interview in the hospital and thought that Austin's speech was slurred. The attorney sought a drug expert to testify on the effects of the administered hospital drugs on Austin's mental function and the impact these drugs may have had on his confession.

A Short History of Drug-Induced Confessions

Alcohol is the oldest drug that is known for producing striking candor and lowering of inhibitions in the consumer.[1] The ability of alcohol to loosen the tongue or assist in truthful confessions was known to the ancients and embodied in the Roman phrase *in vino veritas,* meaning *in wine there is truth.* Flash-forward a few thousand years during the nascent use of anesthetic drugs for relieving the pain of childbirth. In the early 20th century, German obstetricians noticed that women who were administered the drug regimen of morphine (an opioid), and scopolamine[2] (a muscle relaxant) for the pain of childbirth would often begin speaking spontaneously about the intimate details of their private lives.[3]

One particularly outspoken OB/GYN physician from Texas[4] who noticed the effect of morphine and scopolamine in childbirth suggested that injection of morphine and scopolamine might be used in criminal investigations by the police during their interrogation of suspects. Later refinements in the drug regimen found that morphine only induced nausea and sco-polamine alone produced the desired effect of loosening the tongue.[5] The sole use of scopolamine in police interrogations

---

[1] Muehlberger CW (1951) Interrogation under drug influence: The so-called "truth serum" technique. J Crim Law Criminol Police Sci. 42:513–528.

[2] Scopolamine is also known as hyoscine, the latter cited in the SCOTUS case later in the chapter.

[3] Odeshoo JR (2004) Truth or dare?: Terrorism and "truth serum" in the post-9/11 world. Stanford Law Rev. 57:209–255.

[4] *Outspoken from Texas* may be redundant. The Texas physician was Dr. Robert E. House who first published in a medical journal that drugs may be useful for police interrogation of suspects in the early 1920s. See House RE (1922) The use of scopolamine in criminology. Texas State J Med. 18:256–263.

[5] Muehlberger CW (1951) *op. cit.*

The Drug Expert. https://doi.org/10.1016/B978-0-12-800048-9.00014-6

continued throughout the first half of the 20th century. A number of papers were published extolling the usefulness of scopolamine for separating suspects of the crime from true offenders, but also to claim innocence for those suspected of criminal activity.[6] In this regard, use of scopolamine as a "truth serum" and the record of statements made by the person under its influence were equally available at that time to both the prosecutor and the defense.

Scopolamine (*a.k.a.* hyoscine) is an anticholinergic drug, meaning it blocks the action of the endogenous neurotransmitter acetylcholine at the cholinergic receptor site.[7] Acetylcholine and cholinergic receptors of the muscarinic type are the mediators of the parasympathetic side of the autonomic nervous system. The autonomic nervous system (ANS) is a network of neurons and nerve fibers that regulate the body in ways that are *automatic*; controlling heartbeat, respiration, gut movements, sweating, and numerous other bodily functions in a balanced way. The ANS has two separate subsystems with opposing functions: the sympathetic nervous system and the parasympathetic nervous system. We are most familiar with the sympathetic nervous system and its well-known activation in fight or flee situations. The sympathetic nervous system also is the network mimicked by CNS stimulant drugs like methamphetamine and cocaine.[8] The parasympathetic nervous system counteracts the sympathetic nervous system and, through the release of acetylcholine acting on cholinergic receptors, produces a decrease in heart rate, increased saliva secretions, and slowing of the GI tract. Scopolamine relaxes smooth muscle and can relieve cramping and other pains of childbirth.

Scopolamine along with its most clinically used cousin, atropine, is plant alkaloid produced from the family of deadly nightshade plants, including *Atropa belladonna*, and jimson weed.[9] Scopolamine and atropine are called *belladonna* drugs because Italian women at the time of the Renaissance used extracts of the nightshade plant in their eyes to cause pupil dilation, making them appear more attractive and sexually aroused.[10] Atropine is still used today and is indicated to dry up secretions in the mouth and respiratory tract before intubation, for quickening the heat rate in a slow heartbeat block, and for counteracting the toxic effects of insecticide and mushroom poisoning.[11]

Use of scopolamine by arresting officials continued into the early 1950s, in spite of criticism from a legal and pharmacological perspective that began soon after its use as a tool for eliciting "true confessions."[12] The use of scopolamine for drug-induced confessions was surpassed by the newer (at that time) development of barbiturate drugs.[13] The most famous and commonly used barbiturate drug was sodium thiopental branded under the name Sodium Pentothal®. Other barbiturate drugs include pentobarbital, amobarbital, secobarbital, and phenobarbital.[14] Barbiturate drugs act by directly and indirectly increasing the action of the brain's inhibitory neurons and produce sedation and CNS depression.

It is certain that there are many instances of confessions obtained while the suspect is under the influence of powerful mind-altering drugs. As previously mentioned in the introductory chapter, about 1 in 10 persons in the general population abuses drugs. The incidence of drug abuse is closer to 6 or 8 persons out of 10 in the criminal suspect population. It follows that a large majority of arrestees are detained and interrogated while under the influence of drugs. Additionally, there is evidence that drug users undergoing withdrawal from drugs and alcohol are more susceptible to interrogation.[15] Detainees are vigorously questioned and some will give false confessions while under the influence of a drug or two. In these instances, the drug and dose taken by the arrestee remains unknown as there is no mandatory toxicology blood draw for all arrestees.[16] It is likely that in cases of confessions influenced by drug use, the drug expert may help in keeping the confession from entering the evidence stream of the trial

In the rare case, like the index case of this chapter, complete and reliable medical records can be examined to determine if a confession was coerced by concurrent drug use. As elaborated in the next section, confessions obtained under the influence of mind-altering drugs are not considered valid and may be denied entry as evidence in court proceedings.

---

[6] Geis G (1961) The status of interrogation drugs in the United States. J Forensic Med. 8:29–33.

[7] Brenner GM, Stevens CW (2018) *Brenner and Stevens' Pharmacology, 5th Ed.*, Elsevier, Philadelphia, PA, USA.

[8] See Chapters 5 and 8 for profiles of methamphetamine and cocaine, respectively.

[9] Lee MR (2007) *Solanaceae IV: Atropa belladonna*, deadly nightshade. J R Coll Physicians Edinb. 37:77–84.

[10] *Belladonna* is Italian for "b*eautiful woman.*" See Berdai MA (2012) *Atropa belladonna* intoxication: a case report. Pan Afr Med J. 2012; 11: 72. For images see "#bedroomeyes."

[11] *Atropine Sulfate Injection*, at: *www.accessdata.fda.gov/drugsatfda_docs/label/2015/021146s015lbl.pdf.*

[12] Macdonald JM (1955) Truth serum. J Crim Law Criminol. Police Sci. 46:259–263.

[13] Geis G (1961) *Op. cit.*

[14] Barbiturates were also the initial drugs used in the classic three-drug lethal injection protocols for capital punishment. See final chapter 20 *Death Be Not Proud* for more details.

[15] Leo RA (2009) False confessions: causes, consequences, and implications. J Am Acad Psych Law 37:332–343.

[16] Perhaps there should be. A dataset built upon blood levels of specific drugs and charges of particular crimes would be pharmacologically fascinating and helpful in drug policy decisions.

Drug-Induced Confessions and the Drug Expert

The importance of police interrogations for the solving of crime is emphasized by these key considerations: many criminal cases are solved only by confessions of suspects, suspects are not likely to admit their offense without intense police interrogations, and police interrogation techniques are noted by manipulation, cajoling, and other sophisticated methods.[17] As described in the previous section, use of "truth serum" drugs for confession and interrogation has a long history in this country. Although limited jurisdiction battles were surely fought, the only case where the use of "truth serum" in a confession came before the Supreme Court of the United States (SCOTUS) was in 1963.[18]

In the *Townsend v. Sain* case, the defendant was a heroin addict charged with murder. At the first police interrogation, *Townsend* denied any involvement with the crime. Due to his heroin addiction, after a few hours he started to go through opioid withdrawal. Police contacted a physician who injected Townsend with hyoscine, which is not an opioid (the proper type of drug to stave off opioid withdrawal), but an anticholinergic drug like scopolamine used as a "truth serum." Police then interrogated Townsend under the influence of hyoscine and eventually Townsend confessed to the murder and many other crimes. His attorneys later moved to suppress his confession, which was denied by the trial court. After many appeals, it ended up at the highest court of the land where the Justices ruled that the use of a drug-induced confession as evidence at the trial resulted in a due process violation. Chief Justice Warren wrote "*it is difficult to imagine a situation in which a confession would be less the product of a free intellect, less voluntary, than when brought about by a drug having the effect of a truth serum.*"[19]

The upshot is that SCOTUS decided that drug-induced confessions are inadmissible at trial. This was done in the context of drugs given by police departments or their agents, for example, a psychiatrist on the police payroll. It is more common now that the drug will be self-administered by the person giving the confession. Does the source of the drug and the administering party make a difference in the pharmacological effect on memory and thinking that taints the confession? To the drug expert, it doesn't matter; the pharmacological effect on the confession is the same whether forced down his throat or self-injected heroin minutes before apprehension. A drug expert is needed in either case.

Disruption of Thinking and Memory Due to Drugs

Not every drug affects the brain and alters thinking and memory. The penicillin shot given for a case of the *clap* or the insulin injection for the diabetic does not alter the cognitive function of the brain in any significant way. Some drugs improve the cognitive functions of the brain, such as donepezil (Aricept®) used in the Alzheimer's patient, or amphetamines in the normal and nondiseased individual for "brain enhancement."[20] However, there is a large class of drugs that target the brain and produce beneficial *and* adverse effects on brain function. For example, the opioid analgesics like morphine and hydrocodone target pain pathways in the brain and beneficially produce a lack of pain, or *analgesia*. But opioid analgesics also produce many adverse effects including sedation, respiratory depression, and cognitive deficits from the very same targeting of the brain by the opioid drug.

In the chapter case, the drug expert obtained the medical records of the defendant in the hospital burn unit from the client attorney. The defendant was administered the following drugs with the earliest one, morphine, given about 2 h before police interrogation began (see Table 14.1).

The Table produced by the drug expert in this case (below) gives two key pieces of pharmacokinetic data for each drug: the time of peak pharmacological effect, and the time it takes for half the drug amount to be diminished from the body. The latter time, called the elimination half-life ($t_{1/2}$), gives an approximation of the duration of pharmacological effect. If one assumes that the drug concentration in the blood halved from the original level in the blood still exerts a pharmacological effect, the elimination half-life is a good proxy for duration of effect. Of course, the table could be enhanced by adding another column with the *actual* duration of pharmacological action gleaned from the literature, if one is so inclined.

---

[17] Lippman M (2017) *Criminal Procedures.* Chapter 8 *Interrogations and Confessions.* Sage Publishing, Thousand Oaks, CA.

[18] *Townsend v Sain*, 372 U.S at 307 (1963), discussed in Odeshoo JR (2004) Truth or dare?: Terrorism and "truth serum" in the Post-9/11 World. Stanford Law Rev. 57:209–255.

[19] *Townsend v Sain*, 372 U.S at 307 (1963).

[20] There is much interest in brain-enhancing drugs, called *nootropics*, for use in normal persons to enhance their thinking and memory. See Stix G (2009) Turbocharging the brain. Sci. Amer. October, pp. 46–55.

TABLE 14.1 Medications administered to the defendant in the chapter case. The defendant was interviewed at bedside by police and fire chief starting at 10:30 am and lasting until 1:15 pm

Time	Medication given	Dose/Route	Peak effect[a] (min)	Elimination half-life (hour)	Class description
8:15 am	Morphine	1 mg/IV	30–90	1.5–4	Opioid analgesic; central nervous system (CNS) depressant
9:55 am	Risperidone	1 mg/Oral	60–180	20	Antipsychotic psychotropic; CNS depressant
10:09 am	Diphenhydramine	25 mg/Oral	120	2.5	Antihistamine sedative; CNS depressant
10:09 am	Lorazepam	4 mg/IV	10–30	4	Sedative-hypnotic; CNS depressant
10:15 am	Oxycodone	5 mg/Oral	60–100	4	Opioid analgesic; CNS depressant

[a] Peak effect (peak plasma concentration) and drug elimination half-life data from FDA-approved full prescribing information (the "label" as it is known) for each drug and also from the reasonably priced and highly recommended introductory medical pharmacology textbook cowritten by the author.[21]

The adverse effects of opioid analgesics on the brain

The first drug given to the defendant was morphine. Morphine is the gold standard of *opioid analgesic* drugs, indicated for the treatment of moderate to severe pain. It is more generally classified as a CNS depressant. Besides morphine, opioid analgesics include other well-known pain medications such as oxycodone (OxyContin®), hydrocodone (Lortab®, Norco®), and meperidine (Demerol®) and are in the same chemical class as the illegal opioid drug of abuse, heroin.[22] Morphine is available in formulations (drug preparations) for oral, intravenous (IV), intrathecal, and epidural administration. Morphine, like all opioids, works by binding to opioid receptors on pain neurons and inhibiting the activity of the pain neurons. The inhibition of pain neurons produces the analgesia, or relief of pain, that morphine and other opioid analgesics are famous for. All opioids are classified as CNS depressants.

Maximum amounts of morphine in the brain are reached after about 1 to 1.5 h after administration. Morphine remains in the body system for a long time; only half of the morphine is metabolized by 1.5–2 h (elimination half-life), although more sensitive studies extend this half-life to 4 h. In the cerebrospinal fluid (CSF) morphine has an early half-life of 1.5 h and a later phase half-life of 6 h. Morphine is also metabolized in the liver and produces an active morphine metabolite which is 2–4 times more potent than morphine itself. This morphine metabolite has an even longer elimination half-life about double that of morphine itself. This pharmacokinetic information for morphine, as well as the other agents administered to the defendant in this chapter's case, is crucial to determine a drug effect at the time of the police interrogation.

Besides stopping pain, opioids have other adverse effects on the function of the brain.[23] The use of opioid analgesics, including agents such as morphine, hydrocodone, and oxycodone, is associated with cognitive dysfunction following acute and long-term administration in healthy volunteers and chronic pain patients.[24] Although opioids do not produce obvious destruction of nerves and brains cells, cognitive impairment within the context of delirium is considered a neurotoxic effect of opioids.[25] For example, immediate-release morphine added to a chronic opioid treatment showed cognitive adverse effects such as impairments to retrograde (before morphine) and anterograde memory (after morphine) and psychomotor tasks.[26]

[21] Brenner GM, Stevens CW (2018) *Brenner and Stevens' Pharmacology*, *5th* Ed., Elsevier, Philadelphia, PA. Amazon link: *www.amazon.com/Brenner-Stevens-Pharmacology-George-PhD/dp/0323391664*.

[22] Heroin is a brand name, as Bayer introduced as Heroin® following the success of Aspirin® early in the last century. Both trade names have gone the way of Kleenex and lost their trademark with common use. Heroin is nothing more than a morphine molecule with two acetic acid groups added; its chemical name is *diacetyl-morphine*.

[23] There are also non-CNS drugs, that is to say drugs that are not targeted to act in the central nervous system (brain and spinal cord) that can drastically alter the brain. Chemotherapeutic drugs, that is, agents to treat cancer cause a well-recognized brain dysfunction called "chemobrain." See Heflin LH et al. (2005) Cancer as a risk factor for longterm cognitive deficits and dementia. J Natl Cancer Inst. 97:854–856; Wefel JS, Schagen SB. (2012) Chemotherapy-related cognitive dysfunction. Curr Neurol Neurosci Rep. 12:267–275.

[24] Chapman SL et al. (2002) Effects of intermediate- and long-term use of opioids on cognition in patients with chronic pain. Clin J Pain 18:S83–S90.

[25] Lawlor PG (2002) The panorama of opioid-related cognitive dysfunction in patients with cancer: a critical literature appraisal. Cancer 94:1836–1853.

[26] Kamboj SK et al. (2005) The effects of immediate-release morphine on cognitive functioning in patients receiving chronic opioid therapy in palliative care. Pain 117:388–395.

In a large study of chronic pain patients, between 16% and 25% of patients demonstrated worsened performance on neuropsychological and cognitive tests while on opioids.[27]

The defendant was given a second opioid, the potent drug oxycodone, about 15 min before the interrogation began. Oxycodone is an opioid analgesic that has quickly become one of the most commonly prescribed opioids for chronic pain in the United States and Canada mainly due to the aggressive marketing[28] of its controlled-release formulation called OxyContin®. Subjective and psychomotor assessment studies of oxycodone and morphine show that at equal doses, oxycodone produced stronger effects and greater cognitive dysfunction (in terms of psychomotor impairment) than morphine in healthy young volunteers.[29] Single low doses of oxycodone produced a slight but significant cognitive dysfunction characterized but decreased function of working memory in healthy young adults.[30] Comparing oxymorphone and oxycodone, the controlled-release oxycodone (OxyContin®) produced more cognitive and psychomotor impairment than extended-release oxymorphone at equal analgesic doses.[31]

The adverse effects of atypical antipsychotics on the brain

The defendant was administered risperidone (Risperdal®) while in the burn unit before the police interrogation. Risperidone is an *atypical* antipsychotic drug. First of all, a *typical* antipsychotic agent is a drug that acts as an antagonist at dopamine receptors. As you might remember from Chapter 1, in the *Drug Effects on Brain and Behavior* section, dopamine is a major neurotransmitter in the brain and an overabundance of dopamine underlies the pathology of schizophrenia. Therefore it makes sense that the first drug treatment for schizophrenia was typical antipsychotic drugs that block (antagonize) dopamine at its receptors.

Atypical antipsychotics were developed after typical antipsychotic drugs and are more effective at treating schizophrenics who are resistant to previous typical antipsychotics and exhibit the more insidious signs of schizophrenia such as catatonia, abject apathy, anhedonia, and social withdrawal.[32] The atypical antipsychotics like risperidone generally have less serious adverse effects than the typical antipsychotics.

Risperidone (trade name Risperdal®) is FDA approved for the treatment of schizophrenia, for the short-term treatment of acute manic or mixed episodes associated with bipolar disorder in adults, and for the treatment of irritability associated with autistic disorder in children and adolescents aged 5–16 years.[33] It is also more generally classified as a psychotropic agent, that is, an agent that has activity on the brain and mental functions. Antipsychotics are also classified as CNS depressants.[34] Oral administration of risperidone reaches a peak concentration in the blood after about 1 h. Risperidone is mainly metabolized in the liver and yields an active metabolite. Risperidone and its active metabolite remain in the body a very long time. The elimination half-life of risperidone and its active metabolite shows a mean half-life value of 20 h.

The acute effects of risperidone given to normal healthy volunteers produced dizziness in 40% of subjects and sleepiness (somnolence) in 50% of subjects.[35] There was also a decrement in various psychomotor functions (finger-tapping, cursor tracking) and measures of learning and memory. There is some improvement in the prior baseline cognitive abilities of schizophrenics after treatment with risperidone or other antipsychotic drugs,[36] but long-term treatment of schizophrenic patients with typical and atypical antipsychotics for 9 years showed a significant decrement in verbal learning and memory compared to predrug baseline cognitive ability.[37]

[27] Jamison RN et al. (2003) Neuropsychological effects of long-term opioid use in chronic pain patients. J Pain Symptom Manage 26:913–921.

[28] Lexchin J, Kohler JC (2011) The danger of imperfect regulation: OxyContin use in the United States and Canada. Int J Risk Saf Med. 23:233–240.

[29] Zacny JP, Gutierrez S. (2003) Characterizing the subjective, psychomotor, and physiological effects of oral oxycodone in non-drug-abusing volunteers. Psychopharmacology (Berl). 170:242–254.

[30] Friswell J et al. (2008) Acute effects of opioids on memory functions of healthy men and women. Psychopharmacology (Berl). 198:243–250.

[31] Schoedel KA et al. (2010) Reduced cognitive and psychomotor impairment with extended-release oxymorphone versus controlled-release oxycodone. Pain Physician. 13:561–573.

[32] Catatonia is a state of near paralysis and lack of movement; anhedonia ("not hedonia") is a total lack of getting pleasure from life's hedonistic activities.

[33] Risperdal® Full Prescribing Information, Ortho-McNeil-Janssen Pharmaceuticals, Inc. rev. 2009.

[34] In Chapter 18, we shall see that a drug expert was consulted when antipsychotic treatment was withheld from a schizophrenic inmate upon release and who subsequently committed a heinous crime.

[35] Liem-Moolenaar M et al. (2011) Central nervous system effects of the interaction between risperidone (single dose) and the 5-HT6 antagonist SB742457 (repeated doses) in healthy men. Br J Clin Pharmacol. 71:907–916.

[36] Houthoofd SA et al. (2008) Cognitive and psychomotor effects of risperidone in schizophrenia and schizoaffective disorder. Clin Ther. 30:1565–1589.

[37] Husa AP et al. (2014) Lifetime use of antipsychotic medication and its relation to change of verbal learning and memory in midlife schizophrenia – An observational 9-year follow-up study. Schizophr Res. 158:134–141.

The adverse effects of benzodiazepine sedative-hypnotics on the brain

The Defendant was given lorazepam (trade name Ativan®), a sedative-hypnotic agent of the benzodiazepine drug class. Like opioid analgesics, lorazepam is also more generally classified also as a CNS depressant. Lorazepam is chemically and pharmacologically similar to the popular benzodiazepine drugs like diazepam (Valium®) and alprazolam (Xanax®). Lorazepam acts directly in the brain to increase the activity of inhibitory neurons, thereby causing relief of anxiety, promoting sleep, and impairing memory formation and recall of events while under the influence of the drug. Lorazepam given IV is used as a preanesthetic medication, where it produces sleepiness and drowsiness, relieves anxiety, and blocks formation of memory and recall for patients undergoing surgery or other invasive procedures.[38] It is also used to treat epileptic seizures. The duration of action for lorazepam injected intravenously is extremely long lasting. The intended effects of lorazepam injection usually last for 6–8 h. Only half of the administered lorazepam is eliminated in 14.5 h (elimination half-life).

The benzodiazepines (*benzos*), such as diazepam, alprazolam, and midazolam, produce an acute effect on cognitive processing in the brain. For example, literature on the cognitive adverse effects of clonazepam include reports showing that the benzodiazepine clonazepam negatively affected memory and attention in healthy volunteers.[39] As a class, benzodiazepines are famous for producing amnesia, the medical term for loss of memory. Indeed, common outpatient procedures such as colonoscopy rely on the amnesic effects of midazolam to improve the patient experience and assure a return visit in 5 to 10 years for a repeat scope.[40]

The adverse effects of antihistamine sedative-hypnotics on the brain

The defendant was given diphenhydramine as a third medication shortly before the police interrogation. Diphenhydramine is a commonly used antihistamine for the treatment of allergies but also as a sedative-hypnotic. Sold often as Benadryl®, diphenhydramine is available over the counter and in stronger formulations by prescription. Adverse effects on the brain are produced by diphenhydramine injection and include sedation, sleepiness, dizziness, disturbed coordination, fatigue, confusion, restlessness, excitation, and nervousness.[41]

Clinical studies show that diphenhydramine and older first-generation antihistamines significantly decrease alertness, cognition, learning, and memory, and produce impairment with sedation.[42] Diphenhydramine produces greater sedation, drowsiness, and impaired psychomotor performance (such as tracking movement of a cursor with a mouse) compared to the newer, second-generation antihistamines such as levocetirizine.[43] This is due to the second-generation antihistamines which were developed with an inability to cross the blood-brain barrier.

Synergy of CNS depressant drugs

When more than one drug is taken by a person, there is the possibility that the two or more drugs can interact to produce greater effects. Synergy is a common word that also has a specific pharmacological meaning. Synergy occurs when two drugs cause greater pharmacological effects when taken together compared to taken alone. Pharmacological synergy is a common medication interaction used in the clinic, synergy is shown in a number of clinical studies, and drug users often combine drugs for their synergistic effects to get a greater high.[44]

---

[38] It is the authors pet theory that those individuals claiming alien abduction and orifice probing may have experienced inadequate doses of midazolam or other drugs during colonoscopy or other invasive procedures; resulting in fragments of traumatic memories looking for a meaning (doctors as aliens in their garb and masks, machines and digital equipment of the OR remind one of a spaceship, and surgical probing is *probing*).

[39] Dowd SM et al. (2002) The behavioral and cognitive effects of two benzodiazepines associated with drug-facilitated sexual assault. J Forensic Sci 47:1101–1107.

[40] Midazolam is the number one benzodiazepine used for these procedures as it is formulated for IV administration with the brand name Versed®. As benzodiazepines have no analgesic ability, midazolam was often combined with a strong opioid, such as sufentanyl (Sufenta®) for colonoscopy. Nowadays it is more likely the general anesthetic propofol would be given as a sole IV agent; it is a true anesthetic and also returns the colonoscopy patient to reality sooner.

[41] Diphenhydramine Hydrochloride Injection, USP, Full Prescribing Information, BD Rx Inc. rev. 2012.

[42] Simons FE, Simons KJ (2011) Histamine and H1-antihistamines: celebrating a century of progress. J Allergy Clin Immunol. 128:1139–1150.

[43] Verster JC et al. (2003) Acute and subchronic effects of levocetirizine and diphenhydramine on memory functioning, psychomotor performance, and mood. J Allergy Clin Immunol. 111:623–627.

[44] Classic synergistic "eightball" combination for IV drug users is heroin and cocaine. Sigmund Freud is essentially responsible for this combination when he tried to treat heroin addicts by coadministering cocaine. See Jay M (2015) Miracle or Menace?: The Arrival of Cocaine 1860-1900. Int Rev Neurobiol. 120:27–39.

In general, in cases where any CNS drug may be involved, attorneys should examine possible effects of drugs on memory and cognition. An earlier chapter considered the possible effects of psychotropic drugs on eyewitness and victim accounts (see Chapter 10) and the present chapter focuses on the effects of drugs in confession. Both of these scenarios, and many others, may demand the use of a pharmacologist drug expert to enlighten the judge or jury on the adverse effects of drug action.

Involuntary Drug Intoxication

The defendant in the present chapter case was administered mind-altering drugs in the context of medical treatment and then interrogated by the police at bedside. In this regard, drug-induced confession is an example of involuntary drug intoxication. In an erudite review of law and the states of consciousness,[45] a case of an involuntary intoxication defense after a homicide is described. *Ilo Grundberg*, a 57-year-old woman, took the sleep medicine, Halcion®, and shot her 83-year-old mother in the head and killed her. Halcion®, whose generic name is triazolam, is a benzodiazepine drug that was a very popular sleeping medication in the pre-Ambien® days. *Grundberg* was charged with murder and went to trial. However, the state dropped the homicide charges after a court-appointed psychiatrist testified that *Grundberg* killed her mother involuntarily due to an adverse effect of Halcion®. *Grundberg* then went on to bring a civil product liability suit against the makers of Halcion®, the Upjohn Company, for $21 million in damages. Testimony by *Grundberg* revealed that she had been taking Halcion for insomnia for about a year and that she had no memory of the shooting her mother. It was discovered that the Upjohn Company knew that there were about two-dozen reports of murders, attempted murders, and physical threats associated with the administration of Halcion®.[46] *Grundberg's* civil suit was settled out of court before the full trial and the terms of the settlement remain undisclosed.

While the *Grundberg v. Upjohn* case generated a storm of negative press about Halcion® with some countries, including a complete ban in the UK, others found evidence that an involuntary act after drug ingestion is not more likely to occur after Halcion® than any other benzodiazepine drugs.[47] Into this controversy over Halcion® came the development of zolpidem, marketed as Ambien® in 1992. While the following decades saw the rise of Ambien® to the worldwide leader in sleep medicines, reports began to emerge about involuntary acts, including violence and homicide, following the ingestion of Ambien®. Indeed, the next chapter details a case of suicide after the CEO of a Las Vegas casino ingested a prescribed dose of today's number one sleep medication, zolpidem (Ambien®).

The core question of a drug addict self-administering the addicted drug is whether this is a voluntary or involuntary act. The most common answer is quick and easy: the addict has a *choice* whether to take the drug or not, it is a voluntary act. However, if one looks closely, this common belief is based on a moral value and not on the actual scientific evidence, and it is wrong. From animal models, where rats will lever-press cocaine until they die from lack of sleep and food, to humans and the growing opioid epidemic leaving young and old dead bodies in its wake, it is obvious that drug-taking behavior is coerced and therefore involuntary.

Ultimately, any act that occurs after an addicting drug is taken by a drug-dependent individual may be framed as an involuntary drug intoxication. Behavior is controlled by the brain which depends on the function of the brain at the time the behavior is initiated, and the lifelong exposure of the brain to prior drugs and experiences. There is no "ghost in the machine" or separate entity apart from the gooey substance of the brain, no experience or behavior driven by something other than the brain.[48] The brain is.

Those not addicted to drugs may have a hard time understanding the absolute compulsion produced by drug addiction to take addictive drugs. Eating is a good analogous behavior for those non-drug-dependent individual to understand the drive to use drugs by the drug dependent. Imagine going just one day, all day, without eating. Come evening you see a slice of meat pizza (or fruit or vegies for those noncarnivores); it would be extremely difficult to resist eating it. Ergo the presence of the abused drug and the involuntary nature of drug-taking by the drug addict.

The issue of voluntary of involuntary drug use in an addict is taken up in a legal context by Professor Murray, who suggests a middle ground of "*semi-voluntary*" act:

This Comment attacks the assumption that a drug addict's choice to use drugs can be accurately classified as either voluntary or involuntary. Today, reliable research demonstrates that drug addiction is not merely a behavior but an identifiable condition caused by drug usage, genetics, mental illness, and other environmental factors. Scientists have found that a drug addict's choice to use

---

[45] Denno DW (2003) Crime and consciousness: science and involuntary acts. Minnesota Law Rev. 87:269–401.

[46] Denno DW (2003) *Ibid.*

[47] Dinan TG, Leonard BE (1993) Triazolam: As safe as other benzodiazepines. BMJ 306:1475.

[48] Perhaps I should say there is no evidence of a soul or experience of humans that can't be shown to be linked to specific brain regions.

drugs falls into a gray area between voluntary and involuntary. Addicts lose a large amount of control over when they can choose to become intoxicated. As an alternative to the unscientific voluntary/involuntary distinction in the law, this Comment advances the concept of a semi-voluntary act category to describe more accurately a drug addict's choice to use drugs. This category would provide an avenue for a partial affirmative defense that would result in a verdict of not guilty but responsible. This verdict would treat drug addicts who commit crimes while intoxicated with greater nuance and fairness.[49]

The Pharmacist Versus the Pharmacologist Drug Expert

A pharmacist degree prepares one for the *profession of dispensing drugs*. At the present time, a Pharm. D. degree is awarded to those that complete pharmacy school. But this is a relatively new development. In 2005 the American Pharmacy Association and other professional pharmacy groups, including the pharmacy schools, standardized a Pharm. D. degree for all pharmacists as their terminal degree. Before that, it was common for the entry-level pharmacy degree to be awarded after an extended undergraduate program, resulting in the Bachelors of Science—Pharmacology (BSci. Pharm.) degree.[50]

The astute attorney may want to consider a pretrial motion to exclude the testimony of a pharmacist by the opposing party. In this author's opinion, some extremely important pharmacological issues were tainted by the testimony of an unqualified pharmacist, including a lethal injection drug case that reached all the way to the Supreme Court of the United States.[51]

Importantly, there is case law regarding the admissibility of a pharmacist versus a pharmacologist testifying as drug experts. Four federal district court cases will be briefly reviewed to highlight the specific issues. In the earliest case, the Plaintiff, Nancy Wehling brought suit against the makers of Clozaril® (clozapine), an atypical antipsychotic drug used to treat schizophrenia claiming she went into respiratory depression after taking Clozaril® while also on a benzodiazepine.[52] Plaintiff's attorney hired a retired pharmacist and toxicologist whose testimony was challenged by the defendant, Sandoz Pharmaceuticals. The court affirmed the trial court's decision to uphold the motion and the pharmacist was not allowed to testify and the case was dismissed. Some of the reasons provided by the court are instructive to the drug expert and hiring attorneys.

The court found that the pharmacist was unqualified on a number of grounds. It noted that *"[w]ithout prior training, education, or experience in the field, [the pharmacist] review of the literature, after he was retained as an expert witness in this suit, was insufficient to qualify him as an expert on the issues in dispute"* and *"[a]nother significant fact weighing against admitting the testimony is where, as here, the expert developed his opinions expressly for the purposes of testifying."* The teachable moment here is that a pharmacologist drug expert will have all the training, education, and experience in pharmacology that she[53] will automatically qualify as a *bona fide* drug expert. The need for research or literature review of particular drug issues is still paramount for even the world's best drug expert. Every key statement of opinion from the drug expert should be supported by scientific (pharmacological) data; there is too much information and drug data published on a daily basis not to do the research. The court noted that the pharmacist in this case *"is neither a pharmacologist nor medical doctor"* and in the most damning of his unqualifications noted that the pharmacist *"testified that he has no knowledge of how Clozaril® works in the brain, or how it could interact with benzodiazepines."*

In *Newton v. Roche Labs, Inc.,* The Plaintiffs *Newton* are the parents of injured party, their daughter, who claim that the defendant Roche's drug, Accutane® (isotretinoin, a derivative of Vitamin A known as *13-cis-retinoic acid*) caused schizophrenia.[54] The plaintiff's expert, a pharmacist, was rejected as an expert witness due to numerous factors. The Court found that the pharmacist *"does not possess the qualifications to render a causation opinion in this case. Although he holds himself out as a 'doctor' and a pharmacologist, he has never earned an M.D., a Ph.D., or any degree in pharmacology."*[55] The Court found out that the pharmacist's only claim to the title of "doctor" was based upon the completion of a one-year "Pharm.D." program in 1971. In a footnote, the Court revealed that the pharmacist himself stated that the Pharm.D. degree

---

[49] Murray PE (2013) In need of a fix: reforming criminal law in light of a contemporary understanding of drug addiction. UCLA Law Rev. 60:1006–1044.

[50] Vlasses PH (2010) Reflections on a decade of progress in pharmacy education: reasons for celebration. Am J Pharm Educ. 74:174.

[51] The infamous *Glossip* decision concerning the use of midazolam as the first drug in a three-drug lethal execution protocol in Oklahoma. See Chapter 20 for a fuller discussion of this case and other lethal injection drug matters.

[52] A Fourth Circuit decision in *Wehling v Sandoz Pharmaceuticals Corp.*, 162 F.3d 1158, 1998 U.S. App.

[53] A little payback for all the decades of misogynous gender-specific language that still haunts the halls of academia in titles such as "Chairman."

[54] U.S. District Court for the Western District of Texas, *Newton v. Roche Labs, Inc.* 243 F. Supp. 2d 672, 2002.

[55] This same pattern of behavior and misrepresentation by pharmacists was repeated in crucial lethal injection cases arguing the State's use of midazolam, as presented in Chapter 20.

is an entry-level degree and that he intentionally falsely advertised as having a doctorate in pharmacology to attract more interest from lawyers for his consulting business. The pharmacist was sued by a previous plaintiff and paid money to settle the case. Needless to say, the defendant's motion to exclude the pharmacist's testimony was granted and a summary judgment dismissed the case. Incredulously, the same pharmacist rejected in the *Newton* case earlier was hired by new plaintiffs in another case 2 years later.[56]

In *Dellinger v. Pfizer, Inc.,* a similar case involved a pharmacist in the role of a drug expert.[57] Plaintiff *Dellinger* was hospitalized after being prescribed Neurontin® (gabapentin), a central nervous system depressant approved for the adjunct treatment of seizures.[58] *Dellinger* had chronic back pain and his physician prescribed Neurontin® for an "off-label" use. The plaintiff developed acute pancreatitis and pneumonia while in the hospital and had a long period of rehabilitation and recovery. The plaintiff asserted that Neurotin® was the cause of the pancreatitis and pneumonia. The plaintiff's drug expert was a pharmacist. The Pfizer lawyers filed a *Daubert* motion and won. Testimony from the Pharmacist was excluded for being a pharmacist and not a pharmacologist, among other reasons.

The District Court wrote *"Pharmacology can be described as the study of the effect of drugs on living organisms, while pharmacy, on the other hand, can be described as the profession of reading prescription labels and disbursing drugs."* And then the court said, in regard to that expert, *"However, Keys is not a doctor and has a degree in pharmacy, not pharmacology. Without a degree in pharmacology, Keys is not qualified to render a relevant or reliable pharmacological opinion. [You] have to have a degree in pharmacology in order to testify as a pharmacologist."*

The last section provided valuable information for the hiring attorney to consider before hiring a drug expert and fodder to challenge to the opposing party who hired a pharmacist expert. It also provided some real-life examples of adverse effects of prescription drugs altering mental function and the need for the pharmacologist drug expert. Expanding on this topic, the next chapter focuses on a suit brought against the makers of Ambien® for an adverse drug reaction that the plaintiffs claim resulted in a high-profile suicide.

[Narrative continued]

Mr. Diener's medical records were obtained from the Burn Unit during the time of the confession. The drug expert created a timeline of drugs and dosages given within 48 h prior to the police interview. Mr. Diener was administered four types of drugs that have known detrimental effects on thinking and memory: opioids morphine and oxycodone, the benzodiazepine lorazepam, the antihistamine diphenhydramine, and the antipsychotic risperidone. Each of these drugs produces deficits in cognitive functioning, including memory and recall. The drug expert concluded that the administration of morphine, risperidone, diphenhydramine, lorazepam, and oxycodone more likely than not that impacted brain function when Mr. Diener confessed to the police of manufacturing methamphetamine and starting the fire. The defendant's attorney submitted a motion to exclude the confession and the Court excluded its use in the trial. However, there was enough physical evidence gathered from the charred remains of the fire to convict Mr. Diener of possession and manufacture of methamphetamine.

---

[56] United States District Court for the Northern District of New York, *DeVito v. Smithkline Beecham Corp.* U.S. Dist. 2004 WL 3691343.

[57] United States District Court for the Western District of North Carolina, *Dellinger v. Pfizer, Inc.* U.S. Dist. 2006 WL 2057654.

[58] *Adjunct* means along with another typical antiseizure drug. Neurontin® is also approved for the management of postherpetic neuralgia (shingles) in adults.

Chapter 15

Snake Eyes: Gambling with the adverse effects of Ambien®

Sleep Drugs—Drug Laws and Regulations—Approval of New Drugs by the FDA

The Dangers of Ambien® Use—Examining Pharmacokinetics for Drug Dose and Time

The Drug Expert and Big Pharma Litigation

[Narrative]
Ross Martino was a smart, hard-working individual with a successful career in corporate finance. At 45 years-old, his career blossomed from a position as chief financial officer of a waste management firm on the East Coast to the CEO of a major casino in Las Vegas. Mr. Martino recently complained of insomnia to his family physician, attributing his inability to sleep to an upcoming business deal at the casino. His physician prescribed him Ambien CR® at a dose of 12.5 mg per night to help him sleep. One morning, Mr. Martino was found dead by his wife. He had a gunshot wound to the head. There was a pill bottle of Ambien® on the nightstand and a revolver by his hand on the bed. There was no suicide note. Police investigation found no evidence of homicide and the medical examiner listed his death as a suicide. Mrs. Maria Martino, the wife of the decedent, did not believe her husband was suicidal and filed a wrongful death suit against the physician, the physician's practice group, and the makers of Ambien®. Attorneys at a Las Vegas law firm searched the legal databases and found the name of a drug expert who previously testified on the adverse effects of Ambien®. A phone call was made to the drug expert and after a brief discussion, the expert agreed to take the case.[1]

Sleep Drugs

Sleep is a time of rhythmic suppression of the brain's neuronal activity. It is a time every night when one submits to the enduring darkness of unconsciousness, briefly lit by the glimpse of passing dreams. Sleep serves a critical function in health and disease, even if its ultimate teleological reason is not fully understood.[2] Modern medicine rightly treats patients who have trouble falling or staying asleep with a variety of brain activity depressants. Chronic insomnia affects about 10% of the population and sleep medicines like Ambien® are among the best-selling drugs in the industry.[3]

As a group, sleep-inducing drugs fall under the larger class of drugs called sedative-hypnotic drugs. As we learned in the introductory chapter, many sedative-hypnotic drugs used for sleep and for the treatment of anxiety work as CNS depressants by acting at the same receptor used by the brain's own inhibitory neurotransmitter, GABA. In the treatment of sleep, pharmacological inhibition of neurons by sedative-hypnotic drugs in the brain mimics the natural inhibition by GABA during normal, drug-free sleep induction.[4]

---

[1] After hanging up the phone, the drug expert Google'd the attorney's names and their law firm. It was apparent after pulling up a few newspaper articles that the drug expert had unknowingly agreed to work for *mob lawyers*!

[2] The *raison d'etre* for sleep is still unknown. However, learning and recall are associated with better sleep patterns. Dreaming during sleep is crucial. Disrupting rapid eye-movement (REM) sleep, which is associated with dreaming, is detrimental in a dose-dependent way and fatal in the extreme.

[3] Asnis GM et al. (2016) Pharmacotherapy treatment options for insomnia: a primer for clinicians. Int J Mol Sci. 17:50. Ambien® is the #1 drug prescribed for sleep with 44 million or so scripts each year. This ends up being about 4 times more than its closest competitor (Matthew Harper, "*Can a Safer Ambien Make Billions? Merck Aims To Find Out*" Forbes, 10/31/2012).

[4] Saper CB et al. (2010) Sleep state switching. Neuron 68:1023–1042.

The Drug Expert. https://doi.org/10.1016/B978-0-12-800048-9.00015-8

Benzodiazepines, like diazepam (Valium®) or alprazolam (Xanax®), were developed in the 1970s and largely replaced the previously used barbiturate drugs for the treatment of insomnia.[5] Benzodiazepines are much safer to use than barbiturate sedative-hypnotic drugs like secobarbital (Seconal®) and amobarbital (Amytal®). Benzodiazepines and barbiturates both bind to and activate the GABA receptor along with natural GABA in the brain. They both cause greater neuronal inhibition than just GABA alone. However, at the molecular level, barbiturates can produce their effects without the presence of GABA whereas benzodiazepines need GABA present to exert their inhibitory effect. This leads to the well-known "ceiling effect" with benzodiazepines because GABA is limited in the brain, therefore the inhibitory effect of benzodiazepines is limited. Barbiturates do not rely on GABA for their effects therefore they can inhibit neuronal activity to dangerous levels including respiratory depression, coma, and death. Most significantly, unlike barbiturates, it is rare to successfully overdose on benzodiazepines unless combined with other CNS depressants such as alcohol or opioids.[5] This basic pharmacological difference between benzodiazepines and barbiturates was rightly recognized as a stumbling block in the transition from using a barbiturate drug (thiopental or pentobarbital) to using a benzodiazepine (midazolam) in lethal injection protocols.[6] This issue is at the heart of the drug expert cases on lethal injection included in Chapter 20.

Drug therapy for inducing and maintaining sleep

As mentioned in our brief review of drug effects on the brain in Chapter 1, the overactivity of the brain is held in check by inhibitory neurotransmitters, mainly the amino acid-derived *gamma*-aminobutyric acid (GABA). The concentration of GABA in the brain determines whether brain activity increases or decreases. For example, too little GABA and one may experience seizures from overactive neurons. This is why it makes perfect pharmacological sense to use GABA-enhancing drugs to treat epilepsy. On the other hand, too much GABA, or additional GABA-enhancing drugs in the brain, causes the activity of the brain to decrease, producing sedation and sleep. Today, the most commonly used GABA-enhancing drugs are the benzodiazepines. These are best-selling drugs like alprazolam (Xanax®) and diazepam (Valium®) used to treat panic disorders and generalized anxiety among other conditions. Benzodiazepines act on GABA receptors and potentiate the action of GABA to inhibit neuronal activity.[7]

For treating sleep disorders like insomnia, the benzodiazepines are widely used. Since the 1990s, a new class of sedative-hypnotic drugs, known as "z-drugs" were developed. The first "z-drug" and still the number one sleep medicine is zolpidem, marketed by Sanofi as Ambien®. Other "z-drugs" include zaleplon (Sonata®) and eszopiclone (Lunesta®). These drugs have nonbenzodiazepine chemical structures but like Benzos exert their effects by increasing neuronal inhibition at GABA receptors.[8]

Drug Laws and Regulations

The U.S. Food and Drug Administration (FDA) is a federal agency that approves, regulates, and monitors food and drug products, as its name suggests.[9] Except for meat and poultry products,[10] the FDA's jurisdiction includes food products, human and veterinarian drugs, biologicals,[11] and medical devices. The role played more or less by the present-day FDA

---

[5] Asnis GM et al. (2016) op cit.

[6] This pharmacological difference, clearly self-evident to most pharmacologists and anesthesiologists (and medical students) made it all the way up to SCOTUS in *Glossip v. Gross*, 135 S. Ct. (2015). In a typical 5–4 decision, the Justices decided that the use of midazolam did not increase the risk of pain and suffering compared to thiopental or pentobarbital. The opinion of the majority and dissenters is available from the SCOTUS site at: *www.supremecourt.gov/opinions/14pdf/14-7955_aplc.pdf.*

[7] To be precise, they act at GABA$_A$ receptors which are linked to a chloride ion channel. GABA$_B$ receptors are G-protein coupled receptors (GPCRs) and do not mediate the action of benzodiazepines. See Brenner GM, Stevens CW (2018) Chapter 19 Sedative-hypnotic and anxiolytic drugs. In: *Brenner and Stevens' Pharmacology*, 5th Ed., Elsevier, Philadelphia, PA, USA.

[8] To be precise, the "z-drugs" act on the subset of GABA$_A$ receptors containing the alpha 1 subunit. By this subtype selectivity, the "z-drugs" appear to have fewer traditional adverse effects, like REM suppression, tolerance and dependence, and withdrawal, than the Benzos. See Drover DR (2004) Comparative pharmacokinetics and pharmacodynamics of short-acting hypnosedatives: zaleplon, zolpidem and zopiclone. Clin Pharmacokinet. 43:227–238.

[9] Much of this section is based on Nasr A, Lauterio TJ, Davis MW (2011) Unapproved drugs in the United States and the Food and Drug Administration. Adv Ther. 28:842–856 and the FDA website at *www.fda.gov*. A special shout-out to Dr. John P. Swann at the FDA for a fine series of articles on the FDA history and early drug laws at: *www.fda.gov/AboutFDA/WhatWeDo/History/Origin/default.htm.*

[10] The exception to meat and poultry likely reflects the deal made when proto-FDA was moved from the Dept. of Agriculture in 1940 to various federal agencies before ending up in its current home in the Dept. of Health and Human Services in 1980.

[11] Biologicals = biological products, the latter defined by the FDA as "…'biological product' means a virus, therapeutic serum, toxin, antitoxin, vaccine, blood, blood component or derivative, allergenic product, protein (except any chemically synthesized polypeptide), or analogous product." (from Title 42 U.S.C. § 262 - Regulation of biological products).

arose from a single chemist in the Department of Agriculture in 1862 to more than 15,000 federal employees with a $5.1 billion annual budget in 2017.

FDA's drug regulation laws

The first major laws regulating drugs came with the passage of the Food, Drug, and Cosmetic Act (FD&C) in 1938. The FD&C Act for the first time required pharmaceutical manufacturers to show that their drugs were not toxic and safe for human consumption. One year previously, an antibiotic drug was formulated as an elixir containing the poisonous solvent diethylene glycol (antifreeze) and killed 107 people across the United States.

In 1951 the Durham-Humphrey Amendments to the FD&C Act enacted a two-tier approach to drug regulation. There were now nonprescription drugs, also known as over-the-counter (OTC), and there were prescription drugs. Nonprescription drugs are considered safe for the consumer to use without the direct supervision or a prescription from a physician. Prescription drugs need a doctor's prescription and were to be used "under the professional supervision of a practitioner licensed by law to administer such drug."[12]

After another toxic drug event in 1962 with thalidomide use in pregnant women causing severe birth defects, the *Kefauver-Harris Drug Amendments* to the FD&C Act were passed. These amendments mandated that drug manufacturers prove the effectiveness of their drug products as well as their safety before marketing them. Henceforth, the FDA approval of new drugs is done using the dual criteria of safety and effectiveness.

Approval of New Drugs by the FDA

There is nothing intrinsically special about a chemical that becomes a prescription drug. It just so happens that a particular chemical, out of an almost infinite number of other chemicals, hits a pharmacological target within the body and improves a particular medical condition. Of course, there is worldwide pharmaceutical industry looking for these particular chemicals to sell for the treatment of medical conditions. If successful, the particular chemicals are submitted to the FDA for approval and, if successful, become a prescription drug. A prescription drug is nothing but a chemical with a business plan.

The process required for the FDA approval of prescription drugs is simple in the overview.[13] Briefly, the first step is a long period of preclinical research showing that a potential drug has a defined mechanism of action[14] and some preliminary pharmacokinetic data in animals. The drug company then applies for an Investigational New Drug (IND) approval from the FDA if the drug looks promising. When and if the FDA approves the IND, then the drug company can enlist patients in clinical trials and after many years submit a New Drug Application to the FDA. As soon as FDA approval is obtained, the manufacturer can begin to market the product. Part of the FDA process is approval of the Full Prescribing Information (FPI) for the new drug. The FPI is a multipage document that gives the FDA-approved indications, therapeutic effects, and adverse effects, among other information. Because the FPI has the stamp of government approval, physicians who treat for indications not explicitly delineated ("off-label" uses) or use a drug in a manner differing from doses or methods stated in the FPI may be liable to standard of practice claims.[15]

When a new drug is brought to market after FDA approval, the pharmaceutical manufacturer has about 12 years of market exclusivity remaining of the initial 20-year patent, as it takes about 8 years to bring a drug to market.[16] This new drug is given a brand name that is heavily marketed and often becomes known to the general population, like Prozac®, Advil®, Viagra®, among others. This level of drug branding doesn't come cheap; pharmaceutical manufacturers spend about $30 billion dollars per year on marketing drugs to physicians and consumers.[17] After the branded drug's market exclusivity expires, other pharmaceutical companies can apply to the FDA for approval to market a generic version of the branded drug.

---

[12] 21 U.S.C. §353(b).

[13] Conceptually simple maybe. Each step is a multiyear process and *uber* expensive. Only 21% of new drugs that begin human clinical trials end up getting FDA approved, at an average product cost of about $1 billion. See Payette M, Grant-Kels JM (2013) Brand name versus generic drugs: the ethical quandary in caring for our sophisticated patients while trying to reduce health-care costs: facts and controversies. Clin Dermatol. 31:772–776.

[14] Mechanism of action is a simply how the drug works. For example, the mechanism of action of the antihypertensive metoprolol (a *beta*-blocker) is to block $beta_1$-adrenergic receptors which slow the heart rate.

[15] See Chapter 4 *The Power of the Poppy: Overdose from the Opioid Treatment of Cancer Pain* which is centered on a physician using fentanyl (Duragesic®), a powerful opioid analgesic, in the treatment of cancer pain. The drug expert relied heavily on the fentanyl's FPI to prove that the physician was disregarding FDA-approved doses and methods.

[16] Grabowski H et al. (2014) Recent trends in brand-name and generic drug competition. J Med Econ. 17:207–214.

[17] Sarpatwari A et al. (2016) The case for reforming drug naming: should brand name trademark protections expire upon generic entry? PLoS Med. 13:e1001955.

The FDA publishes a list of all approved generic and branded drugs in the United States called the *Orange Book*. The name of the drug manufacturer and the date of drug approval are also given. It is updated in an annual edition each year and supplemental editions on a monthly basis throughout the year. An approved drug may have multiple listings as each dosage form (e.g., tablet or injection solution) and each dosage (e.g., 10 mg or 50 mg tablet) is listed as a separate drug product.[18]

In the United States, all drugs used for medical treatment are approved by the Food and Drug Administration (FDA). Additionally, the FDA approves the prescription labeling information for each drug. Included in the prescribing information is a listing and description of adverse effects. Many clinical studies are also done after the drug is marketed and these studies often reveal additional and sometimes serious adverse effects that were not apparent when the drug was first approved. Additionally, unforeseen problems with some drugs don't occur until they become bestsellers and the number of people taking them reaches into the millions. There are many examples of best-selling drugs that, due to serious adverse effects, are withdrawn from the market including Vioxx®, Accutane®, Baycol®, Meridia®, Hismanal®, Propulsid®, Seldane®, and Darvon®.

The Dangers of Ambien® Use

Like all sedative-hypnotic drugs, zolpidem (Ambien®) shares a number of adverse effects due to its main pharmacological action of depressing neuronal activity. For this reason, the following warning is given in the Full Prescribing Information (FPI) for Ambien®:

> *CNS depressant effects*: Ambien® like other sedative/hypnotic drugs has CNS-depressant effects. Due to the rapid onset of action, Ambien® should only be ingested immediately prior to going to bed. Patients should be cautioned against engaging in hazardous occupations requiring complete mental alertness or motor coordination such as operating machinery or driving a motor vehicle after ingesting the drug, including potential impairment of the performance of such activities that may occur the day following ingestion of Ambien®.[19]

On top of these FDA-approved warnings of the adverse effects of benzodiazepines, Ambien®, and other sedative-hypnotic drugs, other adverse effects of a more unusual nature began to emerge. As early as 1982, *neuropsychiatric* adverse effects were noted with the use of sedative-hypnotic medicines.[20] Adverse effects included delirium, hallucinations, confusion, and agitation with memory impairment. A larger study documented the side effects of anger or violence, impulsivity, self-harming, depression, and manic behaviors with sedative-hypnotic medicines.[21] Sexual fantasies were also reported with sedative-hypnotic use.[22] A review article in 2003 also stressed the sexual nature of behavioral disinhibition (complex behaviors) while under the influence of sedative-hypnotic medicines including numerous cases of masturbation observed by the health care provider.[23] The previous studies focused on adverse effects of older sedative-hypnotic agents, including the benzodiazepines (Xanax®, Valium®, etc.) but not the newer "z-drugs" like zolpidem (Ambien®).

Studies specific to the nonbenzodiazepine, zolpidem (Ambien®), began to appear after the FDA approval of zolpidem in 1992. By 1999, there were already 20 case studies of zolpidem-induced hallucinations in the medical literature.[24] Since then, zolpidem was found to be linked to a growing number of cases of psychosis, delirium, and hallucinations.[25]

---

[18] The 38th edition (2018) of FDA's approved product list can be downloaded as a PDF at: *www.fda.gov/downloads/Drugs/DevelopmentApprovalProcess/UCM071436.pdf*. A search of the *Orange Book* can be done at the FDA website: *www.accessdata.fda.gov/scripts/cder/ob/*.

[19] Ambien® Full Prescribing Information, available from at FDA or Ambien® website.

[20] Ong BY et al. (1982) Lorazepam and diazepam as adjuncts to epidural anaesthesia for caesarean section. Can Anaesth Soc J 29:31–34.

[21] Cole JO, Kando JC (1993) Adverse behavioral events reported in patients taking alprazolam and other benzodiazepines. J Clin Psychiatry 54 Suppl:49–61.

[22] Dundee JW (1992) Advantages and problems with benzodiazepine sedation. Anesth Prog 39:132–7.

[23] Balasubramaniam B, Park GR (2003) Sexual hallucinations during and after sedation and anaesthesia. Anaesthesia 58:549–53.

[24] Toner LC et al. (2000) Central nervous system side effects associated with zolpidem treatment. Clin Neuropharmacol 23:54–58.

[25] Ansseau M et al. (1992) Psychotic reactions to zolpidem. Lancet 339:809; Ben-Hamou M et al. (2011) Spontaneous adverse event reports associated with zolpidem in Australia 2001-2008. J Sleep Res 20:559-568; Brodeur MR, Stirling AL (2001) Delirium associated with zolpidem. Ann Pharmacother 35:1562–1564; Coleman DE, Ota K (2004) Hallucinations with zolpidem and fluoxetine in an impaired driver. J Forensic Sci 49:392–393; de Haas S et al. (2007) Pseudohallucinations after zolpidem intake: a case report. J Clin Psychopharmacol 27:728–730; Elko CJ et al. (1998) Zolpidem-associated hallucinations and serotonin reuptake inhibition: a possible interaction. J Toxicol Clin Toxicol 36:195-203; Hoyler CL et al. (1996) Zolpidem-induced agitation and disorganization. Gen Hosp Psychiatry 18:452–453; Kinnan S et al. (2011) Zolpidem-induced mania in a patient with schizoaffective disorder. Psychosomatics 52:493–494; Kummer L et al. (2012) Zolpidem misuse in two women with no psychiatric history: a crucial role of pleasant visual hallucinations. J Neuropsychiatry Clin Neurosci 24:E32; Markowitz JS, Brewerton TD (1996) Zolpidem-induced psychosis. Ann Clin Psychiatry 8:89–91; Skourides D, Samartzis L (2012) Initiation of illusions after combination of zolpidem and paroxetine in a young woman: a case report. Prim Care Companion CNS Disord 14:p.ii; Tsai MJ et al. (2003) A novel clinical pattern of visual hallucination after zolpidem use. J Toxicol Clin Toxicol 41:869–872; van Puijenbroek EP et al. (1996) Visual hallucinations and amnesia associated with the use of zolpidem. Int J Clin Pharmacol Ther 34:318.

A review of clinical trials before the marketing of Ambien® in the United States showed that zolpidem caused delirium and confusional states in 1.6% of individuals.[26] A larger hospital-based study examined CNS adverse effects in patients who had received 5 or 10 mg zolpidem for the first time.[27] Of 119 patients, 16% experienced central nervous system (CNS) adverse effects, including delirium and confusion, mostly within 8 h of administration. A larger study of 5842 cases of zolpidem exposure found that there was a 2.9% incidence of hallucinations and 3.3% incidence of confusion.[28] Using an odds-ratio approach to analyze voluntarily reported adverse effects of zolpidem use in Australia from 2001 to 2008, zolpidem use increased the likelihood of reporting hallucinations as an adverse effect by 12.9 times compared to other drug groups.[29] In the present-day *Ambien CR® Full Prescribing Information*, the manufacturer reports that in a placebo-controlled clinical trial in adults, there was a 4% incidence of hallucinations and a 3% incidence of disorientation or confusion.

While the previous data differ in their actual incidence of Ambien® users that experience a drug-induced hallucinatory or confusional state, even taking the lower estimate of a 4% hallucination rate, with Ambien® selling at 40 million scripts in a year, hallucination occurs in 1.6 million patients taking Ambien®. Even if hallucinations induced by Ambien® are very rare at a low rate of 0.1%, one would still expect 40,000 hallucinating patients per annum.[30] Some of these are patients[31] who may have harmed themselves or others during a hallucination (see next), or suffered another serious adverse effect as a direct result of buying and taking a physician-prescribed, FDA-approved medication.

Homicide and suicide associated with Ambien® use

Besides the neuropsychiatric adverse effects just noted above, Ambien® use is associated with strange adverse effects called *complex behaviors*. The most commonly observed complex behaviors observed on zolpidem in a large group of patients were sleep-eating, sleepwalking with object manipulation, sleep conversations, sleep driving, sleep shopping, and sleep sex. There was no correlation of these behavioral adverse effects with the patient's age, gender, coexisting diseases, or previous zolpidem use.[32]

It may seem counterintuitive that a sleep medicine and CNS depressant like Ambien® could activate the brain and cause complex behaviors including somnambulism (sleepwalking) when a person is still sleeping. However, not all parts of the brain are quiescent during sleep. For example, the parts of the brain that inhibit movement during sleep are active in normal sleep. It may be that zolpidem also inhibits this part of the brain thereby preventing inhibition of movement and the sleeping person gets up and drives unknowingly to Dairy Queen™ for a Blizzard.™

There is a well-established link between somnambulism (sleepwalking) and violent behavior including homicides (for reviews see Ref. 33) which leads to the third and most serious group of zolpidem adverse effects. Most disturbing is the increasing reports in the medical literature on complex behaviors including homicide and suicide linked to zolpidem (Ambien®). A recent paper reported on two cases of zolpidem-associated homicides in which individuals took 10–30 mg of zolpidem and killed their spouses.[34] Both individuals did not have a history of violence and were unaware of their actions due to the amnesic effect of zolpidem.

An example of suicidal behavior with a high dose of zolpidem was reported in 2010. A 32-year-old man presented to the emergency room after stabbing himself in the hand. The night before he had been agitated and took more than his usual dose of zolpidem and ingested four doses (40 mg). Instead of being calmed he became more agitated and heard voices telling him to stab his hands with a knife (command hallucinations). He stabbed his left hand and tried to stab his right hand but his wife intervened. His hallucinations subsided later after the effects of Ambien® wore off.[35]

[26] Langtry HD, Benfield P (1990) Zolpidem. A review of its pharmacodynamic and pharmacokinetic properties and therapeutic potential. Drugs 40:291–313.

[27] Mahoney JE, Webb MJ, Gray SL (2004) Zolpidem prescribing and adverse drug reactions in hospitalized general medicine patients at a Veterans Affairs hospital. Am J Geriatr Pharmacother 2:66–74.

[28] Forrester MB (2006) Comparison of zolpidem and zaleplon exposures in Texas, 1998-2004. J Toxicol Environ Health A 69:1883–1892.

[29] Ben-Hamou M et al. (2011) Spontaneous adverse event reports associated with zolpidem in Australia 2001-2008. J Sleep Res 20:559–568.

[30] This is where the blockbuster drug has a disadvantage purely by reason of mathematics. Rare adverse effects of a drug used by 10,000 people will probably go undetected but not so when taken by millions of patients.

[31] Or clients depending on your POV.

[32] Dolder CR, Nelson MH (2008) Hypnosedative-induced complex behaviours: incidence, mechanisms and management. CNS Drugs 22:1021–1036; Inagaki T et al. (2010) Adverse reactions to zolpidem: case reports and a review of the literature. Prim Care Companion J Clin Psychiatry 12(6).

[33] Cartwright R (2004) Sleepwalking violence: a sleep disorder, a legal dilemma, and a psychological challenge. Am J Psychiatry 161:1149–5118; Pressman MR (2007) Disorders of arousal from sleep and violent behavior: the role of physical contact and proximity. Sleep 30:1039–1047.

[34] Paradis CM et al. (2012) Two cases of zolpidem-associated homicide. Prim Care Companion CNS Disord 14: Epub 2012 Aug 23.

[35] Manfredi G et al. (2010) Command hallucinations with self-stabbing associated with zolpidem overdose. J Clin Psychiatry 71:92–93.

Suicidal behavior with amnesia after a 10 mg dose of Ambien® was reported in a 37-year-old man who was taking chronic zolpidem at 5 mg per night, then due to increasing problems of insomnia, increased his dose one night to 10 mg.[36] The next day he was brought to the hospital by the police after a call from his wife. He remembers going to sleep at 10:30 pm but had no memory of events that transpired after that. His wife documented that at 1:30 am she heard a gunshot in the basement. His wife confronted him when he walked upstairs, but he was incoherent, and held a gun to his neck. She managed to talk him into setting the gun down but he wanted to go get two more guns in the garage. He was incoherent and disorientated during the whole episode and his wife called the police. Later psychiatric assessment revealed that he had no prior or current diagnosis, and no signs of depression or posttraumatic stress disorder. He denied any history of prior or current suicidal or homicidal thoughts.

A case report associating zolpidem use with suicidal behavior reported in 2011 bears a striking resemblance to this chapter's index case of CEO Ross Martini. A 49-year-old man with no prior psychiatric history was admitted to the hospital with an apparently self-inflicted gunshot wound to the head.[37] The injury was due to a .22 caliber bullet that had been fired left-to-right through both eye orbits resulting in destruction of his right eye and significant damage to the left eye, leaving him totally blind. History was initially obtained from his wife and family, and they denied observing any signs of depression or other indication that he had been considering self-harm. His wife reported that on the night of his injury, he had been watching television and after he had gone to bed, she heard a gunshot and found him wounded. He had an extensive military career, firearms expertise, and collection of high caliber handguns all located in his bedroom and capable of causing much greater damage than the .22 handgun kept on his nightstand. Furthermore, he had been looking forward to an upcoming visit from his son and newborn grandchild who lived in another state. His wife reported that he had recently been started on zolpidem (Ambien®) for insomnia. She did not know if he had taken zolpidem on the night of his admission, and no zolpidem levels had been drawn on admission. The man's mental status improved over the next few weeks and he steadfastly denied shooting himself, noting the last thing he remembered was going to bed that night. He was unable to specifically recall whether he had taken zolpidem that evening. While he vehemently denied any suicidal ideation, he specifically stated that if he had wished to shoot himself, he would certainly have used a larger caliber weapon. Later follow-up at 6 months revealed no additional information indicating that he had attempted suicide, and he continued to deny any deliberate self-harm.

The commonalities found in most of the previous studies are that the recommended dosages of zolpidem (5 or 10 mg) were taken as directed, patients did not previous or after-the-event diagnoses of psychiatric disorders, and that the psychosis, delirium, and/or hallucinations ended with the wearing off of the zolpidem drug effect. The simple observation that psychotic reactions abate after zolpidem is removed from the body is a strong argument for a causal association of zolpidem and psychotic adverse effects.[38]

In the United States, a large study of 5692 household respondents between 2001 and 2003 revealed that prescription use of hypnotics (primarily zolpidem) increased the odds of suicidal thoughts 2.2 times, suicide plans 1.9 times, and actual suicide attempts 3.4 times.[39] A case-controlled study of suicide among the elderly found that even after adjustment for all psychiatric disorders, sedative-hypnotics remained an independent risk factor for suicide, increasing the likelihood by 14 times.[40] Using on odds-ratio approach to analyze voluntarily reported adverse effects of zolpidem use in Australia from 2001 to 2008, it was found that the zolpidem use increased the likelihood of reporting suicidal behavior as an adverse effect by 5.1 times compared to other drug groups.[29]

The incidence of serious adverse effects noted with zolpidem is not indicative of a class effect observed with all the "z-drugs." A 6-year study examined over 5000 instances of adverse effects from the use of zolpidem and from the use of

---

[36] Chopra A et al. (2013) Para-suicidal amnestic behavior associated with chronic zolpidem use: implications for patient safety. Psychosomatics 54:498-501.

[37] Gibson CE, Caplan JP (2011) Zolpidem-associated parasomnia with serious self-injury: a shot in the dark. Psychosomatics 52:88–91.

[38] Causality is thought of differently by scientists and the court. For a scientist, causality is very much linked to a significant difference, meaning 95% or greater certainty. Depending on jurisdiction, the court recognizes contributory causes and primary, sole, or major causes. These are at the certainty level of a "preponderance of evidence" or "more likely than not" and correlate to 51% or greater level of certainty. There are more formal methods for establishing causality of adverse drug reactions (ADR) involving complex algorithms and probability scales. See: Koh Y et al. (2010) Development of a combined system for identification and classification of adverse drug reactions: Alerts Based on ADR Causality and Severity (ABACUS). J Am Med Inform Assoc. 17:720-722; Reps JM et al. (2015) A supervised adverse drug reaction signaling framework imitating Bradford Hill's causality considerations. J Biomed Inform. 56:356–368.

[39] Brower KJ et al. (2011) Prescription sleeping pills, insomnia, and suicidality in the National Comorbidity Survey Replication. J Clin Psychiatry 72:515–521.

[40] Carlsten A, Waern M (2009) Are sedatives and hypnotics associated with increased suicide risk of suicide in the elderly? BMC Geriatr 9:20; Pae et al. (2011) Association of sedative-hypnotic medications with suicidality. Expert Rev Neurother 11:345–349.

zaleplon (Sonata®). They found that there were more CNS side effects after zolpidem use than after zaleplon use.[28] These results confirmed a greater degree of CNS adverse effects after zolpidem exposure compared to zaleplon as noted in previous studies.[41]

Examining Pharmacokinetics for Drug Dose and Time

Pharmacokinetics is the study of drug movement after administration. Pharmacokinetic data about the drug of interest provides a method to compare the drug concentration from the toxicology report with the results obtained in clinical studies using repeated blood sampling and testing for the drug concentration at various times after drug administration. This section uses the real-life chapter case of the zolpidem blood concentrations measured in the decedent as an example methodology. Every time the drug expert is provided with an amount of a drug (in ng/mL) in a blood sample, this amount should be compared with the blood concentrations of the drug at therapeutic levels in a clinical population. While a single value of drug blood concentration is not definitive, it can provide additional information concerning time of drug ingestion and frequency of use. It is an extremely useful exhibit to display the drug concentration of the plaintiff, defendant, or decedent on top of a published time course curve from a clinical study. An example of this method is given in Fig. 15.1.

Zolpidem is available in two main formulations: Ambien® (immediate release) and Ambien CR® (controlled release). All forms of zolpidem are rapidly absorbed after oral administration. Peak zolpidem levels occur in the blood from 30 to 60 min after ingestion and absorption is delayed with food.[42] Following administration of a single 12.5 mg dose of Ambien CR®, the peak blood concentration of zolpidem occurred at 1.5 h after ingestion (Ambien CR® Prescribing Information).

Zolpidem is extensively metabolized in the liver by the CYP3A4 enzyme and produces no active metabolites. The half-life of elimination of zolpidem ranges from 2.4 to 3.5 h.[43] Therapeutic levels of zolpidem in the blood range from 100 to 200 ng/mL, with fatal overdoses of zolpidem greater than 4000 ng/mL in postmortem blood samples.[44] Postmortem redistribution of zolpidem has been noted by differences from cardiac and peripheral sampling sites (1.5- to 3-fold difference), emphasizing the preferred sampling from peripheral sites.[45]

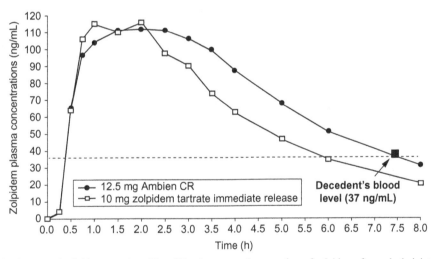

FIG. 15.1 Pharmacokinetic curve of zolpidem over time. Plot of blood concentration over time of zolpidem after oral administration of 10 mg zolpidem immediate release or 12.5 mg zolpidem controlled release (Ambien CR®) formulations. The blood level of zolpidem from the decedent (37 ng/mL) is indicated on the plot by a filled square added by the author. The horizontal dashed line is a 35 ng/mL reference line added by the author. *(Adapted from Fig. 1 in* Ambien CR® Full Prescribing Information *(the "label") approved by the FDA and available on their website.)*

[41] Barbera J, Shapiro C (2005) Benefit-risk assessment of zaleplon in the treatment of insomnia. Drug Saf 28:301-318; Holm KJ, Goa KL (2000) Zolpidem: an update of its pharmacology, therapeutic efficacy and tolerability in the treatment of insomnia. Drugs 59:865-889; Israel AG, Kramer JA (2002) Safety of zaleplon in the treatment of insomnia. Ann Pharmacother 36:852–859; Kurta DL et al. (1997) Zolpidem (AMBIEN): a pediatric case series. J Toxicol Clin Toxicol 35:453–457.

[42] Darcourt G et al. (1999) The safety and tolerability of zolpidem—an update. J Psychopharmacol 13:81-93.

[43] Allard S et al. (1998) Minimal interaction between fluoxetine and multiple-dose zolpidem in healthy women. Drug Metab Disp. 26:617–22; Darcourt G et al. (1999) *Ibid.*

[44] Gunja N (2013) The clinical and forensic toxicology of Z-drugs. J Med Toxicol 9:155–62.

[45] Drummer OH (2004) Postmortem toxicology of drugs of abuse. Forensic Sci Int 142:101–13; Han E et al. (2012) Evaluation of postmortem redistribution phenomena for commonly encountered drugs. Forensic Sci Int 219:265–71.

In most cases when a toxicology report[46] is available, the drug expert needs to interpret the drug concentration by examining a concentration over time curve. These curves are familiar to the drug expert and rather simple in their presentation of data. The vertical line[47] on the graph is the range of concentration of the drug in the blood (see Fig. 15.1). The horizontal line is the time after drug administration, usually expressed in minutes or hours. In the present chapter case, it was important to determine if the postmortem blood concentration of zolpidem (Ambien®) was consistent with Ambien® use as directed by his physician. Otherwise, perhaps the decedent was abusing Ambien® or taking an overdose of Ambien® to commit suicide. The following figure is a graph of the concentration of Ambien® in the blood of patients from a clinical study included in the full prescribing information.[48] The blood concentrations of Ambien® were plotted over time after taking a 12.5 mg tablet of *Ambien CR*®, the controlled release formulation of Ambien®. To show the decedent's level of zolpidem in the present chapter case, a black box and legend is placed onto the image of the graph.[49] As the decedent's level of zolpidem (37 ng/mL) is close to the average concentration obtained in the standard curve after 7.5 h, it is consistent with the decedent taking one Ambien® 12.5 CR tablet the night before his demise.

The Drug Expert and Big Pharma Litigation

Prescribed drugs, also known as prescription medications, are a product like any other manufactured product. Pharmaceutical drug manufacturers, fondly known as *Big Pharma*, are responsible for the safety of their products. Injury from the use of a drug to one party (the plaintiff) can be redressed by filing a civil lawsuit against the drug manufacturer (the defendant). The physician that prescribed the drug is also usually named in a lawsuit. The drug expert can be of service to either side to provide testimony on the presence or absence of a drug's adverse effects.

Pharmaceutical manufacturers are obligated to consumers to make sure that the drug products they sell are reasonably safe when taken as directed.[50] For this reason, the manufacturer must undertake years of research and clinical trials to identify the adverse effects and risks of the drug before it is marketed. FDA approval of the drug is not enough; the manufacturer must also make sure that proper labeling and warnings are included with the drug so that physicians and patients are duly informed of the risks associated with prescribing and taking the medication.

Most pharmaceutical tort cases are *failure to warn* cases. However, in these cases the liability of the drug manufacturer is limited by the *learned intermediary doctrine* as the relationship from the manufacturer is directed to the prescribing physician and not to the consumer. The drug manufacturer is limited as long as it has sufficiently warned the physician of the adverse effects and all the risks associated with prescribing the particular drug. It is the physician that has the duty to warn the patient and be aware of the prescribing dangers as the *learned intermediary*. If the physician is not aware of the dangers, fails to heed the manufacturer's warnings, or does not advise the patient of the drug's risks, then the physician may be found negligent and liable for resulting injuries to the patient.

Pharmaceutical manufacturers can still be sued under four main types of claims: *inadequate warnings*, *breach of warranty*, *design defects*, and *manufacturing defects*. Inadequate warning (or "failure to warn") is the most common liability claim against drug makers and occurs when the information supplied in the drug label (package insert) is not accurate, clear, and/or consistent, and does not convey the degree of risk that the drug may produce. A breach of warranty may occur if the information provided to the physician is proven to be false. Design defects refer to a case whereby the drug maker markets a drug that is inherently unsafe; one that a reasonable drug maker would not have marketed given its risk-to-benefit ratio. A claim of manufacturing defect may occur if the drug product does not meet its specification in terms of its formulation, performance standards, or intended result.[51]

Perhaps the most famous example of a pharmaceutical manufacturing defect occurred with the transdermal (or "patch") formulation of fentanyl, a powerful opioid analgesic. Fentanyl patches, marketed originally as Duragesic®, have a history of manufacturing defects and recalls due to leakage of the fentanyl gel from the drug reservoir in the patch. This can lead to inordinately high doses of fentanyl, with resulting respiratory depression and death.[52] As one can imagine, there were a number of fatalities from leaky gels and subsequent lawsuits filed against the makers of faulty Duragesic® and generic fentanyl patches.

---

[46] See Chapter 10 for further discussion of the Toxicology Report.

[47] The vertical line is also called the "y-axis" or the "ordinate." The horizontal line is known as the "x-axis" or "abscissa."

[48] Available from the manufacturer at *products.sanofi.us/ambien/ambien.pdf*.

[49] The tools to do this in Word are *Insert—Text box*—for legend text, and *Insert—Shapes*—for symbol.

[50] Much of this section is from Jasper MC (2005) Prescription drug litigation, Chapter 10. In: *Prescription Drugs*, Jasper MC, Oceana's Legal Almanac Series: Law for the Layperson, Oceana Publications, Inc., Dobbs Ferry, New York, USA.

[51] Jasper MC (2005) *Ibid.*

[52] FDA Drug Safety Communication (2008) PRICARA™ RECALLS 25 µg/hr DURAGESIC® (fentanyl transdermal system) CII PAIN PATCHES. At: *www.fda.gov/Safety/Recalls/ArchiveRecalls/2008/ucm112374.htm*.

Pharmaceutical tort cases against Ambien®

The adverse effects of Ambien® gained national attention when Congressman Joseph Kennedy (Democrat-Rhode Island) ran into a barrier on the capitol grounds at 2:45 am, telling capitol police that he was late for a vote. He was noted by the officers to act drunk but had no odor of alcohol. Investigation revealed that Kennedy was taking a legal prescription for zolpidem (Ambien®) for the treatment of insomnia. It was likely that an incident of sleep-driving occurred. Drug experts will often consult on Ambien® effects in cases of sleep-driving and motor vehicle accidents.

Since then, an increased number of Ambien lawsuits were filed including a class-action lawsuit of more than 500 Ambien users who gained significant body weight while taking Ambien®. Their claim was "failure to warn" as in most pharmaceutical tort cases. The index case for this chapter included the claim "failure to warn" against the manufacturer as well as "wrongful death" against the health care provider and the clinic where he worked.

In an ideal legal system, the drug expert (and all experts) would be hired by the Court.[53] This would supposedly remove *team* bias or any conscious or subconscious desire to do well for those that pay the drug expert. This would not remove any *personal* bias that the drug expert may have for the parties in the case. This may all be true. However, the drug expert that strays from the consensus of the current research findings and well-supported, evidence-based testimony will be a drug expert no longer.

[Narrative continued]

The drug expert began with a review of the decedent's medical records, pharmacy reports, and other case documents. A thorough search of the medical and pharmacological literature on Ambien®'s adverse effects was done. Numerous studies on the adverse effects of Ambien® were summarized and a thirty-page ligation report was prepared. The blood level of zolpidem in the deceased was consistent with his taking of one Ambien pill on the night before his death as directed. The drug expert concluded that the decedent was taking Ambien® as directed by his physician and not abusing it.

The litigation report showed that there is a convincing amount of case reports and clinical studies showing that a certain numbers of patients taking Ambien® will have adverse effects that may lead to suicide or homicide, sleep-driving, sleep-eating or other bizarre behavior. The case was stalled in the courts with a multitude of motions, banal legal maneuvers, and esoteric manipulations of the law that one would expect in a case of a mega-firm representing the makers of Ambien®. After 4 years, the defendants settled the case for an undisclosed amount.

---

[53] Federal district trial judges under Federal Rule of Evidence 706 can hire and pay for expert witnesses. However they rarely do. *See*: Worthington DL et al. (2002) Hindsight bias, Daubert, and the silicone breast implant litigation: Making the case for court-appointed experts in complex medical and scientific litigation. Psychology, Public Policy, and Law, Vol 8(2), Jun 2002, 154–179.

Chapter 16

Reefer Madness: Driving under the influence of marijuana

The State Legalization of Medical and Recreational Marijuana

Drugged Driving Laws—Marijuana and Driving Impairment

Using Private Drug Testing Laboratories—Training Programs for Drug Experts

[Narrative]

Dave Holland was a 23 year-old male living on his own and working for an auto parts store. One rainy night, after a long session of video games at a friend's apartment, Dave hit a motorcycle rider ahead of him on the downside of a bridge. The rider died of blunt trauma injuries after transport to the hospital. Under the state's Implied Consent Law which mandates a blood sample from any driver involved in a fatality, a blood sample was drawn from Mr. Holland about an hour after the accident and submitted to the state bureau of investigation and forensics lab. The forensics report from the state's toxicology lab reported that the concentration of THC, the main active ingredient of marijuana, was 2 ng/mL. The concentration of THC-COOH, the main inactive metabolite of THC, was 14 ng/mL. A civil case for negligence was filed by the family of the deceased. A lawyer representing the auto insurance company of Mr. Dave Holland contacted a drug expert for assistance in interpreting the levels of THC found in the defendant's blood sample.

In a second case, a tractor-trailer truck ran over a pedestrian at a large highway truck plaza. Mr. Jeff Bailey, the defendant, was driving the truck away from the fuel pumps. The decedent, Mr. José Fernández, was walking back to his car after purchasing a meal from the Subway® restaurant located in the truck plaza. As the defendant drove away from the fueling area and made a left turn, he struck and killed the decedent, hitting him with the passenger side of his vehicle. The decedent was dragged under the wheels of the moving truck until a witness flagged down the defendant and informed him that he ran over a pedestrian. Under the state's Implied Consent Law, the defendant submitted blood samples after the fatal motor vehicle accident with testing done at the state's forensic laboratory. Results of blood samples obtained from the truck driver showed the presence and confirmation of THC at a 10 ng/mL concentration, and its metabolite THC-COOH at a level of 110 ng/mL. A lawsuit was filed by the decedent's wife and family; their lawyer contacted a drug expert to interpret THC blood levels and investigate the potential behavioral impact of smoking marijuana on the operation of a motor vehicle.

The State Legalization of Medical and Recreational Marijuana

In the last decade or two, a *Green Revolution* has swept the populace of many states throughout the nation. This *Green Revolution* is not the one envisioned by 1960s eco-tribes and other environmentalist groups. The green in our case refers to the leaves and flowers of the marijuana plant, and the color of *money*, which is pouring into the cannabis industry and the state's coffers.[1] At the time of this writing, there are 33 states that legalized the possession and use of medical marijuana; 11 states and one district (DC) legalized both recreational and medical marijuana.[2] By the time you are reading this, it is likely the number of states with legal medical and/or recreational marijuana has already increased again.

---

[1] For example, in the first year after legalization of recreational marijuana (starting Feb. 2014), Colorado received $76 million in marijuana taxes. In the year ending Nov. 2018, state revenue from marijuana taxes was over $260 million.

[2] As of Jan 1, 2019, a total of 33 states, the District of Columbia, Guam and Puerto Rico have approved a comprehensive public medical marijuana/cannabis program. Recreational marijuana is legal in the District of Columbia and 10 states: Alaska, California, Colorado, Maine, Massachusetts, Michigan, Nevada, Oregon, Vermont, and Washington. See the National Conference of State Legislators (NCSL) website at: *www.ncsl.org/research/health/state-medical-marijuana-laws.aspx*.

A brief history of marijuana informs the current debate on the legalization of medical and recreational marijuana use. Marijuana use has long roots in human society. Its use has been traced back more than 12,000 years to primitive hunter-gatherers, and notes on medical use go back about 6000 years ago.[3] Marijuana was one of the goods that traveled the Silk Road from China to the Mideast and Europe. It was widely used by the ancient Greek, Roman, and Arabic societies. European imperialism spread marijuana use throughout the known world, eventually ending up in colonial America.

In the American colonies, the growing of hemp was encouraged and even mandated by colonial governments for the making of rope, sails, and clothing. Hemp is the fibrous stalks of the marijuana plant, and it is the dried flowers of the hemp plant that are used as marijuana. In the 1890s, marijuana was a common ingredient in numerous medicinal products and sold openly to the public in corner pharmacies. This all changed with the surge of immigration to the United States after the Mexican Revolution in 1910.[4] Without going into the sordid details, there is/was increasing crackdown on marijuana use fueled in part by racist views of the then-recent Mexican immigrants and the long-standing prejudice against African-Americans.[5] Antimarijuana propaganda proliferated in the 1930s, epitomized by the infamous cringe movie entitled *Reefer Madness*.[6] Eventually, the antidrug movement led to the Controlled Substances Act (CSA) passed in 1970, with marijuana placed along with Schedule I drugs such as LSD and heroin.[7] In this section, we concentrate on the state-based medical and recreational marijuana use laws and their impact on legal cases the drug expert might encounter.

State legalization of medical marijuana

California was the first state to legalize medical marijuana in 1996 after Proposition 215 passed by 55% of the voting populace.[8] Enacted as the *Compassionate Use Act*, it protects patients and defined caregivers who possess or cultivate marijuana for medical treatment approved by a physician from criminal laws which otherwise prohibit possession or cultivation of marijuana.

State laws legalizing marijuana are a bold move by state legislatures, thumbing their nose at the federal government in a show of state sovereignty. However, as previously stated, federal law trumps[9] state law. The CSA was passed by the authority of Congress under the Commerce Clause in the U.S. Constitution which essentially states that the "Congress shall have the Power to regulate Commerce among the several States."[10] The thinking was that illegal and legal drugs are sold (commerce) and shipped across state borders (among the several states) so Congress can make laws and regulate drugs. That the Commerce Clause is at the heart of the CSA was confirmed by SCOTUS in *Gonzales v. Raich*.[11] This case was sent up from the U.S. Court of Appeals for the Ninth Circuit in California, where medical marijuana was legal under state law. Angel Raich was growing marijuana plants for her own medicinal use legally under California's *Compassionate Use Act*, but filed an injunction to prevent criminal charges and to reverse the seizure of her marijuana plants by the DEA. She maintained that Congress does not have the power in the CSA to regulate home-grown marijuana for personal medical use. SCOTUS disagreed and affirmed that the Commerce Clause applies to this case as there is no guarantee that the home-grown marijuana wouldn't pervade the interstate market and that the class activity of growing marijuana has a de facto effect on the natural marijuana market, for example, by reducing the price of marijuana. The feds won the case. The DEA and other federal enforcement agencies can decide at any point to enforce federal drug laws. They can seize and destroy personal stashes of marijuana and also the many acres of commercial marijuana crops. The cannabis industry received about $40 billion dollars in sales in 2018[12] and federal enforcement agencies under present drug laws could justifiably confiscate those monies.

Federal intervention in state marijuana use laws were curtailed during the Obama administration by the issuance of the Cole memo.[13] In 2016 Congress passed laws that supported state sovereignty, enacting the *Rohrabacher-Blumenauer Amendment*, which denies the use of federal funds to "to prevent any of them [States with medical marijuana] from

---

[3] Gessford JB, Knight JJ (2016) Legal "high"-lights in medical and recreational marijuana use by students and employees. Presented at the 2016 School Law Practice Seminar, October 20–22, Portland, OR.

[4] Marijuana timeline, from *Busted: America's war on marijuana*, Frontline, PBS at: *www.pbs.org/wgbh/pages/frontline/shows/dope/etc/cron.html*.

[5] See NPR article at: *www.kqed.org/lowdown/24153/reefer-madness-the-twisted-history-of-americas-weed-laws*.

[6] Movie information from *www.imdb.com/title/tt0028346/?ref_=ttpl_pl_tt*.

[7] Chapter 11 gave further information on the CSA and Anti-Drug Laws in general.

[8] Cambron C et al. (2017) State and national contexts in evaluating cannabis laws: a case study of Washington State. J Drug Iss. 47:74–90.

[9] No reference to #45 intended.

[10] U.S. Constitution, Art. 1, §8, cl. 3. See also Rosenbaum (2011) Law and the public's health. Public Health Reports 126:750–753.

[11] *Gonzales v. Raich*, 545 U.S. 1 (2005). Cited as *Raich* v. *Ashcroft* in lower courts.

[12] *Cannabis capitalism: who is making money in the marijuana industry?* The Guardian, Oct 3, 2018.

[13] Memorandum for US Attorneys: Guidance Regarding the Ogden Memo in Jurisdictions Seeking to Authorize Marijuana for Medical Use. Washington, DC: Office of the Deputy Attorney General James M. Cole; June 29, 2011.

implementing their own laws that authorize the use, distribution, possession, or cultivation of medical marijuana."[14] However, during President Trump's administration, Attorney General Jeff Sessions issued a memo that rescinded prior DOJ memos stating "previous nationwide guidance specific to marijuana enforcement is unnecessary and is rescinded, effective immediately."[15]

Opponents to the legalization of medical marijuana point to the fact that there are three FDA-approved medicines containing THC, the active ingredient of marijuana, or a THC-like analog.[16] Dronabinol is the generic name of THC, with the exact same chemical structure as the naturally made THC in marijuana. Dronabinol is marketed under the brand name of Marinol®, in a formulation of dronabinol (THC) mixed in sesame oil inside a gelatin capsule. Dronabinol is approved for cancer-induced nausea and the anorexia associated with HIV. The Marinol® branding only covers the oral pill form, there is another dronabinol (THC) medicine called Syndros® made only in an oral liquid formulation. Syndros® oral formulation is easier to take and properly dose than Marinol® by cancer patients and other patients suffering from nausea and vomiting.[17] The third cannabinoid drug approved by the FDA for treatment of cancer-induced nausea and vomiting is nabilone (Cesamet®).[18] Unlike Marinol® and Syndros®, nabilone is not the same chemical as THC but is a synthetic THC analog. Synthetic cannabinoids generally exert more adverse effects than THC, and even result in life-threatening toxicity.[19]

Much of the debate for legalizing medical use of marijuana depends on the evidence for its safe and effective use. Medical use of marijuana is not new to humans and was used since the time of the ancients for such purposes as relaxing the uterus in childbirth, treating nausea and vomiting, and for relief of headache and insomnia, among other ailments.[20] A large literature exists in medical and pharmacological journals examining the effects of marijuana on various ailments, often with placebo controls and significant findings. Perhaps the most trusted work was the recent release of a National Academy of Sciences report entitled "The Health Effects of Cannabis and Cannabinoids: The Current State of Evidence and Recommendations for Research."[21] While the most convincing evidence for medical marijuana was found for the treatment of chronic pain, muscle spasm, and the nausea and vomiting that following chemotherapy, the report calls for more research on the beneficial and adverse effects of medical marijuana. For that reason, the National Academies of Sciences support the rescheduling of marijuana from Schedule I to Schedule II so that clinicians and researchers can more readily obtain marijuana for research.

Use of medical marijuana substitutes for the use of alcohol and other drugs. Perhaps one of the most promising results of medical marijuana legalization is the decrease in prescription opioid overdose deaths. Young and old individuals across the country are dropping like flies from an opioid overdose epidemic. Just now, while reading the last sentence and this present one, another person died in the United States from an opioid overdose.[22]

A study in 2014 examined opioid overdose deaths on an annual basis before and after enactment of medical marijuana laws.[23] It was found that legalization of medical marijuana resulted in an average decrease of 25% fewer opioid overdose deaths compared to the number of opioid deaths in the year before enactment. With over 47,600 opioid deaths across the nation in 2017, a federal medical marijuana law might save as many as 12,000 lives per year.[24] Among California medical marijuana patients using marijuana for treatment of pain conditions, 97% of these patients reported that they were able to decrease their use of opioid medications.[25] Medical cannabis was associated with a 64% reduction in opioid use and

---

[14] Gostin LO et al. (2018) Enforcing federal drug laws in states where medical marijuana is lawful. JAMA 319:1435–1436.

[15] Memorandum for US Attorneys: Marijuana Enforcement. Washington, DC: Office of the Attorney General Jeff Sessions; Jan. 4, 2018.

[16] This does not include CBD (cannabidiol) another drug found in marijuana but does not produce the psychoactive effects of THC. CBD is effective in the treatment of epilepsy and other ailments and was recently approved by the FDA (brand name Epidiolex®) for treatment of such.

[17] Badowski ME, Yanful PK (2018) Dronabinol oral solution in the management of anorexia and weight loss in AIDS and cancer. Ther Clin Risk Manag. 14:643–651.

[18] Ware MA et al. (2008) A review of nabilone in the treatment of chemotherapy-induced nausea and vomiting. Ther Clin Risk Manag. 4:99–107.

[19] See Chapter 11 *I Want a New Drug.*

[20] Bostwick JM et al. (2012) Blurred boundaries: the therapeutics and politics of medical marijuana. Mayo Clin Proc. 87:172–186.

[21] National Academies of Sciences, Engineering, and Medicine (2017) The health effects of cannabis and cannabinoids: The current state of evidence and recommendations for research. Washington, DC: The National Academies Press. The National Academies of Sciences is a private, non-profit organization made up of the leading researchers and policy analysts in Medicine, Engineering, and the Sciences.

[22] Opioid overdoses death includes death from heroin (an opioid), morphine, oxycodone, and other prescription opioids, or more likely, fentanyl-spiked "heroin" which is cheap and widely available from Chinese chemical plants.

[23] Bachhuber MA et al. (2014) Medical cannabis laws and opioid analgesic overdose mortality in the United States, 1999-2010. JAMA Intern Med. 174:1668–1673.

[24] Granted the 2017 data already includes states with medical marijuana, therefore a 25% reduction may not be fully realized. Data from the CDC at: *www.cdc.gov/drugoverdose/data/statedeaths.html.*

[25] Reiman A et al. (2017) Cannabis as a substitute for opioid-based pain medication: patient self-report. Cannabis Cannabinoid Res. 2:160–166.

improved quality of life with less adverse effects among chronic pain patients.[26] A study of Medicare prescriptions for seniors in states with medical marijuana saw a significant decrease in prescriptions for opioid medications as well as drugs to treat depression, anxiety, nausea, psychoses, seizures, and sleep disorders.[27]

State legalization of recreational marijuana

The arguments for medical marijuana are easily understandable and well defined. The reasons to legalize the recreational use of marijuana are less clear. A major concern is an increase in adolescent use of marijuana after legalization. Rates of adolescent marijuana use have not uniformly increased in states after legalizing recreational marijuana, with Colorado showing no increase and Washington showing a slight increase.[28] However, traffic fatalities with positive marijuana toxicology tests increased after legalization in Colorado.[29] Also, the ER admittance of children with marijuana intoxication increased by over 30% in states that legalize recreational marijuana.[30] Most pediatric intoxications result from edibles, often in the form of THC-infused gummy-bears, cookies, and the like. State regulators might consider banning edibles in candy and cookie formulations. The crucial fact comparing opioids and cannabinoids is that THC overdose does not and cannot produce fatality, in stark contrast to opioid drugs which kill pretty easily. Using medical marijuana instead of opioid pain-killers totally removes any possibility of overdose harms for the individual user and cohabiting family members. Dose escalation over time, or drug tolerance, occurs quite readily with the use of chronic opioids whereas increased cannabinoid doses over time are not observed.[31]

There appears to be a further decrease in opioid mortality after a state moves from medical marijuana use laws to both medical and recreational marijuana laws.[32] A study of opioid deaths revealed that "broader access to medical marijuana facilitates substitution of marijuana for powerful and addictive opioids."[33] Like after medical marijuana laws (above), prescription opioid use as tracked by Medicare records was reduced by over 30% following the legalization of recreational marijuana.[34]

Pharmacologically speaking, it would be better for the many people with symptoms that cannabis can treat, like chronic pain, to smoke a marijuana joint than take a pharmaceutical pill that might produce a severe and fatal addiction.[35] Legalization of recreational marijuana lowers the threshold for using marijuana in a medicinal way, especially for the multitude of individuals in our lop-sided society who cannot afford $150 or $250 needed to obtain a medical marijuana card.

Drugged Driving Laws

There is only one drug whose level in the blood can be reliably correlated with driving impairment. That drug is alcohol. Alcohol is the most researched drug in the world, and a multitude of alcohol studies over the last 100 years shows a clear relationship between blood alcohol concentrations and driving impairment.[36]

Excluding alcohol, which has a legally set impairment level of 0.08% BAC (blood alcohol concentration) there are no scientifically accepted levels of impairment for blood concentrations of other legal and illegal drugs. As early as 1985, the National Institute on Drug Abuse recognized that, except for ethanol, the determinations of drug concentrations in body fluids are of limited value for establishing driving impairment.[37] This report concludes that although psychoactive drugs are the types of prescription and illegal drugs most commonly thought to cause impairment, their mere presence in the blood or other body fluids cannot be construed as evidence of impairment. A report from the National Safety Council in 2004 similarly acknowledged that "there is no clear correlation between blood drug concentrations and impairment for

---

[26] Boehnke KF et al. (2016) Medical cannabis use is associated with decreased opiate medication use in a retrospective cross-sectional survey of patients with chronic pain. J Pain 17:739–744.

[27] Bradford AC, Bradford WD (2016) Medical marijuana laws reduce prescription medication use in Medicare part D. Health Aff. 35:1230–1236.

[28] Hasin DS (2018) US epidemiology of cannabis use and associated problems. Neuropsychopharmacol. 43:195–212.

[29] Bondallaz P et al. (2016) Cannabis and its effects on driving skills. Forensic Sci Int. 268:92–102.

[30] Kim HS, Monte AA (2016) Colorado cannabis legalization and its effect on emergency care. Ann Emerg Med. 68:71–75.

[31] MacCallum CA, Russo EB (2018) Practical considerations in medical cannabis administration and dosing. Eur J Intern Med. 49:12–19.

[32] Livingston MD et al. (2017) Recreational cannabis legalization and opioid-related deaths in Colorado, 2000-2015. Am J Public Health 107:1827–1829.

[33] Powell D et al. (2018) Do medical marijuana laws reduce addictions and deaths related to pain killers? J Health Econ. 58:29–42.

[34] Shi Y et al. (2019) Recreational marijuana legalization and prescription opioids received by Medicaid enrollees. Drug Alcohol Depend. 194:13–19.

[35] Don't get me wrong, THC is an addictive drug, just not as addictive as the other ones. For example, nicotine is often found to be the most addicting drug, with transition to drug dependence a whopping 67.5% for nicotine users, 22.7% for alcohol users, 20.9% for cocaine users, and 8.9% for cannabis users. Lopez-Quintero C et al. (2011) Probability and predictors of transition from first use to dependence on nicotine, alcohol, cannabis, and cocaine: results of the National Epidemiologic Survey on Alcohol and Related Conditions (NESARC). Drug Alcohol Depend. 115:120–130.

[36] See next chapter for more information on alcohol and driving.

[37] National Institute on Drug Abuse (NIDA) (1985) Consensus report. Drug concentrations and driving impairment. Consensus Development Panel from NIDA. JAMA 254:2618–2621.

many drugs."[38] The report concluded that in "DUI cases involving alcohol, a clear understanding has developed over the past 50 years regarding the relationship between increasing blood concentration and impairment. The same cannot be said for drugs." In 2003 a report from the U.S. Department of Transportation entitled "State of Knowledge of Drug-Impaired Driving" confirmed that there is a lack of correlation between illicit drug concentrations and psychomotor impairment.[39] They concluded that experts in the field do not agree on specific blood concentrations of psychoactive drugs that could be designated as evidence of impairment. In a 2009 report to Congress, the National Highway Traffic Safety Administration stated that "The ability to predict an individual's performance at a specific dosage of drugs other than alcohol is limited."[40] Indeed, at a 2012 joint meeting of the Office of National Drug Control Policy (ONDCP) and the NHTSA, experts realized that determining threshold levels of drug concentrations for impairment is nearly impossible and that "the determination of such thresholds for even the common impairing drugs would require decades of research."[41] In spite of the wide acceptance that the sufficient studies have not yet ripened to yield reliable data, governments have imposed drugged driving laws that include blood levels of commonly used drugs. With regard to marijuana, a summary of a 2015 NHTSA Expert Panel on Legalization/Decriminalization of Marijuana states that in crafting new drugged driving laws, "Avoid per se levels. The science does not support them."[42]

Per se drugged driving laws

Per se (Latin for "by itself") drug laws impose charges of driving while under the influence of drugs when a driver's blood sample contains a given concentration of a drug or the detection of *any* amount of drug, the latter being the special case of a *zero per se* law. As an example of the first type of *per se* law, it is illegal to drive with a blood alcohol concentration (BAC) at or above 0.08%. This BAC level is consistent in all state jurisdictions, U.S. districts, and territories as a bright line dividing nonimpaired from alcohol-impaired drivers. For other drugs, the states may have different *per se* laws concerning the same drug. For example, both Colorado and Washington set their marijuana *per se* drugged driving laws at a THC blood level of 5 ng/mL (nanogram per milliliter). But for Oklahoma, with a *zero per se* law in place such that detection of *any* amount of a Schedule I controlled substance, like THC, is punishable as driving under the influence. The text of the Oklahoma statute is given as follows:

§47-11-902. Persons under the influence of alcohol or other intoxicating substance or combination thereof - Penalty - Enhancement.

A. It is unlawful and punishable as provided in this section for any person to drive, operate, or be in actual physical control of a motor vehicle within this state, whether upon public roads, highways, streets, turnpikes, other public places or upon any private road, street, alley or lane which provides access to one or more single or multi-family dwellings, who:

1. Has a blood or breath alcohol concentration, as defined in Section 756 of this title, of eight-hundredths (0.08) or more at the time of a test of such person's blood or breath administered within two (2) hours after the arrest of such person;

2. Is under the influence of alcohol;

3. **Has any amount of a Schedule I chemical or controlled substance**, as defined in Section 2-204 of Title 63 of the Oklahoma Statutes, or one of its metabolites or analogs in the person's blood, saliva, urine or any other bodily fluid at the time of a test of such person's blood, saliva, urine or any other bodily fluid administered within two (2) hours after the arrest of such person;

4. Is under the influence of any intoxicating substance other than alcohol which may render such person incapable of safely driving or operating a motor vehicle; or

5. Is under the combined influence of alcohol and any other intoxicating substance which may render such person incapable of safely driving or operating a motor vehicle.

---

[38] National Safety Council (NSC) (2004) Priorities and Strategies for Improving the Investigation, Use of Toxicology Results, and Prosecution of Drug-Impaired Driving Cases (available on website).

[39] Department of Transportation (DOT) (2003) State of Knowledge of Drug-Impaired Driving (available on website).

[40] National Highway Traffic Safety Administration (NHTSA) (2009) Drug-Impaired Driving: Understanding the Problem and Ways to Reduce It: A Report to Congress (available from website).

[41] Office of National Drug Control Policy (ONDCP) (2012) Roundtable on the Role of Drug Testing Technology in the Drugged Driving Criminal Justice Process: The Challenge, a Vision and a Path Forward (available on website).

[42] 2015 NHTSA Expert Panel on Legalization/Decriminalization of Marijuana on DWI—Highlights. At: *www.ghsa.org/sites/default/files/2017-06/ncrep_062617.pdf*.

B. The fact that any person charged with a violation of this section is or **has been lawfully entitled to use alcohol or a controlled dangerous substance or any other intoxicating substance shall not constitute a defense against any charge of violating this section.**

[bold added][43]

As noted before by numerous high-level agencies, there is not yet enough research or results to set a reliable *per se* limit on any drug except alcohol. States with a draconian *zero per se* drugged driving law however, go too far as THC can be detected in the blood for weeks after last use. As technology improves, smaller and smaller amounts may be detectable until the point of smoking a joint months ago may be detectable in suspect individuals.

It may also be obvious to the reader that the *Green Revolution* will increase the need for drug experts in every state that legalizes medical and/or recreational marijuana. There may also be cases of medical malpractice against a physician who recommended medical marijuana use and adverse effects occurred. Most cases will likely center on the use of marijuana and driving impairment. This is the topic of the next section.

Marijuana and Driving Impairment

While the previous policy statements show that the medical and scientific consensus at the present time does not allow a correlation of THC or any drug blood levels to the degree of driving impairment, there are clinical studies which examine performance on tasks thought to be needed for driving. In one study, marijuana smoking impaired one performance test (tracking) but not motor reaction or cognitive tests at levels between 2 and 5 ng/mL THC.[44] Another review noted that increasing THC blood levels above 5 ng/mL impairs automatic performance but there was no change in tests requiring cognitive control until a level of THC at 10 ng/mL is reached.[45]

One review on marijuana and driving suggested that a THC level in the blood of 7–10 ng/mL was equal to a blood alcohol concentration (BAC) of 0.05%.[46] While 0.05% BAC is below the legal limit of alcohol use and driving in the United States (set at 0.08%), there are clear signs of driving impairment at 0.05% BAC and a significant number of lives could be saved by lowering the legal limit to 0.05% BAC.[47]

Another study noted that an elevated risk of motor vehicle accidents in marijuana users occurs at a THC threshold of 6 ng/mL.[48] Other reviews have suggested that an elevated risk of impaired driving does not occur until THC levels are >10 ng/mL.[49] The risk of a motor vehicle accident (MVA) with injury was doubled in the first 2 h after smoking marijuana but there was no increased risk of MVA injury after 3 h.[50] This study went on to report that MVAs where the driver was only positive for THC and no other drugs, the median blood THC level was 12 ng/mL. In 84% of the apprehended drivers, the blood THC levels were equal to or greater 5 ng/mL.

The State of Washington, among the first states to legalize the use of recreational marijuana, set a *per se* legal limit for THC of 5 ng/mL. Colorado has a permissive inference law also at a level of THC at 5 ng/mL.[51] A systematic review of the science behind establishing THC limits and driving laws suggests that legal limits for THC in blood samples should range from 7 to 10 ng/mL. This range "safely avoids misclassification of drivers presenting with THC residues from previous cannabis use."[52]

In summary, marijuana use can cause driving impairment at THC blood levels >5–10 ng/mL. This is consistent with Colorado and Washington state driving laws setting THC legal limits at 5 ng/mL. In the first chapter case, the driver that hit the motorcycle gave a blood sample that yielded a THC blood level of 2 ng/mL. This low level of THC is not associated with driving impairment or elevated risk in epidemiological studies. In the second case of this chapter, the trick driver that killed

---

[43] Universal Citation: 47 OK Stat § 47-11-902 (2014).

[44] Ramaekers JG et al. (2006) Cognition and motor control as a function of Delta9-THC concentration in serum and oral fluid: limits of impairment. Drug Alcohol Depend. 85:114–122

[45] Grotenhermen F et al. (2007) Developing limits for driving under cannabis. Addiction 102:1910–1917.

[46] Neavyn MJ et al. (2014) Medical marijuana and driving: a review. J Med Toxicol. 10:269–279.

[47] Fell JC, Voas RB (2006) The effectiveness of reducing illegal blood alcohol concentration (BAC) limits for driving: evidence for lowering the limit to .05 BAC. J Safety Res. 37:233–243.

[48] Grotenhermen F et al. (2007) *Op cit.*

[49] Armentano, P (2013) Should per se limits be imposed for cannabis? Equating cannabinoid blood concentrations with actual driver impairment: practical limitations and concerns. Humboldt J Social Relat. 35:45–55.

[50] Hartman RL, Huestis MA (2013) Cannabis effects on driving skills. Clin Chem. 59:10.1373/clinchem.2012.194381.

[51] Lee D et al. (2015) Plasma cannabinoid pharmacokinetics after controlled smoking and ad libitum cannabis smoking in chronic frequent users. J Anal Toxicol. 39:580–587.

[52] Grotenhermen F et al. (2007) *op cit.*

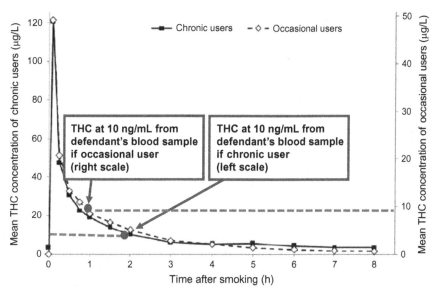

FIG. 16.1 Blood concentrations of THC in chronic and occasional users after smoking a standard marijuana cigarette (joint). Smoking began at time "0" on the horizontal axis and THC concentrations for Chronic users *(solid square symbols)* is on the left vertical axis and for Occasional users *(open diamonds)* on the right vertical axis. The truck driver's THC concentration is added as a *solid circle; boxes* and *dashed lines* also added. *Note*: μg/L=ng/mL. *(Reproduced from Toennes et al. (2008)[53].)*

a pedestrian gave a THC level of 10 ng/mL. This driver was likely impaired and more importantly, was within the window of marijuana's acute pharmacological effect as shown next.

Time of last marijuana use

Often the blood sample is obtained hours after an event so the court will be interested in the levels of THC at the time of the incident. There are two methods that can be used by the drug expert to determine the time of last marijuana use and the levels of THC at the time of the incident.

The first is a graphical method based on blood levels of THC obtained from clinical studies with volunteers smoking marijuana. Measurement of THC in the blood at various times after marijuana use was used to construct a concentration-time curve (see Fig. 16.1). One of the best studies examined both chronic users of marijuana and occasional users of marijuana, as THC is eliminated from the blood differently in these two groups of users.[53] The figure from that seminal paper is presented as follows and shows the blood concentrations of THC in chronic and occasional users after smoking a standard marijuana cigarette (joint). Superimposed on the figure are the data-points of the THC level of 10 ng/mL *(filled circles)* which was the level of THC obtained from the blood of the truck driver in our second case of this chapter.

The use of THC levels after smoking marijuana in both chronic and occasional smokers allows a good estimate of the range of time that marijuana was last used. In our example shown in the following figure, one can say that a level of 10 ng/mL equates with last use of marijuana from 1 to 2 h ago. In other words, no matter if the truck driver was a chronic user of marijuana or just an occasional smoker, it is more likely than not that he smoked marijuana 1–2 h before the blood draw, which is within the period of acute pharmacological effects of marijuana, and within the time of the incident. The low level of blood THC (2 ng/mL) in the chapter's first case ends up being at least 4–5 days after marijuana use (data not shown on graph).

The second method is more like that done for retrograde calculation of blood alcohol[54] and uses pharmacokinetic models and equations that were established and tested previously in clinical studies. In this method, the blood concentrations of THC alone, or THC and THC-COOH, are entered into equations. The equations yield estimates, in hours, from the time of marijuana use until the time of blood sampling. This method was developed by Marilyn Huestis and her colleagues and

---

[53] Toennes SW et al. (2008) Comparison of cannabinoid pharmacokinetic properties in occasional and heavy users smoking a marijuana or placebo joint. J Anal Toxicol. 32:470–477.

[54] See next Chapter.

vetted with clinical data.[55] While this method was verified with concurrent clinical determinations of THC levels over time, the confidence interval (range of values that are within 95% certainty) can be quite large and impractical when applied to a real case.

The first graphical method above usually works well for THC levels and any drug level versus time issues, as pharmacokinetic blood concentration over time curves like that found before are available for nearly all drugs. The graph also makes for a great exhibit in the courtroom as it is visually striking and can be explained to the jury by the drug expert.

Using Private Drug Testing Laboratories

One of the most important pieces of data for all criminal and civil cases impacted by drug use, which are many, is a toxicological report of drugs detected and quantified in a blood sample from the party of interest. In criminal cases, blood samples are often obtained during autopsy with a resulting toxicology report. A blood sample is obtained from the driver in a fatal MVA case under Implied Consent Law in many states. As elaborated in Chapter 8, there are two types of drug results: the first or preliminary drug test results and the second and confirmatory drug test results. As detailed in that chapter, preliminary drug tests are not probative and state and federal statutes[56] generally mandate a second and confirmatory drug test to posit a result. Certainly as a drug expert, testimony should be based on confirmed drug tests with attempts to force interpretation of preliminary drug test results thwarted.

The drug expert may facilitate the process to obtain forensic drug testing of the defendant's or decedent's blood sample. The hiring attorney may need assistance obtaining independent forensic testing to refute drug test results from state forensic laboratories offered by the prosecution. State jurisdictions, and different state agencies within that jurisdiction, vary on the length of time that the forensics lab must retain a parallel sample for use by the defendant or a civil party. In Oklahoma, the Office of the Chief Medical Examiner forensics laboratory puts a *hold status* of a blood sample for 5 years, whereas the Oklahoma State Bureau of Investigation, Forensic Science Center, vials of blood from *blood kits* used primarily for DUI or DWI purposes are retained for only 60 days.[57] Smart attorneys will be cognizant of the hold status of blood samples in their jurisdiction and the various state agencies and will consider timely consultation with a drug expert to interpret the test results and the possibility of getting an independent test done.[58]

There are a number of forensic drug testing laboratories across the country. The largest one is National Medical Services (NMS) Labs in Willow Grove, PA.[59] According to bloomberg.com, NMS Labs, Inc. has 2000 state, county, and city law enforcement and medical examiner clients in North America. NMS Labs performs more than half of all postmortem toxicology tests in the United States. Their forensic testing division is well versed in chain-of-custody procedures needed in criminal and civil cases. A partial listing of drug tests available by NMS Labs is listed in Appendix L.

Training Programs for Drug Experts

There is not a specific training program for drug experts at this time.[60] The book in your hands is the only resource at present for aspiring drug experts and attorneys who hire them. However, as a drug expert is a subclass of expert witnesses in general, there are many resources (books, DVDs, etc.) and programs available for the training of an expert witness. One organization is called SEAK (Skills, Education, Achievement, and Knowledge) and was founded over 30 years ago by an attorney.[61] Besides offering a number of books and DVDs on expert witness training and business, SEAK holds frequent workshops and seminars on various topics of interest to the budding expert witness. According to their website, SEAK is the world's leading provider of expert witness training and texts. SEAK has trained over 20,000 doctors, lawyers, nurses,

---

[55] Huestis MA et al. (2005) Estimating the time of last cannabis use from plasma delta 9-tetrahydrocannabinol and 11-nor-9-carboxy-delta^9-tetrahydrocannabinol concentrations. Clin Chem. 51:2289-2295. The equation for calculating the prior time of use from only the THC blood level is given in the paper by Model I: $\log t = -0.698 \log [\text{THC}] + 0.687$ (t = time in hours). Model II: $\log t = (0.576 \log [\text{THC-COOH}]/[\text{THC}]) - 0.176$, uses both THC and THC-COOH to calculate prior time of marijuana use. The calculation of the error variance is also given.

[56] Federal drug workplace rules are a good starting point for standards of drug testing.

[57] Toxicology Quality Manual (2017) Oklahoma State Bureau of Investigation (OSBI), Forensic Science Center.

[58] This was done in the case presented in Chapter 6 *Hairs of the Innocent*. The second drug test showed that the girl did not consume (eat or smoke) marijuana during her weekend stay with her father.

[59] At: *www.nmslabs.com*.

[60] Hopefully there will be training sessions soon. A website and organization was launched with the publication of this book. See *www.drugexpert.org* and join the effort.

[61] On the web at: *www.seak.com*.

expert witnesses, and other professionals. They also publish an expert witness directory that, for a fee, expert witnesses can include their contact information and areas of expertise.

[Narrative continued]

In the first case, the driver had a THC level of 2 ng/mL which the drug expert opined was too low enough to suggest that marijuana-induced impairment contributed to the MVA. Studies of marijuana driving impairment generally agree that the threshold for marijuana impairment is most likely above 5 ng/mL. A THC level of 2 ng/mL is the baseline level of THC in a chronic marijuana smoker as shown on the THC blood concentrations over time graph. This low THC level is found after 4–5 days post-marijuana use and long after the time of acute marijuana effects. Based on this finding elaborated in the drug expert's litigation report and during a deposition, the parties reached an agreement and a settlement was made.

In the second case, a blood sample from the truck driver obtained 1 h after the pedestrian fatality yielded a level of THC at 10 ng/mL and THC-COOH at 110 ng/mL. There is much scientific data to support driving impairment after marijuana use when the THC blood concentration is over 5–7 ng/mL. Additionally, because the blood level was obtained 1 h after the accident, the drug expert was able to testify that the THC level was higher at the time of the fatal MVA. The high levels of THC show that, more likely than not, the defendant was intoxicated with marijuana at the time of the accident. The estate of the decedent was able to obtain a large settlement from the employer of the truck driver.

Chapter 17

A Visit to the Dram Shop: Tequila shots and a traffic fatality

Dram Shop Law for the Drug Expert—Driving Under the Influence of Alcohol

The Use and Misuse of the Breathalyzer

Retrograde Calculation of Blood Alcohol Concentrations

Drug Recognition Experts—Marketing of the Drug Expert

[Narrative]
One evening, Mr. Henry Battler stopped at McKinneys, an Irish pub, and consumed five tequila-based alcoholic drinks over a three hour period. At approximately 1:30 am, Mr. Battler left the pub and proceeded to drive home. A mile from the pub, Mr. Battler ran a stop sign and crashed into the driver's side of a crossing vehicle. The driver was critically injured and died later that night at the hospital. A blood sample was obtained from Mr. Battler 90 min after the MVA which resulted in 0.72% BAC. The family of the decedent filed a civil lawsuit against Mr. Battler for wrongful death, and against the pub, in violation of the state's dram shop laws regarding the serving of alcohol to intoxicated patrons. The attorney hired by the decedents sought the counsel of a drug expert to calculate the BAC of Mr. Battles at the time of the fatal motor vehicle accident.

Dram Shop Law for the Drug Expert

"Dram shop" is an old 18th century English term for bars or pubs that sold alcohol. In London, gin was sold by the spoonful and called a "dram."[1] Dram shop laws, known more formally as commercial host liability laws, arose from the religious pressure exerted by the Temperance Movement in the mid-19th century.[2] The first statutes were in response to saloons profiting from selling alcohol to known habitual drunkards. The societal cost of alcoholism was recognized in the destruction of families. Alcoholics were demonized with religious zeal. The first dram shop statutes were limited in scope and unused during Prohibition. After Prohibition ended, these earlier statutes were either repealed or ignored. Up until the 1960s, commercial host liability was adjudicated by common law (case law)[3] which held that the drinker was entirely responsible for his actions and any resulting harms.

During the 1960s, state courts began to establish common law such that the drinker and the establishment that served the drinker were jointly held liable for resulting harms.[4] The gradual shift to include serving establishments in lawsuits represented the growing awareness that alcoholism was not simply a moral failure of a drunk but a chronic disease called alcoholism. Courts were also sensitive to the fact that many plaintiffs were unable to receive just compensation for their harms from an individual drinker. Courts also ruled that an injured victim was entitled to compensation when the alcohol retailer acted in a negligent and illegal manner.[5]

---

[1] Roberts JR and Dollard D (2010) Alcohol levels do not accurately predict physical or mental impairment in ethanol-tolerant subjects: relevance to emergency medicine and dram shop laws. J Med Toxicol. 6:438–442.

[2] Mosher JF et al. (2013) Commercial host (dram shop) liability. Am. J Prev Med. 45:347–353.

[3] As opposed to statutory law created by legislators.

[4] Mosher JF et al. (2013) *Op cit.*

[5] Strategizer 57 Reducing alcohol-related harms through Commercial Host, Community Anti-Drug Coalitions of America (CADCA) in partnership with the Center on Alcohol Marketing and Youth (CAMY) at JHSPH, available at: *www.camy.org/_docs/resources/reports/alcohol-availability/strategizer-57-commercial-host-liability.pdf.*

The Drug Expert. https://doi.org/10.1016/B978-0-12-800048-9.00017-1

At present, 42 states and the District of Columbia have a dram shop law in effect,[6] but they vary greatly in terms of liability, eligible parties, and other factors among the different states. It is not easy to prove that the alcohol vendor (bartender, e.g.) was negligent by serving an intoxicated patron. Some states have elements of proof that a plaintiff must meet in order to invoke the Dram Shop Act.[7] For example, there must be proof of sale of alcohol to the patron, injuries suffered by the patron, a proximate cause linking the alcohol sale and intoxication, and that alcohol intoxication was at least a contributing factor to any third-party damage.

Some states have only civil liability laws, whereas other states have both civil and criminal liability statutes for violating dram shop statutes.[8] While dram shop liability and social host liability (see later) are usually brought to court as civil suits, in cases of an innocent party's death from the behavior of an intoxicated person, both civil and criminal charges may be brought against him[9] and the retail establishment or bar that provided the alcohol. Only 10 states allow intoxicated patrons to sue the alcohol establishment if they only injure themselves. Dram shop liability laws are primarily designed to protect innocent third parties, like a person in another car killed by the intoxicated patron after leaving the bar.[10] Research shows that dram shop laws significantly reduce deaths due to drunk drivers.[11] Advocates for increasing the effectiveness of dram shop laws suggest a National Dram Shop Act that sets in place standards of liability, definitions, and penalties.[12]

Depending on the level of intoxication, it may not be easy to prove that the dram shop owner or bartender-server should have known the patron was inebriated and therefore not serve him alcohol. Studies show that experienced bartenders only correctly identified an intoxicated subject 25% of the time, even after watching them go up and down a staircase.[13] Nine out of 12 bartenders continued to serve a subject whose BAC was greater than 0.10%. Early studies show that 30 New Jersey police officers did worse than the bartenders in recognizing intoxicated persons, even after subjecting them to a field sobriety test. Later studies showed police officers were accurate only in detecting alcohol intoxication at higher BAC levels, above 0.12% BAC.[14]

Physicians were also not accurate in detecting alcohol intoxication levels by using clinical exams.[15] Surprisingly, one of the most reliable indicators among the physicians group was the smell of alcohol on the breath. This indication was shown to be reliable even in alcohol-tolerant individuals.[16]

Dram shop laws are gaining broader application as evidenced by the recent Oklahoma Supreme Court decisions for the plaintiff against a convenience store owner for selling beer to a presumably intoxicated buyer who then killed someone in an MVA.[17] There is also strong evidence and a call for dram shop laws to be enforced against valets so that they will not give car keys to an inebriated patron leaving an alcohol-serving establishment.[18]

Like dram shop liability, social host liability laws are also found in 33 states.[19] Social host liability laws hold the hosts of private functions, like a house party or pool party, liable for injuries (or death) caused by their negligence in serving alcohol to an inebriated guest, or not stopping an intoxicated guest from operating a motor vehicle. Although not as common as drug expert involvement in dram shop cases, a drug expert is also needed in a social liability case, for either the plaintiff or the defendant.

---

[6] Those states without dram shop laws are Delaware, Kansas, Louisiana, Maryland, Nebraska, Nevada, South Dakota, and Virginia.

[7] List taken from the Illinois Dram Shop Act. Findlaw.com at: *dui.findlaw.com/dui-laws-resources/dram-shop-laws.html.*

[8] NCSL website at: *www.ncsl.org/research/financial-services-and-commerce/dram-shop-liability-state-statutes.aspx.*

[9] Gender-specific language intended here as men are responsible for 4 in 5 incidences (81%) of alcohol DUIs. Young men of the ages 21–34 are responsible for 32% of all drunk driving accidents even though they represent only about 11% of the population. From the CDC at: *www.cdc.gov/vitalsigns/DrinkingAndDriving.*

[10] From Insureon, a food and beverage insurance company, at: *www.foodservices.insureon.com/portals/0/liquor-liability-insurance.pdf.*

[11] Scherer M et al. (2015) Effects of dram shop, responsible beverage service training, and state alcohol control laws on underage drinking driver fatal crash ratios. Traffic Inj Prev. 16:S59–S65.

[12] Cafaro TW (2006) You drink, you drive, you lose: or do you? Gonzaga Law Rev. 42:1–28.

[13] Rubenzer S (2011) Judging intoxication. Behav Sci Law 29:116–137.

[14] Rubenzer S (2011) *Op cit.*

[15] Kumar A et al. (2018) The clinical evaluation of alcohol intoxication is inaccurate in trauma patients. Cureus 10(2): e2190. DOI 10.7759/cureus.2190.

[16] Bond J et al. (2014) Exploring structural relationships between blood alcohol concentration and signs and clinical assessment of intoxication in alcohol-involved injury cases. Alcohol Alcoholism 49:417–422.

[17] Sexton C (2018) Analyzing the Oklahoma Supreme Court's peculiar expansion of dram shop liability [Boyle v. ASAP Energy, Inc., 408 P.3d 183 (Okla. 2017)]. Washburn Law Journal Online 58:1–10.

[18] Mezger M (2015) Keys please: making valets refuse to give a drunk driver his keys after a night in the bar. Available at SSRN: *ssrn.com/abstract=2659256* or *http://dx.doi.org/10.2139/ssrn.2659256.*

[19] As of 2015, there were 33 states that mandate social host liability through common law or state statutes. Like dram shop law, there is variability in those states with 4 states that limit the damages, 4 states which limit who may be sued, and 11 states that require stricter negligence standards than usual. *The September 2016 Report to Congress on the Prevention and Reduction of Underage Drinking, Policy Summary titled Social Host Liability.*

Driving Under the Influence of Alcohol

Surely there were people operating a horse while under the influence of alcohol, but that was probably not a huge problem. But the convergence of the availability of mass-produced automobiles and the repeal of Prohibition caused an epidemic of alcohol-related motor vehicle accidents in 1930s.[20] In 1938 an influential study was published in the Journal of the American Medical Association (JAMA) that used a breath alcohol testing instrument called the *Drunkometer* to show that the risk of a motor vehicle accident was 6 times greater at a BAC of 0.10% and 25 times greater at 0.15% BAC.[21] This early testing technology developed into the portable breath alcohol detectors used today, such as the Breathalyzer discussed in the next section.

There is no question that consumption of alcohol impairs the ability to drive a car (operating a motor vehicle). Since the 1938 JAMA paper mentioned before, there have been hundreds of papers published examining the relationship between blood alcohol concentration (BAC) and driving performance measurements using simulation and on-the-road methods in clinical studies. With almost 100 years of research, it can be stated with certainty that increased BAC is strongly associated with increased crash risk and with more serious injury and fatality.[22] Impairment is seen in a number of different tests including reaction time, tracking, and more complex measures from driving simulator studies like lane deviation and obstacle avoidance. Impairment due to alcohol is not the same and does not occur at the same dose for all cognitive tasks.[23] Generally speaking, more complex tasks are impaired by alcohol at lower BAC than simple tasks.[24]

The overwhelming evidence for driving impairment after alcohol consumption is clear and convincing. Because of this, alcohol is the only drug that has a scientifically reliable and justified *per se* blood levels for establishing impairment (0.08% in the United States, but lower in most European countries and Japan). Even this *per se* limit of 0.08% alcohol in the blood may be too high; there are signs of driving impairment at 0.05% BAC and a significant number of lives could be saved by lowering the legal limit to 0.05% BAC.[25] The drug laws establishing a *per se* limit in blood samples for other drugs besides alcohol were discussed in the previous chapter. The most common method to measure BAC in intoxicated drivers is by a law enforcement officer employing an Alcohol Breath Testing device (Breathalyzer). Data on Breathalyzer accuracy and reliability are presented in the next section.

The future is now and legal scholars have already opined on the ramifications of semiautonomous and fully autonomous cars on drunk driving laws. This proactive approach to prepare legally for the future is admirable given the speed at which new technology is thrown upon us. Semiautonomous vehicles are defined as automated cars which signal a *take-over* by the driver when certain situations arise, like lane changing onto the shoulder in a work-zone. A recent study using semiautonomous cars found that 0.08% BAC produced significant delays in the take-over times, but not at 0.05% BAC.[26] Therefore current alcohol driving laws could be applied to semiautonomous cars. Those that desire to imbibe alcohol and drive will have to wait until the availability of fully autonomous cars where no take-over by a human is needed, wanted, or even possible.

Laws against alcohol use and the operation of a motor vehicle need not be limited to earth-bound cars and vehicles. It was recently reported that the State of New Jersey passed a law punishing "drunk droning," a DUI statute for those operating a drone.[27] It seems like it would be hard for law enforcement to identify a drone being flown under the influence of alcohol given the baseline swaying flight and the ultimate crashing of most drones flown by sober operators personally observed by this author.

The Use and Misuse of the Breathalyzer[28]

Blood sampling for alcohol content was introduced in Chapter 9, and other drugs that interfere with the determination of the blood alcohol concentration (BAC) were detailed there. In this section, we examine the use and possible misuse of the roadside alcohol breath tester.

---

[20] Swartz J (2004) Breath testing for prosecutors: targeting hardcore impaired drivers. American Prosecutors Research Institute (APRI) Alexandria, VA, USA.

[21] Holcomb RL (1938) Alcohol in relation to traffic accidents. JAMA 111:1076–1085. According to this article, police methods used at that time to detect alcohol intoxication included properly enunciating the phrase "Methodist episcopal" and examining a hand-writing sample.

[22] Charlton SG, Starkey NJ (2015) Driving while drinking: performance impairments resulting from social drinking. Accident Anal Prevent. 74:210–217.

[23] Dry MJ et al. (2012) Dose-related effects of alcohol on cognitive functioning. PLoS ONE 7: e50977.

[24] Charlton SG, Starkey NJ (2015) *Op. cit.*

[25] Fell JC, Voas RB (2006) The effectiveness of reducing illegal blood alcohol concentration (BAC) limits for driving: evidence for lowering the limit to .05 BAC. J Safety Res. 37:233–243.

[26] Wiedemann K et al. (2018) Effect of different alcohol levels on take-over performance in conditionally automated driving. Accident Anal Prevent. 115:89–97.

[27] McFarland et al. (2018) Drinking and droning is now illegal in New Jersey. CNN online, posted 4/20/2018.

[28] *Breathalyzer* was once a trademarked name but now has become a genericized trademark like *Kleenex*, *Xerox*, *Aspirin*, and *Heroin*, among others, which were all trademarked names at one point.

In 1954 a new portable Alcohol Breath Testing device was tested and sold, called the Breathalyzer.[29] There are now a number of devices for evidentiary breath alcohol testing used in every county in the United States and around the world.[30] The National Highway Traffic Safety Administration (NHTSA) in the U.S. Dept. of Transportation (DOT) sets the standards for breath alcohol testing and publishes an *Approved Evidential Breath Measurement Devices* on their website.[31] States have their own list of approved breath alcohol testing devices and their own rules on testing.

The detection of breath alcohol using breath testing devices is accomplished by two different detection methods: electrochemical (EC) fuel cell detection and infrared wavelength (IR) detection. The EC fuel cell detector is an older technology that works by measuring the oxidation energy produced by the exhaled ethanol and converting this chemical energy into an electrical current. The greater the electrical current, the greater the breath alcohol content (BrAC). Newer Breathalyzers with IR detectors work by measuring the amount of infrared light absorbed by ethanol in the air sample; the more IR waves[32] absorbed, the greater the amount of ethanol present in the breath.[33]

Typically, the cheaper EC breath testers are used as preliminary breath testers and IR breath testers are used for evidentiary breath testers. As it can be difficult for police to detect alcohol impairment by physical observation and field sobriety tests alone (especially in an alcohol-tolerant individual) a handheld device that uses EC detectors resulting in a BAC[34] over 0.08% provides the police with the grounds to arrest a driver and obtain an evidentiary breath alcohol test using a device with an IR detector or a blood sample.[35] From an analytical point of view, the disadvantage of EC detector devices is that it measures only a single point of data (obtained from the end of the exhalation) whereas in an IR detector device, the BrAC is measured as a smooth curve over the whole exhalation breath.

There are clear rules in obtaining an evidentiary breath test by the feds and states. The Code of Federal Regulations[36] states that the first breath alcohol test is a screening test which must be followed by a blank air test yielding a 0.00 reading and a second confirmation test 15 min following the screening test. If this exact procedure is not followed, the alcohol test is considered to have a "fatal flaw" and "that the test was cancelled and must be treated as if the test never occurred."[37] This is in accord with scientific studies that show duplicate samples in agreement within predetermined standards (within 0.02 BAC, for example) are needed to insure precision as the actual biological/sampling component is the largest source of measurement variability.[38]

The manufacturers of Breath Alcohol Testers certify the accuracy of their model as meeting the DOT specifications for breath alcohol readings, namely, that the readings at 0.020% BAC and 0.040% BAC are within ±0.005% BAC.[39] The allowable interval between calibration verification tests should not exceed 30 days or 50 tests, whichever comes first. A log of these calibration verifications needs to be maintained as proof that these verifications are completed at these minimal intervals. This record-maintaining, strict calibration, and operational procedures are taken seriously by the courts; a recent Oklahoma Supreme Court case overturned the Appeals Court reversal of the trial court decision due to lack of records and procedures with the use of a Breathalyzer.[40]

The actual breath alcohol concentration (BrAC) tabulated by the Breathalyzer is not equal to the blood alcohol concentration (BAC). The software within the Breathalyzer automatically calculates the BAC from the BrAC by multiplication of the BrAC with a conversion factor and displaying the BAC. The conversion factor of 2100:1 (also called a partition ratio) was set by law following the advice of a federal panel, called the Committee on Alcohol and Other Drugs in 1976.[41] The conversion factor 2100 is widely accepted and written in the laws and regulations of alcohol breath testing of the states.

---

[29] Swartz J (2004) *op cit.*

[30] Its use varies widely as well as how many drivers take the alcohol breath test. In the United States, most states have implied-consent laws which make refusal of taking a Breathalyzer test result in the loss of a driver's license or other administration act. Other countries, like Britain and Canada, make refusal of a breath alcohol test equivalent to the crime of driving above the BAC limit. See: Voas RB et al. (2009) Implied-consent laws: A review of the literature and examination of current problems and related statutes. J Safety Res. 40:77–83.

[31] At: *www.transportation.gov/odapc/Approved-Evidential-Breath-Measurement-Devices*.

[32] Or photons. We don't want to forget that light is both a wave and a bunch of particles called photons.

[33] American Prosecutors Research Institute (APRI) (2004) Breath testing for prosecutors: targeting hardcore impaired drivers. *www.ndaa.org/wp-content/uploads/breath_testing_for_prosecutors.pdf*.

[34] The breath alcohol concentration (BrAC) obtained by the Breathalyzer is automatically displayed as BAC, using a conversion factor that is discussed further below.

[35] Wigmore JG (2013) Breath Alcohol, in *Encyclopedia of Forensic Sciences* (Second Edition) Elsevier, pp. 313–317.

[36] CFR Title 49: *Transportation. Part 40 – Procedures for Transportation Workplace Drug and Alcohol Testing Programs.*

[37] CFR, Title 49. Part 40 §40.267.

[38] Gullberg RG (2006) Estimating the measurement uncertainty in forensic breath-alcohol analysis. Accred Qual Assur 11: 562–568.

[39] The Intoxilyzer Instrument Quality Assurance Plan (ver. 1.42 dated 08-01-2000), obtained from Ms. Pam Hagan, CMI, Inc.

[40] *Muratore v. State ex rel.* Dept. of Public Safety, case Number 111586, decided 01-28-2014.

[41] Okorocha O, Strandmark M (2012) Alcohol breath testing: is there reasonable doubt? Syracuse J Sci Tech Law 27:124–144.

However, the use of a standard 2100:1 ratio is not scientifically valid, as this ratio differs between individuals and ranges from 900 to 3700 to 1 among test subjects. This is one of the problems with alcohol breath testing results used in a legal setting. Other problems are briefly highlighted next.

Given that the Breath Alcohol Tester device is maintained and calibrated as needed, and that the breath alcohol technician performs the Breath Alcohol test as mandated, there are still a number of studies that demonstrate a large degree of variance in correlating breath alcohol levels with blood alcohol levels. Comparing devices that use the newer IR detection versus the older EC detection showed that the EC detector devices had the largest analytical variability.[42] In a study comparing the breath alcohol levels to standard blood alcohol analysis, it was noted that there was bias to the BrAC values compared to BAC values and that the bias increased as the BAC levels increased.[43] In general, there are many problems with Breath Alcohol Test devices including the blood-breath alcohol partition ratio (how much blood alcohol crosses into the lungs), blood water content (variability among individuals in hematocrit), breathing rate (hypo and hyperventilation), and body temperature (8.62% increase in breath alcohol level with 1 degree increase in body temp), to name some.[44] Another study found that the breath alcohol values might range from 23% below to 19% above the blood alcohol values.[45] For these reasons even Breath Alcohol Test devices using IR detection are recommended only as screening devices and the best evidentiary measurement is from a blood draw to determine BAC.[46]

Besides the Breathalyzer and other such BrAC devices, there are a number of new roadside devices for drug detection in development. Much effort is going into the development of an oral fluid test (spit tester) for the detection and quantification of nonalcoholic drugs. The holy grail of roadside drug testing devices, with a huge market, is a roadside drug tester for the active ingredient of marijuana, THC, and its metabolites.[47] The advancing *Green Revolution*, invading even the reddest and most conservative states like Oklahoma, creates a large demand for roadside detection of marijuana smokers who unwisely get into the driver's seat while high.

Retrograde Calculation of Blood Alcohol Concentrations

We know from pharmacokinetics, the study of the time course of a drug in the body, that a drug (and remember, alcohol is a drug) goes through a cycle of increasing and decreasing concentrations in the blood and target tissues like the brain. Alcohol is absorbed through the gut and to a first approximation, reaches peak levels in the blood within 1 h (see Fig. 17.1). Alcohol, or more precisely ethanol, is eliminated at a constant rate from the body due to the saturation of the liver enzymes that metabolize ethanol.[48] The precise elimination rate for ethanol differs according to nutritional status, diet, concurrent food intake, frequency of alcohol intake, gender, individual genetics, and ethnicity.[49] However, it has been suggested that 0.010%–0.025% BAC/h is an accurate range of ethanol elimination for the vast majority of individuals.[50]

As shown in Fig. 17.1, after alcohol reaches its peak in the blood, alcohol concentration gradually decreases over time due to metabolism and excretion. Because alcohol freely passes into the brain, nearly the same time course would also model the amount of alcohol in the brain over time. Logically, given a curve of alcohol concentrations in the blood over time such as the one shown later, if one knew the BAC (blood alcohol concentration, in %) at one point on the curve, one could calculate the curve backwards to get the BAC at a point in time prior to the time the BAC was obtained.[52]

Calculation of the BAC backwards in time, called retrograde calculation of BAC, is a standard method to determine the BAC at the time of a motor vehicle accident.[53] The Defendant's blood samples were taken approx. 90 min or 1.5 h after the MVA. This number (1.5) is important as it is needed for the formula used to calculate BAC at the time of the accident (see Fig. 17.2). Because of the amount of alcohol research done over the decades, there are reliable formulae for the backwards

[42] Gullberg RG (2008) Employing components-of-variance to evaluate forensic breath test instruments. Sci Justice 48:2–7.

[43] Morey TE et al. (2011) Measurement of ethanol in gaseous breath using a miniature gas chromatograph. J Anal Toxicol. 35:134–142.

[44] Lablanca DA (1990) The chemical basis of the Breathalyzer. J Chem. Educat. 67:259–261.

[45] Jones AW (1993) Pharmacokinetics of ethanol in saliva: comparison with blood and breath alcohol profiles, subjective feelings of intoxication, and diminished performance. Clin Chem. 39:1837–1844.

[46] Rose S, Furton KG (2004). Variables affecting the accuracy and precision of breath alcohol instruments including the Intoxilyzer 5000. Georgia DUI Law, A Resource for Lawyers and Judges. ISBN 0-03271-6296-1.

[47] One could argue it might have been wiser to first have a roadside tester for cannabis-impaired driving before the legalization of recreational marijuana use.

[48] Cederbaum AI (2012) Alcohol metabolism. Clin Liver Dis. 16:667–685.

[49] Chan LN, Anderson GD (2014) Pharmacokinetic and pharmacodynamic drug interactions with ethanol (alcohol). Clin Pharmacokinet. 53:1115–1136.

[50] Jones AW (2010) Evidence-based survey of the elimination rates of ethanol from blood with applications in forensic casework. Forensic Sci Int. 200:1–20.

[51] Kovatchev B et al. (2012) *In silico* models of alcohol dependence and treatment. Front Psychiatry 3:4.

[52] Calculation of the BAC forward in time is also possible (anterograde calculation) however, tables of the BAC for men and women according to drinks and weight are available for this purpose. See Chapter 12 *Where There's a Will, There's a Way*.

[53] Posey D, Mozayani A (2007) The estimation of blood alcohol concentration: Widmark revisited. Forensic Sci Med Pathol. 3:33–39.

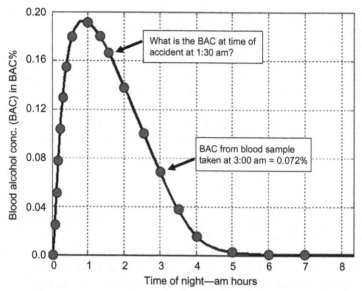

FIG. 17.1 Typical time course of BAC annotated with the specific BAC obtained from the driver in this chapter's case. The patron served by the bar had a BAC of 0.072% at the time of the blood draw, but the accident occurred 1.5 h earlier. *(Figure adapted from Kovatchev et al.)[51]*

$$BAC_{\text{at time of accident}} = BAC_{\text{of blood sample}} + (T_{\text{time elapsed (h)}} \times E_{\text{elimination rate per hour, \% BAC}})$$

FIG. 17.2 Equation for retrograde calculation of BAC.

or retrograde calculation of BAC. It has been stated that using alcohol elimination rates ranging from 0.010%/h to 0.025%/h will be accurate for the vast majority of individuals.[54] These low and high range values for the alcohol elimination rates are used below and plugged into the standard formula for retrograde calculation.[55]

The formula for calculating BAC back to the time of the motor vehicle accident is shown above in Fig. 17.2.

In the present case, the patron BAC from the blood draw was 0.072% and the time elapsed from obtaining the blood sample and the MVA was 1.5 h, which are plugged into the previous equation. Two values are used for E (elimination rate) in the equation: 010% elimination per hour and 0.025% elimination per hour. Calculations for these two values give 0.087 and 0.1095. Truncated to the usual two decimals for BAC,[56] the patron in this case had a calculated BAC ranging from 0.08% to 0.10% BAC at the time of the accident. This BAC is above the legal limit of alcohol intoxication when driving (0.08% BAC) and portrays how blood BAC may be below the legal limit for alcohol intoxication at the time of the blood draw but at or above the BAC limit at the time of the accident. See Appendix M for the complete calculations and formulae.

Drug Recognition Experts

As noted before in the context of bar patrons, recognition of alcohol intoxication is not an easy or reliable task. Even harder is the recognition of intoxication from other drugs besides alcohol in impaired drivers. The Drug Recognition Expert (DRE) is a law enforcement officer who passed a certification class. A brief history of the DRE program is next.

Like many new ideas that originate in California and metastasize to the rest of the country, the Drug Evaluation and Classification Program was developed by the Los Angeles Police Department (LAPD) in the early 1970s. LAPD officers noticed that many drivers were apprehended for impaired driving but didn't blow an intoxicating level of alcohol and

---

[54] Jones AW (2010) *Op. cit.*

[55] Standard formula from American Prosecutors Research Institute (2003) Alcohol toxicity for prosecutors: targeting hardcore impaired drivers. APRI, Alexandria, VA. At: *www.ndaa.org/wp-content/uploads/toxicology_final.pdf.*

[56] Note that truncation is not the same as "rounding off." Rounding off 0.079% BAC yields 0.08% whereas truncating to two decimal points yields 0.07%. This can obviously make a difference in drink driving cases. I have testimony from our state's forensic toxicologist that they officially truncate to two decimals in their toxicology reports. It may be different in other jurisdictions but is something the detailed drug expert should know.

escaped prosecution.[57] Drivers who failed a field sobriety test (e.g., walking toe-to-toe, touching fingers to nose with eyes closed) but had low or nonexistent BAC were problematic. Such drivers were sometimes brought to a physician for evaluation, but physicians were reluctant to participate due to for various reasons including their lack of knowledge of specific drug effects and drug-impairment effects on driving, and the onus of trial testimony. Sargent Studdard of the LAPD approached narcotics officer Leeds. They did drug research, consulted with experts, and developed the first methods for training and certifying a police officer as a Drug Recognition Expert (DRE). Eventually Officers Studdard and Lee got further support from the LAPD and the National Highway Traffic and Safety Administration (NHTSA, a federal agency).

The DRE officer is certified by the Drug Evaluation and Classification (DEC) Program, established in 1987 by the International Association of Chiefs of Police (IACP)[58] and the NHTSA of the U.S. Department of Transportation. Instead of relying on a pharmacologist or toxicologist expert witness, who are busy and expensive, certified DREs already employed by law enforcement agencies can provide DRE reports and testify in courts in cases of drug-impaired drivers. The ultimate goal of the DRE program is to "help prevent crashes, deaths, and injuries caused by drug-impaired drivers."[59]

The DRE program is touted as a success, and there are some studies that examined DRE accuracy. Using a selected and verified sample of marijuana-impaired drivers, researchers found that DRE correctly identified marijuana-using drivers from control drivers.[60] Indications such as pulse, blood pressure, and pupil size were significantly different in marijuana drivers compared to control nondrug using drivers. Further studies in marijuana drivers showed that red eyes, droopy eyelids, altered speech, tongue coating, and the smell of marijuana were the best indicators of marijuana intoxication.[61] Unlike the earlier study however, these authors did not find a good correlation between pulse and blood pressure and marijuana use (THC blood levels) in this study.

The DRE evaluation consists of a number of tests and indications, taking about an hour to complete, and consisting of over 100 items (indications) to note. Research on the effectiveness of DRE drug evals and accuracy of drug identification shows that DREs are more accurate when only one drug is used by the driver and when drug levels are in the higher range.[62] Sensitivity of DRE evaluations differs for the different classes of drugs, ranging from 91% for PCP (angel dust) to 60% for marijuana to 19% for CNS stimulants in one study.

A Drug Recognition Expert is a law enforcement agent who has completed specialized training in the recognition of drivers operating under the influence of drugs. DRE reports are sometimes included in the official reports, but with the widespread use of blood kits and toxicology lab analysis, the role of the DRE is more limited. The proof is in the pudding, so to speak, in this case *blood* pudding.[63] The toxicological analysis of the drug-impaired driver's blood sample, if confirmed and quantified, provides the scientific and legal standard for any drug detected in a putative drug-impaired driver.

The testimony of the DRE can be overvalued by the jury if they are not told that the DRE is a police officer who completed a short course in drug detection. The defense attorney should employ a drug expert when the prosecution plans to present the DRE report or testimony. In cases where a drug expert is pitted against a DRE, the drug expert's attorney must make clear that the DRE only received training in detecting which type of drug the driver may have been using. The DRE has little foundation in pharmacology or toxicology and this can be shown during cross-examination. The major contrast is that the true drug expert does not work for a law enforcement agency and, just like police lab forensic toxicologists, DREs may have a conflict of interest between their testimony and their employment.

The complete 7-day course curriculum is available from the Maine.gov website.[64] The class handout provides examples of DRE reports for each class of drug recognized. DRE materials also contain the indicators and measures made by DRE investigators. These charts at the end of the class handout are useful for the prosecution and the defense as the strength

---

[57] Participant manual for Drug Recognition Expert class (2018) National Highway Traffic Safety Administration (NHTSA), Transportation Safety Institute (TSI) and International Association of Chiefs of Police (IACP).

[58] The IACP accredits DRE programs and offers DRE instructor training.

[59] Declues K et al. (2016) A 2-year study of Δ^9-tetrahydrocannabinol concentrations in drivers: examining driving and field sobriety test performance. Forensic Sci. 61:1664–1670.

[60] Hartman RL et al. (2016) Drug Recognition Expert (DRE) examination characteristics of cannabis impairment. Accid Anal Prev. 92:219–229.

[61] Declues K et al. (2018) A two-year study of Δ^9-tetrahydrocannabinol concentrations in drivers; Part 2: Physiological signs on Drug Recognition Expert (DRE) and non-DRE Examinations. J Forensic Sci. 63:583–587.

[62] Beirness et al. (2007) Evaluation of the drug evaluation and classification program: a critical review of the evidence. Traffic Inj Prev. 8:368–376.

[63] Blood pudding is actually made up of blood sausages in which goat or pig blood is obtained at slaughter and filled into sausage sleeves and boiled. It is a dish they (*still*) serve in the UK. Order it next time you are across the pond if you dare.

[64] *www.maine.gov/dps/bhs/impaired-driving/dre/documents/2018DRE7-DayFullParticipantManual.pdf.*

of the defendant's DRE report might depend on the signs of drug effects noted. Each of the criteria used by DREs can be examined with the DRE during direct or cross-examination and each item is amenable to the input of a drug expert.

Marketing of the Drug Expert

The marketing of the drug expert is simple because in most cases there is no marketing. There are companies, of course, that the drug expert can pay to list their name and description of expert services in a database for attorneys looking for an expert witness.[65] In the author's experience, most referrals come from queries to the state bar association email *listserver* or truly word of mouth between attorneys. Other experts also note that word-of-mouth referrals are the most likely source of continuing expert witness jobs. When asked why a certain drug expert was recommended by an attorney to another attorney, respondents told one author that "he or she wrote a good report."[66] Writing a good report was the number one reason for a personal recommendation, with "giving a good deposition" and "easy to work with" distant second and third reasons. This confirms the importance of producing a good if not great report when asked to do so.[67]

Like many career-advancing moves, the toughest part for a pharmacologist moving into the drug expert business is getting the first shot at it. Those interested should note such medico-legal interests on their faculty homepage, constructed so that the words "drug expert" will catch a high-ranking link in a Google search. It is also a good idea to tell your faculty colleagues, and any attorneys in the area, that you are interested in serving as a drug expert. Finally, the pharmacology department chair may field a request for a drug expert from an attorney so the pharmacologist-*cum*-drug expert should definitely let the department chair know of this career interest.

[Narrative continued]

Mr. Battles entered the criminal judicial system to meet his fate on charges of vehicular homicide while driving under the influence of alcohol. The parents of the driver struck by Mr. Battles filed civil suit against the public establishment, McKinneys, which served Mr. Battles the five tequila-based drinks before the deadly car crash that killed their daughter. They claimed that the bartender at McKinneys should not have served Mr. Battles due to his obvious intoxication. Retrograde calculation of the driver's BAC from the time of the blood sample to the time of the accident showed that he likely had a BAC ranging from 0.08% to 0.10% when he struck and killed their daughter. The case was decided in favor of the plaintiffs but the trial court's decision was overturned on appeal. McKinneys celebrated the appellate verdict with a 2-for-1 special on tequila shots on the following Friday night.

---

[65] I have not used this marketing approach so unsure of its success in obtaining more drug expert gigs. An example of an expert witness database is available on the SEAK website at: *www.seakexperts.com*.

[66] Field DL (2013) *The Expert Expert: The Path to Prosperity and Prominence as an Expert Witness*. iUniverse Publishers, Bloomington, IN, USA.

[67] Key aspects of litigation report writing are discussed in Chapter 4 and a report excerpt is included in Appendix D.

Chapter 18

The Devil Made Me Do It: Rape after prison release of an untreated schizophrenic

Antipsychotic Treatment of Schizophrenia—Treatment of Mental Illness in Prison

Postrelease Treatment of Mentally Ill Offenders

Psychedelic Drugs Used in Psychiatry—The Drug Expert and the Nonuse of Drugs

[Narrative]

Robbie Jones is a 23-year old white male first diagnosed with schizophrenia after admission to a psychiatric hospital three years ago and was treated with antipsychotic drugs. He quickly improved and was released from the inpatient unit. However, Robbie was not compliant in taking his antipsychotic medications and soon after release from the hospital was convicted of assault with a deadly weapon and incarcerated for 2 years. In state prison, Robbie's mental illness was described as "chronic paranoid schizophrenia" and he was given antipsychotic drugs that he took on a regular basis. About two months before his release, Robbie refused to take his prescribed antipsychotic drugs stating "he felt better and didn't need them." The prison psychiatrist did not begin proceedings for involuntary medication nor enable Robbie to continue antipsychotic medications upon his release from prison. The prison psychiatrist wrote in the discharge health summary report that Robbie had "No identified health problems, routine care only. Medications needed: ranitidine (Zantac®) for gastric reflux." Robbie was released from prison and went to live with his single mother in a double-wide mobile home.

About a month after Robbie moved into the trailer park, an 8-year old child was molested and raped in a nearby mobile home. The child was in the care of her mother's live-in boyfriend at the time of the incident while the mother was at work. The boyfriend became the prime suspect and after many months in custody, was exonerated by DNA evidence. Canvassing of the mobile park residents led to suspicions of Robbie Jones, who according to his mother, left for Seattle to stay with some friends. Local police notified the Seattle PD and Robbie was identified and taken into custody following a routine traffic stop. DNA evidence obtained from a swab of Robbie's cheek matched the DNA from semen in the rape kit. Robbie was charged with first-degree rape of a victim younger than 14, lewd molestation, and first-degree burglary. He was facing a life sentence in prison if convicted.[1]

A Public Defender was appointed to Mr. Robbie Jones. The PD contacted a local drug expert to examine the prison medical records with regards to antipsychotic treatment and to determine if the lack of antipsychotic treatment after his release contributed to the resulting heinous criminal behavior.

Antipsychotic Treatment of Schizophrenia

Schizophrenia is a scary mental disease. It is a severe mental illness highly prevalent among our population, with age of onset in young adults in their late teens and twenties. Schizophrenia is a psychiatric disorder that inflicts about 1 person in 100. Think of that prevalence rate the next time you are in a room of a hundred people at a lecture or a sporting event with thousands of people.[2] It is a mathematical reality that schizophrenics are among us, walking down the street beside us. Symptoms of schizophrenia include voice hallucinations, delusions, and psychotic episodes.[3] The etiology or cause of schizophrenia is not entirely known, though there are some genetic components, environmental factors, and precipitating drug mechanisms implicated.[4]

---

[1] The rape of a child was a capital crime in many states until SCOTUS decided in *Kennedy v. Louisiana*, 554 U.S. 407 (2008), that the Eighth Amendment's Cruel and Unusual Punishments Clause prohibits a death sentence for the rape of a child when the child did not die.

[2] Average number of fan attendance at a Chicago Cubs baseball game at Wrigley Field during the season they won the World Series in 2016 was 39,906 fans. One-percent prevalence of schizophrenia yields 399 schizophrenics in the crowd, assuming they like the Cubs as much as the general population.

[3] Brenner GM, Stevens CW (2018) *Brenner and Stevens' Pharmacology, 5e*, Elsevier, Philadelphia, PA, USA.

[4] Brown AS (2011) The environment and susceptibility to schizophrenia. Prog Neurobiol. 93:23–58.

The Drug Expert. https://doi.org/10.1016/B978-0-12-800048-9.00018-3

As shown in the introductory chapter of this book, untreated schizophrenics often commit crimes that put them in the national news spotlight.[5] It is clear, however, that schizophrenia can be successfully treated with drugs. Antipsychotic medications effectively reduce the intensity of the psychotic hallucinations, albeit with some adverse effects.[6] Indeed, as discussed later, the adverse effects of antipsychotic drugs are a major issue in the legality of forced antipsychotic medication of institutionalized schizophrenics.

Tragically, in the United States, about half of the people who need pharmacological treatment for psychiatric disorders do not receive needed medications. The treatment gap for most mental illnesses ranges from about 40%–60%, with about 36%–47% of persons with schizophrenia and psychosis remaining untreated.[7] Patient groups advocate for the reclassification of schizophrenia from a mental illness to a neurological disease which would increase funding for research and treatment.[8]

A study of almost 300 schizophrenic patients showed that mentally ill patients were 5 times more likely to have been convicted of violent crimes, 2.5 times more likely to commit property crimes, and 3 times more likely to commit drug law crimes than the general population.[9] Another study found that mental health patients were 3 times more likely to be arrested compared to nonmental health patients.[10] Although mental health proponents may not like to publicize these findings for fear of further demonizing people with psychiatric disorders, it is clear that the treatment gap and lack of pharmacological treatment in persons with a severe psychiatric disorders pose a risk of harm to themselves and to society. Especially for those unfortunate souls inflicted with schizophrenia.

The good news is that patients with mental illness receiving adequate psychotropic medications no longer pose an increased threat to society. One study found that among a large group of 517 stabilized outpatients diagnosed with a psychiatric disorder, only 4% had a history of homicide attempts.[11] Another study found that with medication and other treatment, most persons with stable mental illnesses do not exhibit an increased risk of violence.[12] Antipsychotic drugs appear to restore the dysfunctional brain in persons with schizophrenia to normalcy. How they do that is the topic of the next subsection.

Antipsychotic drugs and their mechanism of action

To a first approximation, schizophrenia is one of the easiest mental illness states to effectively treat with drug therapy.[13] Schizophrenics have too much dopamine in their brains, due to high levels of this neurotransmitter being released from dopamine neurons. Increased dopamine in the synapse leads to too much dopamine binding to dopamine receptors. Activation of dopamine receptors leads to abnormal changes in the brain circuitry and expression of schizophrenic behavior. As all addictive drugs produce a release of dopamine into the nucleus accumbens, the schizophrenic in this regard could be likened to a nonstop cocaine abuser. It is easy to understand then how schizophrenia and chronic cocaine or methamphetamine abuse share common psychotic symptoms as they are biochemically linked to excess dopamine. The psychosis and aggression produced by increased dopamine in the schizophrenic is mirrored in the psychosis and aggression induced by amphetamine and methamphetamine abuse in the meth addict. Legal issues surrounding methamphetamine use in homicide cases are the topic of Chapter 15 *Speed Kills*.

Logically, the main action of using drugs to treat schizophrenia is to block the overabundance of dopamine produced in the schizophrenic brain. The drugs used to treat schizophrenia are called antipsychotic drugs, although antipsychotic drugs also have additional indications or uses. For the most part, antipsychotic drugs act as dopamine receptor antagonists, blocking the overabundance of dopamine that occurs in the schizophrenia brain.[14] Particular antipsychotic drugs that may be familiar to the reader include chlorpromazine (with the well-known trade name of Thorazine®), a zombifying older antipsychotic drug with potent sedative properties; haloperidol (Haldol®), the widely used agent that brought schizophrenics

[5] *The more heinous the crime, the sicker the perpetrator.*

[6] Muench J, Hamer AM (2010) Adverse effects of antipsychotic medications. Am Fam Physician. 81:617–622.

[7] Kohn R et al, Saxena S, Levav I, Saraceno B (2004) The treatment gap in mental health care. Bull World Health Organ. 82:858–866.

[8] Letter from Linda Stalters, CEO of Schizophrenia And Related Disorders Alliance of America, to CDC Director Robert R. Redfield, MD, August 28, 2018.

[9] Modestin J, Ammann R (1996) Mental disorder and criminality: male schizophrenia. Schizophr. Bull. 22: 69–82.

[10] Link B et al. (1992) The violent and illegal behavior of mental patients reconsidered. Amer Sociol Rev. 57:275–292.

[11] Asnis GM et al. (1997) Violence and homicidal behaviors in psychiatric disorders. Psychiatr Clin North Am. 20:405–425.

[12] Rueve ME, Welton RE (2008) Violence and mental illness. Psychiatry 5:34–48.

[13] Other easily understandable mental illnesses at the reductionist level include anxiety disorders (due to lack of GABAergic inhibition) and depression (due to lack of sufficient serotonin and norepinephrine neurotransmission).

[14] Brenner GM, Stevens CW (2018) *Op cit.*

back into the community but is tainted by adverse effects; and the newer atypical antipsychotic risperidone, famous for late-night commercials soliciting Risperdal®-injured parties. For persons undergoing involuntary or forced medication (see later), long-acting intramuscular depot injection of antipsychotics are used.[15]

Besides their use in treating the psychosis of schizophrenia, there is a more recent trend to expand the marketplace of antipsychotic drugs for treatment of other nonpsychotic mental illness. For example, the FDA-approved indications for a newer atypical antipsychotic called aripiprazole (Abilify®), added the treatment of manic episodes associated with bipolar I disorder, an add-on treatment for major depression, and in children, for treatment of irritability associated with autistic disorder.[16] Aripiprazole is also indicated for the treatment of Tourette's syndrome,[17] confirming research studies showing its effectiveness in children.[18] Current studies on risperidone to control aggression in youth suggest that it may also get approved for conduct disorders in unruly children.[19]

Treatment of Mental Illness in Prison

The history of the treatment of the mentally ill in this country is not pleasant.[20] In colonial America, historical records show that schizophrenics and other severely mentally ill persons were treated as criminals and locked up in jails and prisons. This practice continued for decades until the pioneering efforts of the nurse Dorothea Dix in Boston. Nurse Dix exposed the degrading conditions that schizophrenics and other insane persons experienced in prisons, writing "*I come as the advocate of helpless, forgotten, insane and idiotic men and women; of beings, sunk to a condition from which the most unconcerned would start with real horror.*"[21] Dix's reform efforts throughout the United States led to the establishment of 75 public psychiatric hospitals by 1880 and most insane persons were transferred from prisons into the new insane asylums[22] at that time.

For more than 100 years, the idea that insane persons did not belong in prison but rather in mental hospitals for protection (asylum) and treatment carried the day. This all changed in the 1960s and 1970s with the emptying and closure of state mental hospitals and the release of truly insane persons into the community without adequate health care. The majority of patients released from insane asylums, without further antipsychotic treatment, relapsed into psychosis, displayed aberrant behavior, and committed bizarre acts that led to misdemeanor or felony charges, most ended up back in jail or prison.

Today, county jails and state and federal prisons are the largest mental health care facilities in the United States.[23] It is estimated that about 20 percent of prisoners have serious mental illness, diagnosed as psychiatric disorders (e.g., schizophrenia and bipolar disorder).[24] Another 20 percent or so require some form of psychiatric care during incarceration for less severe mental illness.

Forced medication of captured schizophrenics with antipsychotics

The Supreme Court of the US (SCOTUS) made a landmark decision in *Estelle v. Gamble* (1976)[25] that held "*deliberate indifference*" by the prison staff to an inmate's serious medical problem (severe illness or injury) constitutes cruel and unusual punishment under the 18th Amendment.[26] It is a constitutional right of inmates to receive medical care. In some cases, involuntary or forced medication will be needed in an institutionalized patient or inmate to protect himself, the prison staff, and other inmates.

---

[15] Cournos F et al. (1991) Outcome of involuntary medication in a state hospital system. Am J Psychiatry 148:489–494.

[16] *Abilify® Full Prescribing Information* (2016) Otsuka Pharmaceutical Co., Tokyo, Japan. At: *www.abilify.com*.

[17] Tourette's syndrome or disorder is noted by frequent motor tics and vocal outbursts of obscenities (*coprolalia*). For popular comedic depiction, see Murray, Bill (1991) *What About Bob?* (in bedroom scene faking Tourette's). Buena Vista Pictures, Walt Disney Company, Burbank, California.

[18] Sallee F et al. (2017) Randomized, double-blind, placebo-controlled trial demonstrates the efficacy and safety of oral aripiprazole for the treatment of Tourette's disorder in children and adolescents. J Child Adolesc Psychopharmacol. 27: 771–781.

[19] Demirkaya SK et al. (2017) A retrospective study of long acting risperidone use to support treatment adherence in youth with conduct disorder. Clin Psychopharmacol Neurosci. 15: 328–336.

[20] Much of this information comes from Torrey et al. (2014) The treatment of persons with mental illness in prisons and jails: a state survey. Joint report of the Treatment Advocacy Center and the National Sheriff's Association.

[21] Torrey et al. (2014) *Ibid.*

[22] Asylum is from the Greek word *asylon* (άσυλο) meaning *refuge*, a place of protection.

[23] Ford M (2015) Atlantic Monthly, June 8.

[24] Dlugacz H and Wimmer C (2013) Legal aspects of administrating antipsychotic medications to jail and prison inmates. International J Law Psych. 36:213–228.

[25] *Estelle v. Gamble*, 429 U.S. 97 (1976).

[26] Rold WJ (2008) Thirty years after *Estelle v. Gamble*: A legal retrospective. J Correction Health Care 14:11–20.

The Supreme Court of the United States (SCOTUS) ruled in the *Washington v. Harper (1990)*[27] that involuntary administration of antipsychotic drugs to schizophrenic inmates is constitutional as long as the prisons hold an administrative hearing for that determination. The Code of Federal Register outlines the procedures for forced medication of antipsychotics to psychotic inmates in federal prisons.[28] An administrative hearing is held, with notification to the inmate (at least 24 hours before the hearing) and providing date, time, place, and purpose of the hearing. This notice to the inmate must also include an explanation of the reasons for involuntary psychiatric medication. The inmate has the right to present evidence and witnesses and to have a staff representative for assistance. If the inmate does not request a representative, the medical director of the institution must appoint one. The hearing is conducted by a psychiatrist who is not the attending psychiatrist and was not consulted for the original diagnosis. The attending psychiatrist must present clinical data and determine that the inmate presents a threat of *ongoing* danger of harm to himself[29] or others, poses a serious threat of property damage to the facility or the secure running of it, or is so "gravely disabled" that the inmate is no longer functioning (catatonic schizophrenia, for example). The psychiatrist overseeing the hearing must write a written report of the initial decision, which can be appealed. However, an administrative hearing is waived if the inmate presents an immediate threat of the same three criteria noted before for ongoing threat. Essentially, this may mean that an untreated schizophrenic in prison first undergoes forced antipsychotic medication without an administrative hearing under the *immediate* clause, then forced medication continues after the hearing to handle the *ongoing* threats of untreated schizophrenia.

The issue of forced antipsychotics drugs to gain competency to stand trial came to light in the recent case of United States *v. Loughner* in 2011.[30] Jared Lee Loughner was charged with multiple counts of murder for the Tucson, AZ mass shooting that killed 6 people, including US District Judge John Roll, and attempted murder for the permanently injured Congresswoman Gabrielle Giffords and 13 others.[31] He was initially declared incompetent to stand trial by the district court and sent to the federal forensic medical facility and given antipsychotic drugs by force. Loughner's public defenders filed a preliminary injunction to cease forced medication, and on appeal the Ninth Circuit upheld the forced medication of Mr. Loughner which was then continued. After about a year of involuntary medication, Loughner was found fit to enter a guilty plea and was sentenced to seven consecutive life sentences plus 140 years with no chance of parole.[32]

Most importantly, involuntary or forced medication of schizophrenics and other psychotic individuals works. Early studies showed the effectiveness of forced medication to schizophrenics and other severely mentally ill persons. In schizophrenic patients given a single dose of a long-acting antipsychotic drug,[33] a two-week follow-up noted a significant improvement of their psychotic symptoms and all patients were accepting antipsychotic treatment voluntarily.[34] Other studies along the same line concluded that "*the treatment refusal of every patient in our sample was influenced by [their] psychosis.*"[35] Reasons for the refusal of medicine by psychotic patients include the belief that nothing was wrong with them and that the medication was poison. After involuntary antipsychotic treatment, most patients thought that having forced antipsychotic medication was a good thing.[36]

A more recent study of forced antipsychotic treatment in mentally ill inmates showed that forced medication reduced the number of severe disciplinary charges and reduced all charges compared to the year before they were given involuntary antipsychotic treatment.[37]

---

[27] *Washington v. Harper*, 494 U.S. 210, 223 (1990).

[28] 28 CFR 549.46, at *www.law.cornell.edu/cfr/text/28/549.46*.

[29] Gender-specific terminology intended here. Most prison inmates are males and schizophrenia is more common in males than females.

[30] *United States v. Loughner*, No. 11–10339 (9th Cir. 2012).

[31] Bacigal RJ, Tate MK (2014) *Sidebar*, page 62. In: *Criminal Law and Procedure: An Overview, 4th Ed.*, Delmar Cengage Learning, Clifton Park, NJ.

[32] Some might argue that a more fitting outcome would be continued commitment in a medical treatment facility and continued administration of antipsychotic medications. Certainly schizophrenics are innately insane in spite of apparent masking of symptoms with antipsychotic drugs.

[33] Antipsychotic drugs available as long-acting depot formulations include fluphenazine and haloperidol. They are called depot injections because the drug formulation is oil based and deposited into a major muscle mass where it enters the bloodstream at a steady pace. These drugs have a long duration of action (1 week or more) allowing for once-weekly injections ideal for forced medication protocols.

[34] Keisling R (1983) Characteristics and outcome of patients who refuse medication. Hospital and Community Psychiatry 34:847–848.

[35] Schwartz HI et al. (1988) Autonomy and the right to refuse treatment: patients' attitudes after involuntary medication. Hosp Commun Psychiatry 39:1049–1054.

[36] Greenberg WM et al. (1996) Patients' attitudes toward having been forcibly medicated. Bull Amer Acad Psych Law 24:513–524.

[37] Salem A (2015) Nonemergency involuntary antipsychotic medication in prison: effects on prison inpatient days and disciplinary charges. J Am Acad Psychiatry Law 43:159–164.

Postrelease Treatment of Mentally Ill Offenders

In terms of numbers, there are as many as 50,000 mentally ill patients in state forensic hospitals, about 100,000 persons with serious mental disease in jails, and more than a quarter of a million (250,000) inmates with serious mental illness in prison.[38] At some point, most of these individuals will be released from their institutions and return to their communities.

Failure to treat schizophrenics with antipsychotic medications leads to a fourfold increase in the relapse rate and suicide, and increased risk of violent behavior.[39] Additionally, nontreatment of schizophrenics leads to an increased use of emergency psychiatric services and hospitalization, and increased arrests and instances of substance abuse. On the other hand, treating schizophrenics with antipsychotic medications improves executive function (planning and thinking of consequences), attention and memory, and other cognitive processes. A recent cohort study of released mentally ill prisoners found that postrelease treatment with antipsychotics led to a significant reduction of violent reoffending.[40] One study found in a large group of 517 stabilized outpatients with a psychiatric disorder that only 4% reported a history of homicide attempts.[41] With treatment, most persons with stable mental illnesses do not exhibit an increased risk of violence.[42]

Guidelines and regulations from federal and state agencies, and standards from the American Bar Association, highlight the need for postrelease treatment of severely mentally ill patients. The federal Substance Abuse and Mental Health Services Administration (SAMHSA), part of the Public Health Service, states in their Treatment Improvement Protocol[43] entitled "*Continuity of offender treatment for substance use disorders from institution to community*":

Incarcerated substance-users have high rates of coexisting mental health disorders; it is crucial for these offenders that medication orders and files are transferred. **Careful reassessment of the inmate's medication is required upon release to the community** [bold added].

The American Bar Association (ABA) Standards for Criminal Justice-Treatment of Prisoners, 3rd Edition (2011)[44] codifies the regulations for the treatment of prisoners in the United States.

Standard 23-6.5 Continuity of care
(a) A correctional agency should ensure each prisoner's continuity of care, including with respect to medication, upon entry into the correctional system, during confinement and transportation, during and after transfer between facilities, **and upon release**. A prisoner's health care records and medication should travel with the prisoner in the event of a transfer between facilities, including facilities operated by different agencies.
Standard 23-8.9 Transition to the community
(d) When a prisoner with ongoing medical or mental health care needs is released to the community, correctional authorities should make reasonable efforts to:
  (i) **identify and arrange for community-based health care services, including substance abuse treatment; and**
  (ii) **ensure that all health care treatment and medications provided to the prisoner during the term of imprisonment will continue uninterrupted, including, if necessary, providing prescription medication or medical equipment for a brief period reasonably necessary to obtain access to health care services in the community**; providing initial medically necessary transportation from the correctional facility to a community health care facility for continuing treatment; or **otherwise addressing the prisoner's serious immediate post-release health care needs.** [bold added]

---

[38] Cuddeback GS et al. (2016) Enrollment and service use patterns among persons with severe mental illness receiving expedited Medicaid on release from state prisons, county jails, and psychiatric hospitals. Psychiatr Serv. 67:835–841.

[39] Erickson SK (2007) Legal fallacies of antipsychotic drugs. J Am Acad Psychiatry Law 35:235–246.

[40] Chang Z et al. (2016) Association between prescription of major psychotropic medications and violent reoffending after prison release. JAMA 316:1798–1807.

[41] Asnis GM et al. (1997) Violence and homicidal behaviors in psychiatric disorders. Psychiatr Clin North Am. 20:405–25.

[42] Rueve ME, Welton RS (2008) Violence and mental illness. Psychiatry (Edgmont) 5:34–48.

[43] Center for Substance Abuse Treatment (1998) Continuity of offender treatment for substance use disorders from institution to community: Treatment Improvement Protocol (TIP) Series 30. Substance Abuse and Mental Health Services Administration, Public Health Service, Rockville, Maryland. DHHS Publication No. (SMA) 98–3245

[44] Available at:*www.americanbar.org*.

More specific to the chapter case, state departments of corrections have policies for the treatment of mentally ill offenders after their release. The Oklahoma Department of Corrections (OKDOC) has policies for the treatment of offenders with mental illness upon release from the care and custody of the OKDOC. One such policy is Section-06 Classification OP-060901, under Pre-Release Planning and Reentry Process[45]:

---

1. The administrator of mental health operations (AMHO) will ensure that proper discharge planning activities, **resources and support are available for offenders with serious mental illness** and offenders with other complicated and/or chronic mental health disorders. The AMHO) will troubleshoot, monitor and evaluate discharge plans.
   a. The AMHO serves as **a liaison with the Department of Mental Health and Substance Abuse Services (ODMHSAS) staff in the placement of Integrated Services discharge managers in facilities with mental health units** (JHCC, MBCC and OSP).
   b. The Integrated Services discharge managers **will coordinate the mental health reentry planning for offenders with serious mental illness discharging to the Tulsa or Oklahoma County areas.** ODMHSAS discharge planners will work in conjunction with ODMHSAS funded community mental health center based Reentry Intensive Care Coordination Teams (RICCT). **RICCT staff provides in-reach services to offenders with serious mental illness.** [bold added]

The OKDOC officials could not produce evidence that any of their own policy procedures were followed in the index case of this chapter. The drug expert insisted that the continued pharmacological treatment of the defendant with antipsychotics would have likely prevented the incident before the court.

Psychedelic Drugs Used in Psychiatry

LSD is a psychedelic drug that was popularized during the 1960s by groups such as the "*hippies*." One of the most potent drugs that affect the brain,[46] LSD is the acronym for lysergic acid diethylamide, a synthetic drug discovered accidentally to have bizarre psychedelic effects by the German pharmaceutical chemist Albert Hoffman in 1943.[47] Psychedelic drugs produce visual hallucinations (as opposed to the auditory hallucinations of schizophrenia), persistence of after images ("traces"), and synesthesia (crossing over of the senses, for example, sounds may be seen or colors may be heard).[48] Hallucinogens also produce effects described as deeply religious and mystical, of losing one's ego with a sense of self-dissolution, and becoming at one with God, Nature, or the Universe.

Before LSD use in the 1960s, hallucinogenic drugs from plants and mushrooms were used to induce altered states of consciousness in religious ceremonies and healing rituals by pre-Columbian Mesoamerican cultures, like the Mayans and Aztecs.[49] Mescaline is psychedelic drug found in the peyote cactus. During the late 1950s and 1960s, counterculture thinkers and artists began to self-experiment with peyote buttons, or ingest oral doses of synthetic mescaline which was then available. One self-described account of the pharmacological effects of mescaline was published as the influential book *Doors to Perception* by Aldous Huxley.[50]

Even though mescaline is a DEA Schedule I controlled substance, peyote is used to this day, legally, by members of the Native American Church. Surprisingly, the Native American Church won the right to use this drug in religious ceremonies with the passage of the *American Indian Religious Freedom Act* in 1994.[51]

Psilocybin is the active hallucinogenic drug in "*magic mushrooms*." Like LSD and mescaline, psilocybin is thought to produce its strong psychedelic effects by acting on the brain's serotonin system. Psilocybin has been synthesized and is the most popular hallucinogenic drug recently tested for its utility in treating mental illness (see later).

---

[45] *doc.ok.gov/Websites/doc/Images/Documents/Policy/op060901.pdf.*

[46] Potency is measured by how much drug you need to get an effect. With LSD, a mere 25 μg (micrograms) is enough to send a person on an 8-hour trip. A microgram of drug is smaller than the period at the end of this sentence and weighs 1 millionth of a gram. A gram is about the weight of a small paperclip.

[47] An amazing description of Dr. Hoffman's first accidental LSD experience is recounted in: Hoffman A (1980) *LSD – My Problem Child*. McGraw-Hill Book Company, New York City, NY, USA.

[48] Brenner GM, Stevens CW (2018) *Op. cit.*

[49] Cartod-Artal FJ (2015) Hallucinogenic drugs in pre-Columbian Mesoamerican cultures. Neurología 30:42–49.

[50] Huxley A (1954) *The Doors of Perception*. Chatto & Windus, London, UK . Aldous Huxley is the grandson of Sir Thomas Huxley quoted in Chapter 7. Aldous Huxley is most famous for his dystopian novel *Brave New World* published in 1932.

[51] Prue B (2014) Prevalence of reported peyote use 1985–2010 effects of the American Indian Religious Freedom Act of 1994. Amer J Addict. 23:156–161.

Unlike the hallucinogenic drugs, ketamine is an analog of phencyclidine (PCP, "*angel dust*") and is classified as a *dissociative anesthetic*. Ketamine is an FDA-approved drug, used to induce anesthesia and in some cases, to be used as the sole anesthetic.[52] Ketamine injection (Ketalar®) is an older drug and approved before 1982 and has a wide margin of safety and unintentional administration ten times greater than the therapeutic dose led to complete recovery.[53]

Therapeutic use of hallucinogens and ketamine

After the passage of the *Controlled Substances Act* in 1970 (see Chapter 11) research into the therapeutic effects of hallucinogenic drugs came to a halt.[54] More recently, there has been a resurgence of clinical studies examining the putative beneficial effects of psychedelic drugs. Most clinical studies of the effectiveness of hallucinogenic drugs in treating mental illness, including schizophrenia, were done using LSD and psilocybin. These hallucinogenic drugs were shown to have efficacy in treating nicotine and alcohol addiction, depression, and end-of-life anxiety.[55] Besides their well-known action on the serotonin system in the brain, psychedelics disrupt normal neural connections and provide novel functional brain associations helpful in a number of psychiatric disorders.

Microdosing

A recent phenomena is the use patterns of illegal controlled substances, primarily hallucinogens, is called *microdosing*.[56] Microdosing is the pattern of use whereby very low doses of psychedelic substances are taken periodically, usually every other day or every third day. Scientific studies of microdosing are limited but users report that microdosing enhanced creativity and open-mindedness and reduced negative attitudes and negative emotions. It is likely that further studies of microdosing for the purpose of psychiatric therapy will be forthcoming.

The Drug Expert and Nonuse of Drugs

While the rampant use of drugs in the United States is linked to crime, the crime that occurs by lack of drug use appears greater in intensity and magnitude. At the time of this writing, cable news stations are reporting the on-air slaying of two journalists in Virginia. This follows other nationwide reports of shootings in movie theaters, military bases, colleges, high schools, and is epitomized by the most horrific slaying of 20 schoolchildren at Sandy Hook Elementary School in Newtown, Connecticut.[57] In all of these cases, the assailant was found to suffer from mental illness, with most cases ending with the assailant committing suicide after his horrendous act. These acts and countless others are due to the lack of drugs, more specifically, the lack of treatment of mental illness by effective and available psychotherapeutic drugs such as antidepressants and antipsychotics.

The State, as guardian and health care provider during the inmate's stay, does not guarantee continuing care once the inmate is released. Without treatment, the mentally ill, and especially the schizophrenics, are likely to recidivate and land back in prison.

Insane persons, like florid schizophrenics and psychotic manic-depressives, are essentially wards of the state or should be if no responsible family member or caretaker is available. Adequate mental health facilities, and not ersatz treatment center such as jails or prisons, should be available and reinstitutionalization should occur when needed. Antipsychotic

---

[52] Induction of anesthesia is the beginning of the general anesthesia process and can be accomplished by a strong sedative or a general anesthetic drug. The difference between induction of anesthesia and maintaining general anesthesia are paramount in the case of using midazolam as a lethal injection agent. See Chapter 20 *Death Be Not Proud* for a full discussion of anesthesia.

[53] Ketalar® (ketamine hydrochloride for injection), full prescribing information, Par Pharmaceutical, April 2017.

[54] Nichols DE et al. (2017) Psychedelics as medicines: an emerging new paradigm. Clin Pharm Ther. 101:209–219.

[55] Kyzar EJ et al. (2017) Psychedelic drugs in biomedicine. Trends Pharm Sci. 38:992–1005.

[56] Polito V, Stevenson RJ (2019) A systematic study of microdosing psychedelics. PLoS ONE 14(2): e0211023.

[57] The Sandy Hook shootings finally triggered a response from the President and Congress to write legislation to close the "gun show loophole" which remains a venue to legally obtain guns without a background check. Even after such a national tragedy, the Senate failed to pass by just 6 votes a bipartisan gun-control bill that would have expanded background checks to gun-show purchases. Teresa Welsh, *Gun Control Bill Hits a Wall ... But Just For Now?* U.S. News and World Report, April 18, 2013.

medications should be encouraged or if needed, forced upon those meeting the criteria for their use. Long-acting antipsychotic medications, consisting of a depot intramuscular injection every 2 to 4 weeks, are effective in controlling the symptoms of schizophrenia and restoring normalcy in those pained individuals.[58]

[Narrative continued]

A motion was made by the State to keep the drug expert from testifying, however the judge ruled against the motion and the drug expert was allowed to testify at trial during the sentencing phase. The drug expert outlined the Defendant's medical history and antipsychotic use prior to his last incarceration. Testimony was also given on the State's Department of Corrections' Policy on continuing mental health treatment for released offenders, the efficacy of antipsychotic treatment for schizophrenia, and the statistics of crimes committed by untreated schizophrenics. The State argued that the Defendant stopped antipsychotic treatment one month before his release and therefore did not need further treatment upon release. The Defendant's drug expert countered that a schizophrenic patient is not the best judge of needing treatment and forced medication procedures should have been done to keep the defendant on the antipsychotic medications while in the prison and community mental health programs contacted after his release. The Court sentenced Mr. Jones to 30 years for the Burglary count and life without a chance for parole for the First Degree Rape (child under 14) count to run consecutively.

---

58 Correll CU et al. (2016) The use of long-acting injectable antipsychotics in schizophrenia: evaluating the evidence. J Clin Psychiatry 77(Suppl. 3): 1–24.

Chapter 19

Dead Men Tell No Tales: Drug levels in a drowned, a decayed, and a dumpster corpse

Insurance Claims and Drug Use

Drug Detection in Fluid From the Eyeballs and Other Places

Postmortem Detection of Alcohol and Methamphetamine

Fetal Remains and Maternal Drug Use

The Toxicologist and the Pharmacologist Drug Expert

[Narrative]

John Plano was a 23-year old college grad from a well-to-do family in South Tulsa. One weekend at Grand Lake, he rented a speedboat and met his friends on the lake. After tying up to a flotilla of moored vessels, he stepped across to the next boat to meet-up with his friends. He soon returned to his boat and took a dive into the waters from the bow. His friends became worried, then very agitated when they didn't see him surface. They called the Grand Lake Water Patrol who responded within 10 min and began searching the waters. After 4 h of searching and darkness approaching, the search crews stopped for the night. Three days later, a fisherman reported a dead body floating in a cove near the scene of the accident. The decedent, Mr. Plano, was identified as the corpse from dental records and autopsy. The toxicological results showed that alcohol and THC was present in fluid samples from the eyeball (vitreous humor) but none from samples of heart or liver. On the basis of this finding, the insurance company refused payment of the decedent's life insurance policy, on the grounds that the insured party was impaired by drugs at the time of the accident. The parents of the insured sued the insurance company with the assistance of a private law firm. The law firm consulted with a local drug expert regarding the detection of alcohol in vitreous fluid, and the insurance company's denial due to drug impairment based on these results.

In a separate case, the decayed body of a woman was discovered in an apartment by the manager after a neighbor complained of a foul odor. A full autopsy was done with no signs of trauma or obvious pathology. Toxicology was done on putrefied liver samples and the amounts of two prescription drugs and one OTC drug were quantified. On the basis of this toxicology report, the deceased life insurance company refused to pay the death benefit to her mother due to alleged suicide of the insured. The mother sought legal assistance and her attorney contacted a local drug expert to interpret the findings of the toxicology report.

In a third case, a shoebox containing fetal remains was discovered in a dumpster by a homeless person. Toxicology of the fetal remains was limited to a decayed liver sample which gave methamphetamine and amphetamine levels in the fetal liver samples. The mother was tracked down and arrested for murder. A national organization for legal rights of pregnant women contacted a local drug expert to opine on the interpretation of the methamphetamine and amphetamine levels found in the fetal remains.

Insurance Claims and Drug Use

Private life insurance and accidental death insurance arose as a response to the *Industrial Revolution*, and primarily the new transportation network of railroads.[1] One of the first accident death insurance companies was formed in response to accidents and injuries that occurred with railroad travel in England. In 1863 the Travelers Insurance Company was the

---

[1] Scales AF (2000) Man, God and the Serbonian bog: the evolution of accidental death insurance. 86 Iowa L. Rev. 173.

first company to issue accident policies in the United States.[2] The name *"Travelers Insurance"* is apt and points out to the moorings of the present life insurance and accidental death and dismemberment (AD&D) policy stemming from the special case of persons using the modern conveyances of the time. Nowadays, life insurance is packaged with AD&D policies and coverage is continuous and independent of traveling or not.[3]

While any death results in the same outcome to the deceased and surviving loved ones (i.e., the insured is dead) all manner of death does not automatically trigger the death benefit. For example, life insurance companies cannot pay out claims from a husband who takes out a large policy on himself with his wife as beneficiary, then kills himself so his wife can live comfortably the rest of her life. Like all insurance companies, life insurance companies do not want to pay *any* death benefits if they don't have to; such is the case in every for-profit industry.[4] For that reason, there are a number of circumstances when death benefits are excluded.

For example, the group Life Insurance and AD&D plan[5] offered to employees of the OSU Medical School in Tulsa lists the following death benefit exclusions (bold added):

Accidental Death and Dismemberment Exclusions

ReliaStar Life does not pay benefits for loss directly or indirectly caused by any of the following:
- *Suicide or intentionally self-inflicted injury, while sane or insane.*
- *Physical or mental illness.*
- *Bacterial infection or bacterial poisoning. Exception: Infection from a cut or wound caused by an accident.*
- *Riding in or descending from an aircraft as a pilot or crew member.*
- *Any armed conflict, whether declared as war or not, involving any country or government.*
- *Injury suffered while in the military service for any country or government.*
- *Injury which occurs when you commit or attempt to commit a felony.*
- **Use of any drug, narcotic or hallucinogenic agent –**
  - *unless prescribed by a doctor.*
  - *which is illegal.*
  - *not taken as directed by a doctor or the manufacturer.*
- **Your intoxication. Intoxication means your blood alcohol content meets or exceeds the legal presumption of intoxication under the laws of the state where the accident occurred.**

Because the use of alcohol, prescription drugs, OTC drugs, and/or illegal drugs is so common among insured individuals (as it is in all people, see Chapter 1), life insurance companies will often deny death benefits if there is any sign of drug use in the deceased. It is often the job of the drug expert to assist the insurance companies (rarely) and the plaintiffs filing suit against them (commonly), when issues of drug use in the deceased arise.

Drug Detection in Fluid From the Eyeballs and Other Places

The ideal postmortem sample for detection of drug use is a vial of femoral blood. Blood is the easiest to use, as the methodology for blood sampling in the living can be applied to blood sampling in the dead. Peripheral bold samples, such as from the femoral vein, also give the best comparison of drug levels between the living and the dead. Nearly every drug, if taken by humans, has a research paper or two on the pharmacokinetics of that drug and corresponding blood levels and time course of those levels. Most drugs approved by the FDA in the last few decades also include peak blood concentration of a drug in the full prescribing information.

Vitreous humor fluid samples for postmortem detection of drugs

When femoral blood cannot be obtained from a corpse due to decapitation, dismemberment, or fractionation, there is one place in the body that contains fluid encapsulated in a sealed container: the eyeball. The eyeball holds its shape due to the vitreous humor. *Humor* is an old word for fluid, as in the *four humors of the body*.[6] Vitreous humor is a clear, colorless fluid

---

[2] Travelers Insurance Company, with its iconic red umbrella logo, is still going strong today.

[3] For instance it is said that most home accidents occur in the bathroom. The insured in that case is would not be considered in a state of conveyance from one place to another, i.e., travelling.

[4] Like health care, perhaps insurance companies should be embedded in a nonprofit structure.

[5] *Your Group Life Insurance Plan*, for OSU employees, from ReliaStar Insurance Company, subsidiary of the Dutch ING financial group.

[6] Early Greek medicine identified the four humors of the body as blood, yellow bile, black bile, and phlegm.

filling the main chamber of the eye. Vitreous humor can be sampled by using a syringe and needle and inserting about 1 cm into the eyeball and slowly withdrawing the vitreous fluid.[7] Because of its blood supply, the vitreous humor also reflects a drug's concentration in the peripheral blood, although the relationship between vitreous fluid and blood levels of a drug is not clear (see later). For this reason, vitreous humor samples are often used for forensic analysis, especially in decayed or decomposing human bodies.[8]

Studies comparing the use of vitreous fluid or femoral blood samples for use in routine drug screening showed that drug screens in femoral blood resulted in twice as many positive drug tests in blood than vitreous fluid.[9] This suggests that vitreous fluid, either by its restricted blood flow and lower drug concentrations or other biological processes, is not as good as blood for routine drug detection in postmortem samples.

The vitreous fluid sample taken from the drowned man in the first narrative case of this chapter yielded a vitreous alcohol concentration of 0.10%, which was the basis of the insurance company denial of death benefits to the parents of the dead man. There were no other samples obtained in that case.

Liver samples for postmortem detection of drugs

The liver could easily qualify as the number one internal organ in the abdomen. It is the only internal organ that can regenerate itself, and among its many roles, acts as the gatekeeper of all foreign substances that enter the body. Food and drugs taken orally are absorbed in the stomach and small intestine and immediately enter a special blood vessel pathway called the hepatic portal system. Drugs that are given by the IV route, directly in the bloodstream, quickly end up in the liver due to its large blood flow. The liver is also the number one site for drug metabolism.

Putrefied liver tissue taken from the decedent described in the second chapter case was analyzed by GC-MS and three drug substances were detected and quantified.[10] The toxicology report from the Medical Examiner's Office reported zolpidem (Ambien®) at 4.5 μg/g (micrograms per gram of liver tissue), carisoprodol (Soma®) at 200 μg/g, and diphenhydramine (Benadryl®) at 30 μg/g in the putrefied liver samples of the decedent. On the basis of these findings, the insurance company denied benefits to the dead woman's spouse, asserting that the presence of these drugs showed that the decedent purposely overdosed on these medications and committed suicide.

Decomposed liver samples from the fetal remains found in third chapter case were also sampled and tested for drugs. The fetal liver tissue had a methamphetamine concentration of 3.0 μg/g and amphetamine was detected but not quantified. On the basis of this finding, the state's toxicologist opined that the mother's use of methamphetamine caused intrauterine fetal demise.

Other tissue sources for postmortem drug detection

The kidney, brain, and muscle are also used for postmortem drug detection.[11] These samples are often used when blood cannot be obtained. Samples can be used from these tissues but they also contain large amounts of lipids (fats) which interfere with the analytic methods used in toxicology. However, there is limited data to compare postmortem and premortem drug concentrations to aid in interpretation of results from these samples.

More rarely, bone, hair, and fingernail samples are used for the postmortem detection of drugs, especially in decomposed corpses. Bone tissues are especially useful if the body has undergone severe decomposition, exsanguination, or skeletonization.[12] Examination of bone tissue in a completely skeletonized corpse revealed significant levels of the opioid fentanyl. The amount of fentanyl was found to be dependent on the type of bone tissue examined (legbone *vs.* vertebrae) and area of the bone (outer tissue *vs.* bone marrow).[13] Hair sampling for drug detection is noninvasive and can be obtained in the living and the dead. As discussed in Chapter 6 *Hairs of the Innocent*, drug detection in hair has a long window of detection as drugs in hair are interwoven into the hair matrix as the hair grows. In postmortem hair samples, depending on the length of the hair,

[7] Yee L et al. (2000) Chiral high-performance liquid chromatographic analysis of fluoxetine and norfluoxetine in rabbit plasma, urine, and vitreous humor using an acetylated beta-cyclodextrin column. J Anal Toxicol. 24:651–655.

[8] Metushi IG et al. (2016) Assessment and comparison of vitreous humor as an alternative matrix for forensic toxicology screening by GC-MS. J Anal Toxicol. 40:243–247.

[9] Metushi IG et al. (2016) *Ibid.*

[10] Gas chromatography-mass spectrometry, the standard method for identifying and quantifying forensic drug samples. See Chapter 5.

[11] Margalho C et al. (2011) Illicit drugs in alternative biological specimens: A case report. J Forensic Legal Med. 18:132e135.

[12] Orfanidis A et al. (2018) Alprazolam and zolpidem in skeletal tissue of decomposed body confirms exposure. J Forensic Sci. http://dx.doi.org/10.1111/1556-4029.13890.

[13] Lafrenière NM, Watterson JH (2009) Detection of acute fentanyl exposure in fresh and decomposed skeletal tissues. Forensic Sci Internat. 185:100–106.

exposure to drugs in the deceased may be determined for the past 6 months or longer. However, this precludes use of hair samples to ascertain immediate or acute drug effects in the deceased. Hair is also an ideal matrix for drug detection in ancient humans, like cocaine metabolites found in Northern Chilean mummies dating back to 2000 BCE.[14] In a more recent case, antipsychotic drugs were detected in the fingernails and toenails of an unidentified and bloated corpse.[15] Drug testing helped investigators determine the identity of the corpse as it narrowed their search to a long-term user of antipsychotic medicines.

As mentioned, liver, kidney, brain, and most of the other tissues samples noted before, as well as vitreous fluid samples from the eye, cannot be obtained in living patients. Therefore the data from toxicological tests using these postmortem samples cannot be directly compared to reference data of drug and alcohol levels measured in living subjects. The drug expert is often the person to make this key point in the trial to avoid the overinterpretation by other experts. Existing data correlating any drug levels obtained postmortem from drug levels in living beings is extremely limited.

Postmortem Detection of Alcohol and Methamphetamine

Postmortem blood samples are ideally taken from a peripheral site, with the femoral vein in the leg considered the "*gold standard*" in medicolegal and forensic research.[16] In analytical toxicology guidelines, it is stated that drug levels from postmortem blood samples are most reliable when the interval between death and postmortem sampling is short, and blood samples are collected from a peripheral site, preferably the femoral vein.[17] Under ideal conditions, because postmortem blood samples can be compared to peripheral blood samples obtained in living patients, an attempt at correlating therapeutic and toxic (or intoxicating) levels of drugs and ethanol can be made.[18]

As introduced in Chapter 8, postmortem redistribution (PMR) of drugs occurs when a drug's concentration in the blood is different before and after death. This is important as nearly all of the data on the blood level of a drug and any adverse or toxic effects are based on blood levels in living subjects (antemortem samples). Depending on the drug, PMR can artificially increase blood concentrations when postmortem processes draw drugs from tissues in to the blood. Conversely, the process of PMR can decrease blood levels of a drug after death by the stoppage of blood circulation and drug absorption into fat tissue. For many drugs, PMR processes can be negligible with no change in antemortem and postmortem levels.[19]

In any event, in many cases the drug expert only has postmortem drug concentration data and is asked to form an opinion. Some opinions can be made when the drug levels are *in extremis*, for example, super-high levels of a drug might easily relate to drug concentrations found in forensic studies of documented suicides using the drug at issue.[20] Many cases yield astonishing low levels of drug in postmortem samples, supporting a nonexistent role of acute drug use in the decedent.

Vitreous fluid sample for alcohol determination

With all the instances of alcohol mentioned in this book, the reader might be tempted to leave the coffee shop and head to a nearby bar.[21] However, the postmortem redistribution of alcohol is an important topic to bring up because so many people drink alcohol and drive, or jump off a boat, and end up dead that reports of postmortem alcohol levels often find their way to the drug expert's desk.

Because a femoral blood sample is considered the most reliable site of sampling for forensic interpretation (see earlier), much forensic research compares the ethanol concentration from vitreous fluid to ethanol concentration from femoral blood

---

[14] Cocaine metabolites were found in these hair specimens. Baez H et al. (2000) Drugs in prehistory: chemical analysis of ancient human hair. Forensic Sci Internat. 108:173–179.

[15] Chen H et al. (2014) Determination of clozapine in hair and nail: the role of keratinous biological materials in the identification of a bloated cadaver case. J Forensic Leg Med. 22:62–67.

[16] Launiainen T, Ojanperä I (2014) Drug concentrations in post-mortem femoral blood compared with therapeutic concentrations in plasma. Drug Test Anal. 6:308–316.

[17] Flanagan RJ, Connally G, Evans JM (2005) Analytical toxicology: guidelines for sample collection postmortem. Toxicol Rev. 24:63–71.

[18] Also have to consider postmortem redistribution of the drug, discussed in the next section below. See also: Skopp G (2004) Preanalytic aspects in postmortem toxicology. Forensic Sci Int. 142:75–100.

[19] For an excellent article on PMR by a leading expert in the area, see Drummer and his colleagues, *e.g.* Gerostamoulos D, Beyer J, Staikos V, Tayler P, Woodford N, and Drummer OH (2012) The effect of the postmortem interval on the redistribution of drugs: a comparison of mortuary admission and autopsy blood specimens. Forensic Sci Med Pathol.8:373–379.

[20] Obviously there are some caveats in comparing levels of a postmortem drug in a legal case and drug concentrations reported in forensic studies. For example, most drugs have quite a large lethal blood concentration range which can provide little information in comparing a single value from a real case.

[21] Drug-craving cues like the numerous mentions of alcohol in this book are based on actual data. Neuroimaging shows that craving areas of the brain become activated ("light up") in response to pictures of crack cocaine in abstinent users, another proof that addictive drug use alters the brain.

samples.[22] These studies show that the ratio of vitreous fluid alcohol to femoral blood alcohol is highly variable. Some cases show a high ratio of vitreous fluid alcohol to femoral blood alcohol, other the opposite, with a low ratio of vitreous fluid alcohol to femoral blood alcohol. The ratio of vitreous ethanol to blood BAC is highly variable when the level of ethanol in the blood is less than 0.10% BAC. The concentration of ethanol in the vitreous fluid is typically higher than that in femoral blood; however, the relationship between vitreous fluid and heart blood is not clear.[23]

An early study made a mathematical model to prediction of blood alcohol concentration (BAC) from the alcohol concentration in the vitreous fluid but concluded that *"the prediction interval is too wide to be of real practical use."*[24] They continued that previous authors provided simple conversion factors to estimate BAC from vitreous alcohol *"without taking into account the uncertainty of the prediction for an individual subject."* Another study of 62 deceased subjects found that ethanol concentrations in the vitreous fluid did not have a significant correlation to peripheral BAC.[25]

Expert authors in the field suggested more studies are needed before vitreous fluid ethanol can make reliable predictions of BAC.[26] They outlined the studies needed: a large population of cases where the time and amount of alcohol consumed before death was known, the time of death, and the time of postmortem sampling was known. Other authors found that the ratio between vitreous ethanol concentration and blood BAC is so variable that a *rule-of-thumb* practice is to take half the vitreous alcohol concentration to estimate the BAC.[27]

In the present chapter case of the drowned corpse, the insurance company denied benefits largely based on the alcohol level from a single sample of vitreous fluid. From a single determination of 0.12% vitreous fluid alcohol, the insurance company claimed the decedent's BAC was greater than 0.08% and that he was intoxicated. This violated the *no intoxication* clause of the life insurance policy. The claim of intoxication was made by the insurance company in spite of both the report from the medical examiner and the official death certificate note an accidental death by drowning with no contributing factor or other significant factor of alcohol intoxication.

Postmortem redistribution of alcohol

Postmortem redistribution of drugs and ethanol results when the drug or ethanol diffuses from higher concentrations to areas of lower concentrations in the corpse following the disruption of cellular membranes.[28] Postmortem redistribution of drugs and ethanol makes it impossible to determine with certainty the actual drug or ethanol content in the person before they died. It is well established in the forensic pharmacology literature that ethanol undergoes postmortem redistribution.[29] Postmortem redistribution of ethanol is also caused by trauma to the deceased in the manner of death. Traumatic injuries to the torso are known to increase BAC.[30] Other studies show that specimen site variability (e.g., heart blood versus femoral blood) is due to postmortem redistribution of ethanol.[31]

Postmortem production of ethanol

After a person dies, a process of accelerated microbe growth begins in many tissues of the body. These microbes, mostly bacteria, yeast, and fungi, have been identified in postmortem tissues and are known to produce alcohol as part of their natural metabolism.[32] This process is called the "postmortem production of ethanol" or "endogenous ethanol production" (inside the body, as opposed to exogenous ethanol from a few drinks). Ethanol synthesis by microbes is observed in the early stages of decomposition or putrefaction.[33] Postmortem production of ethanol can lead to ethanol level as high as

[22] Caplan YH, Levine B (1990) Vitreous humor in the evaluation of postmortem blood ethanol concentrations. J Anal Toxicol. 14:305–307; Kugelberg FC, Jones AW (2007) Interpreting results of ethanol analysis in postmortem specimens: a review of the literature. Forensic Sci Int. 165:10–29.

[23] Honey D et al. (2005) Comparative alcohol concentrations in blood and vitreous fluid with illustrative case studies. J Anal Toxicol. 29:365–369.

[24] Pounder DJ, Kuroda N (1994) Vitreous alcohol is of limited value in predicting blood alcohol. Forensic Sci Int. 65:73–80.

[25] Mackey-Bojack S et al. (2000) Cocaine, cocaine metabolite, and ethanol concentrations in postmortem blood and vitreous humor. J Anal Toxicol. 24:59–65.

[26] Sylvester PA et al. (1998) *Op cit.*

[27] Jones AW, Holmgren P (2001) Uncertainty in estimating blood ethanol concentrations by analysis of vitreous humour. Clin Pathol. 54:699–702.

[28] Kugelberg FC, Jones AW (2007) *Op cit.*; Pélissier-Alicot AL et al. (2006) *Op cit.*; Drummer OH (2004) Postmortem toxicology of drugs of abuse. Forensic Sci Int. 142:101–113.

[29] Kugelberg FC, Jones AW (2007) *Op cit.*; Iwasaki Y et al. (1998) On the influence of postmortem alcohol diffusion from the stomach contents to the heart blood. Forensic Sci Int. 94:111–118.

[30] Winek et al. (1995) The role of trauma in postmortem alcohol determination. Forensic Sci Int. 71:1–8.

[31] Can et al. (2012) Importance of sampling sites for postmortem evaluation of ethyl alcohol. Forensic Res. 3:7.

[32] Lewis RJ et al. (2004) Ethanol formation in unadulterated postmortem tissues. Forensic Sci Int. 146:17–24.

[33] Boumba VA et al. (2008) Biochemical pathways generating post-mortem volatile compounds co-detected during forensic ethanol analyses. Forensic Sci Int. 174:133–151.

0.22 g/dL (0.22% BAC).[34] Postmortem production of ethanol is not rare but common. All 9 accident victims showed post-mortem production of ethanol in an FAA-investigation accident.[35] Importantly, this study also showed that postmortem production of ethanol can occur in bodies stored at 4°F, as is commonly done in the morgue.

It is often stated that a vitreous humor fluid sample is less likely to undergo postmortem production of ethanol due to its isolated location in the eyeball.[36] However, research shows that fluid samples from the vitreous fluid can show evidence of postmortem production of ethanol.[37] Through postmortem redistribution, any microbial production of ethanol elsewhere would also be freely available to distribute to the vitreous humor fluid. Drug concentrations have been noted to undergo postmortem increases in the vitreous humor fluid samples, which was attributed to dehydration.[38] Additionally, the vitreous humor contains glucose (a sugar) which is known to be used for the postmortem production of ethanol by microbes.[39] Also, there are a number of other substrates besides glucose that microbes can use for the postmortem production of ethanol including amino acids, fatty acids, and glycerol.[40]

According to some investigators, postmortem BAC analysis has an unacceptable high rate of specimen site variability.[41] Vitreous fluid alcohol concentration did not correlate well without high variability when compared to BAC obtained from femoral and heart blood samples. There is high variability in the value of BAC depending on where the blood is sampled from the body. Studies show that even the left side of the heart may yield significantly different BAC values than the right side of the heart in postmortem determinations of ethanol concentration.[42]

Postmortem redistribution of methamphetamine

One study measured antemortem (while subject was still alive) and postmortem levels of methamphetamine and amphetamine in blood samples. Methamphetamine and amphetamine concentrations in peripheral blood samples were 1.5 to 2 times greater in the postmortem samples compared to the antemortem samples.[43] In this study, antemortem samples were taken 7–22 min prior to a declaration of death at the hospital, and the postmortem samples 5–30 h after death at autopsy.

As mentioned earlier, obtaining samples after death for forensic analysis for drugs is confounded by postmortem redistribution (PMR) of drugs. Methamphetamine undergoes extensive PMR and methamphetamine is concentrated in the liver. Human and primate studies with direct imaging show that the liver and kidneys are organs with the highest uptake of methamphetamine. In humans, about a quarter (23%) of the total methamphetamine dose was concentrated in the liver in live imaging studies.[44]

Fetal Remains and Maternal Drug Use

Estimates of illicit drug use[45] during pregnancy vary widely in the medical literature. Maternal use of illicit drugs is self-reported by about 5%–10% of pregnant women. However, universal drug testing in high-risk populations (low socioeconomic status) reveals a higher rate of 10%–40% illicit drug use during pregnancy.[46]

In general, maternal use of illicit drugs during pregnancy may place the fetus at risk for problems including low birth weight, small head circumference, increased preterm delivery, and other developmental complications.[47] With the use of illicit drugs, the evidence or data is insufficient or too variable to ascertain with certainty drugs that produce ill effects on the fetus and at what drug concentrations. Furthermore, clinical studies that take into account the confounding factors such

---

[34] Skopp G (2004) Preanalytic aspects in postmortem toxicology. Forensic Sci Int. 142:75–100.

[35] Lewis et al. (2004) *Op. cit.*

[36] de Martinis BS et al. (2006) Alcohol distribution in different postmortem body fluids. Hum Exp Toxicol. 25:93–97.

[37] de Lima IV, Midio AF (1999) Origin of blood ethanol in decomposed bodies. Forensic Sci Int. 106:157–162.

[38] Skopp G (2004), *Op. cit.*

[39] Kugelberg FC, Jones AW (2007) Interpreting results of ethanol analysis in postmortem specimens: a review of the literature. Forensic Sci Int. 165:10–29.

[40] Boumba VA et al. (2008) Biochemical pathways generating post-mortem volatile compounds co-detected during forensic ethanol analyses. Forensic Sci Int. 174:133–151.

[41] Sylvester PA et al. (1998) Unacceptably high site variability in postmortem blood alcohol analysis. J Clin Pathol. 51:250–252.

[42] Pélissier-Alicot AL et al. (2006) Comparison of ethanol concentrations in right cardiac blood, left cardiac blood and peripheral blood in a series of 30 cases. Forensic Sci Int. 156:35–39.

[43] McIntyre IM et al (2013) Antemortem and postmortem methamphetamine blood concentrations: three case reports. J Anal Toxicol. 37:386–389.

[44] Volkow ND et al. (2010) Distribution and pharmacokinetics of methamphetamine in the human body: clinical implications. PLoS One 5:e15269.

[45] Includes the abuse of prescription drugs, like opioids, as well as the standard drugs like marijuana, coke, etc.

[46] Farst KJ et al. (2011) Drug testing for newborn exposure to illicit substances in pregnancy: pitfalls and pearls. Int J Pediatr. 2011:951616. doi: 10.1155/2011/951616.

[47] Rayburn WF (2007) Maternal and fetal effects from substance use. Clin Perinatol. 34:559–571.

as poverty, poor nutrition, lack of prenatal care, and so on, from actual drug use-related factors are limited, sometimes inconsistent, or does not exist in the few studies that were done.

A study from 2009 examined admission at federally funded drug treatment centers and found that in 1994, methamphetamine use accounted for 8% of admitted pregnant women.[48] In 2006 treatment for methamphetamine was the reason given by 24% of pregnant women. While the increase in the meth-using mothers reporting for treatment may have been due to the success and growth of the treatment program in targeting methamphetamine users, the use of methamphetamine during pregnancy remains a significant health issue. The next section reviews clinical studies with respect to methamphetamine use and adverse drug effects on the fetus.

Methamphetamine effects on the fetus

In a comprehensive clinical study of all pregnancies in California from 2005 to 2008, the medical records of 8542 women who used methamphetamine during pregnancy were compared with over 2 million women who did not use methamphetamine.[49] Preterm birth, defined as delivery of less than 37 weeks, was present in 23.4% of meth users compared to 8.9% in the control group of nonuser pregnancies. However, there was not a significant increase in preterm death of the neonate, occurring in 2.1% of meth-using mothers and in 1.6% in nonusing mothers. Two important conclusions come from this study: preterm death is not increased by maternal use of methamphetamine and that earlier delivery that occurs due to methamphetamine use is not reflected in a greater death rate of preterm neonates. These data also show that even with methamphetamine use, 76.6% of neonates are born at full-term, proving that methamphetamine is more likely to have no effect on the fetus. Finally, the data show that preterm death or intrauterine fetal demise (IUFD) occurs at a rate essentially the same in the meth-exposed and non-meth-exposed fetus, and is rare at only 2.1% of meth using mothers and 1.6% of nonusing mothers. The previous study also noted that methamphetamine use may have been protective against gestational diabetes.

Other studies note an increase in preterm births and low birth weight of neonates born to mothers who used methamphetamine during pregnancy.[50] As noted in this paper, when assessing the impact of illicit drug exposure during pregnancy, there are numerous other confounding factors to take into consideration and rule out before the effects can be attributed solely to the drug action. These include concurrent use of tobacco and alcohol, use and access to prenatal care, polydrug exposure, prescription drugs, insurance coverage, nutrition, and socioeconomic status to name a few. These other factors are associated with methamphetamine use per se.

A large clinical study of methamphetamine effects on intrauterine growth of neonates exposed to methamphetamine during pregnancy was done using a target group of 204 mothers who used methamphetamine compared to 3501 mothers who did not.[51] This study employed a sophisticated multivariate analysis that factored in the covariates of neonate gender, prenatal care visits, household income, socioeconomic status, mother's weight gain, mother's age, partner status, and race. Additionally, cooccurrence of methamphetamine and maternal tobacco, alcohol, and marijuana use was considered. In the final analysis, there was a significant decrease in the overall size of neonates at birth in meth-using mothers than nonusing control group. However, there were no significant differences in average birth weight of babies from meth users or control mothers. The researchers found no instances of IUFD attributed to the use of methamphetamine in meth-using mothers.

Surprisingly, in this chapter's third case, no blood or urine samples were obtained from the accused mother for drug testing after she was apprehended. Hair samples from the mother would have been ideal in that drug use during the time of pregnancy could have been analyzed. Without evidence of maternal use of methamphetamine during the pregnancy, it is not possible to conclude with certainty that prenatal exposure of methamphetamine was a contributing factor in the intrauterine fetal demise.

Methamphetamine in fetal liver samples

There are few studies of fetal liver tissue and methamphetamine. One study examined the incidence of fetal drug exposure in Alabama from 2004 to 2011 using toxicological records from the Alabama Department of Forensic Sciences.[52] The

---

[48] Terplan M et al. (2009) Methamphetamine use among pregnant women. Obstet Gynecol. 113:1285–1291.

[49] Gorman MC et al. (2014) Outcomes in pregnancies complicated by methamphetamine use. Am J Obstet Gynecol. 211:429.e1–7.

[50] Ladhani NN et al. (2011) Prenatal amphetamine exposure and birth outcomes: a systematic review and meta-analysis. Am J Obstet Gynecol. 205:219.e1–7.

[51] Nguyen D et al (2010) Intrauterine growth of infants exposed to prenatal methamphetamine: results from the infant development, environment, and lifestyle study. J Pediatr. 157:337–339.

[52] Kalin JR (2014) Incidence of fetal drug exposure in Alabama: 2004-2011. J Forensic Sci. 59:1029–1035.

authors found that out of 15,600 total fatalities (all ages) with postmortem toxicology screens, only 39 cases were from fetal or neonate deaths. Of these 39 cases, 22 were positive for any drug and only 7 were positive for methamphetamine or amphetamine. Liver samples were available from 2 cases with methamphetamine levels of 1.2 µg/g and 2.3 µg/g. However, in the first positive meth case, five other drugs were detected, including the opioid hydrocodone. In the second positive meth case, the conclusion was that the manner of death was undetermined. The authors concluded that placental insufficiency, miscarriage, and IUFD are natural occurring events (unrelated to drug use) and that fetal/neonate death *"is often deemed drug-related only by virtue of a positive toxicological finding."*

A small forensic report examining 8 cases of maternal methamphetamine use and fetal demise reported only a single case of intrauterine fetal demise (IUFD) where fetal liver samples were obtained. In this one case, a toxicology analysis reported a methamphetamine level of 0.52 µg/g and amphetamine level of 0.04 µg/g in the fetal liver sample. In that single case the manner of death was given as *"IUFD, with findings consistent of asphyxia in the presence of maternal methamphetamine abuse."*[53] However, there were no supporting studies to confirm the pathologist's finding and no physical evidence of asphyxia.

The detection of amphetamines in the liver samples is not that uncommon. The liver concentrates methamphetamine and amphetamine, and other drugs, as the liver is the site of drug metabolism. There are also binding sites for methamphetamine and amphetamines on the cells of the liver tissue.[54] In postmortem studies, liver tissues were found to have 6–7 times higher concentrations of methamphetamine and amphetamine than peripheral blood.[55] In another study, liver concentrations of methamphetamine ranged from about 2 to 9 times that of peripheral blood.[56]

A forensic study in apparent suicides by drug overdose examined amphetamines found in adult liver samples.[57] The authors noted that in 6 out of 13 postmortem liver samples, false positive concentrations of amphetamines were found in liver samples that were not found in blood or other biological samples of the deceased. This could be the result of a large number of other drugs and medicines that can give a false positive methamphetamine result. The authors also state that it is known that amphetamines can be generated spontaneously from body substances in the liver and that this can occur in decomposing liver tissue. All the previous studies were done in adult postmortem tissue samples. There are no studies comparing blood to liver methamphetamine concentrations in a fetus or neonate.

One study examined illicit drug and metabolites found in maternal hair samples in conjunction with drugs and metabolites found in fetal tissue remains in a group of 60 women undergoing elective abortion.[58] There was not a good correlation between maternal use of illicit drugs as reflected in the hair samples and levels of illicit drugs found in the fetal tissue samples. The authors also noted that there is a large variability in the movement of drugs through the placenta and placental metabolism of drugs. *Placentopharmacology* and the workings of the placenta are still not well understood.

A single measurement of the concentration of methamphetamine from liver samples which may be from 2 days to 1 week or more in a decomposing fetus does not support a determination of death due to methamphetamine toxicity. There are no such toxic levels known for methamphetamine in liver samples in adults and certainly no studies of possible toxic levels of methamphetamine in liver tissue samples obtained from fetal remains. At present, there is no scientific basis for asserting that a certain amount of methamphetamine in the decayed liver sample of the fetal tissues was the cause of death of the discarded fetus.

The Toxicologist and the Pharmacologist Drug Expert

Toxicology is the study of the toxic effects of drugs, chemicals, or other substances on living organisms. A toxicologist may have an undergraduate, masters, or PhD degree. The label of "toxicologist" is therefore broader than the label of "pharmacologist"[59] which was adjudicated to be indicative of a person holding a PhD in Pharmacology, that is, a Professor of Pharmacology. Not that there is anything wrong with being a toxicologist, some of my best friends are toxicologists. It's just that the level of training and experience, and therefore expertise on drugs, can vary drastically in a toxicologist drug

[53] Stewart JL, Meeker JE (1997) Fetal and infant deaths associated with maternal methamphetamine abuse. J Anal Toxicol. 21:515–517.

[54] Jones AL, Simpson KJ (1999) Review article: mechanisms and management of hepatotoxicity in ecstasy (MDMA) and amphetamine intoxications. Aliment Pharmacological Ther. 13:129–133.

[55] McIntyre IM (2015) A "theoretical" post-mortem redistribution factor (F_t) as a marker of post-mortem redistribution. Eur J Forensic Sci. 2:24–26.

[56] McIntyre IM et al. (2011) Postmortem methamphetamine distribution. J Forensic Res 2:122–125.

[57] Sutlovic D et al. (2017) Amphetamine in post-mortem liver sample? Peertechz J Forensic Sci Tech. 3:1–4.

[58] Falcon M et al. (2012) Maternal hair testing for the assessment of fetal exposure to drug of abuse during early pregnancy: Comparison with testing in placental and fetal remains. Forensic Sci Int. 218:92–96.

[59] See Chapter 14, section entitled *"The Pharmacist versus the Pharmacologist Drug Expert."*

expert in contrast to the solid, lumbering, and extensive multiyear training (including toxicology) for the PhD pharmacologist drug expert.[60]

Of course, a PhD level Toxicologist would be no less acceptable than a PhD pharmacologist, and may be a better choice depending on the toxic drug issue at hand. It is important to recognize the different types of toxicologists that the drug expert or attorney may encounter in various cases. The toxicologist who signs off on investigative reports and is director of the state forensic laboratories in my home state is a PhD Toxicologist with a PhD in Toxicology from a pharmacology and toxicology program. The head of the Tulsa police forensics laboratory is a Toxicologist with a Master's Degree in Toxicology. The lab technician at the largest medical toxicology lab in town is an undergraduate with a major in Toxicology and a bachelor's degree. All three persons are commonly referred to as a toxicologist and have the title of "Toxicologist" next to their name, but their levels of expertise, skill sets, and areas of knowledge vary widely.

The type of a degree that the expert witness earned rightly matters to attorneys as shown in sociological studies carried out by surveys and experimental legal cases.[61] Experimental case results show that type of degree, as well as the actual testimony, years of experience, and testifying history are among the top four characteristics that attorneys assess in deciding to employ an expert witness. The number of publications and the expert's fee are lesser ranked considerations. In the survey data, particular aspects underlying expert witness credibility that were ranked most important by attorneys were, in order, perceived trustworthiness, communication skills, and conclusions to be offered in testimony and report.

The toxicologist in the chapter case on fetal remains detected methamphetamine and amphetamine in a liver sample from the fetal remains and opined that use of methamphetamine by the mother caused fetal death. He did not present any report or evidence from the medical literature to support his testimony. The drug expert wrote a detailed report with over thirty references from clinical research and forensic studies. The drug expert concluded that there is no reliable data to compare the level of detected methamphetamine in a decayed fetal liver sample to a toxic level in the blood that would kill a fetus.

[Narrative continued]

The drug expert researched several journal articles on the postmortem distribution of alcohol and findings from other forensic cases. It was found that estimates of alcohol levels and impairment from analysis of postmortem vitreous humor is unable to predict blood levels at the time of the accident. There was only one sample and that was obtained 72 h after the accident. Additionally, a literature search showed that the correlation of ethanol levels between vitreous humor samples and blood samples was not established. The judge found the drug expert's testimony persuasive and made a judgment against the insurance company. Eventually, after many requests from their attorney, the parents of the decedent received full benefit from the insurance company.

In the second case of the putrefied liver, there were two prescription drugs and one OTC drug detected and quantified from decayed liver samples. There was no evidence from pharmacy records that the prescription drugs were being abused. The OTC drug was relatively non-toxic, containing the antihistamine diphenhydramine. The drug expert concurred with the medical examiner in that there was no toxicological evidence to assert that the woman's death was nothing but accidental. After a long delay, the dead woman's mother received the death benefits from the insurance company.

In the third chapter case with the fetal remains, the drug expert found that false positives of methamphetamine and amphetamine are not rare due to other drug cross-reactions on the assay, that the liver concentrates methamphetamine, and that there were no conclusive studies of fetal methamphetamine and toxicity. There was no evidence that the mother used methamphetamine while she was pregnant. Methamphetamine toxicity to the fetus leading to intrauterine demise (IUFD) is not clearly established in the literature of forensic or clinical studies. Largely due to the drug expert's report, the second degree murder charge was dismissed. The mother still has charges pending related to the stillbirth and her drug use during pregnancy.

---

[60] After a 4-year undergraduate biology degree and a 3-year American Peace Corps in Nepal *tour-of-duty*, I spent 3 years at U of IL at Chicago for my M.S. in Biomedical Sciences, 4 years for Ph.D. in Pharmacology at Mayo Clinic, and 2 years postdoc at U of MN before finally getting my first job as Assistant Professor of Pharmacology here at OSU. That was 30 years ago.

[61] Wechsler HJ et al. (2015) Attorney beliefs concerning scientific evidence and expert witness credibility. Int J Law Psychiatry 41:58–66.

Chapter 20

Death Be Not Proud: The pharmacology of lethal drug executions

Let Me Be Perfectly Clear—Capital Punishment by Lethal Drug Injection

Lethal Drugs From Compounding Pharmacies

The Supreme Court of the United States and Lethal Injection Drugs

Alternative Methods of Execution—Epilogue and Conclusions

[Narrative]

Right now about 3000 condemned inmates sit in death row awaiting death by lethal injection. The triple-drug lethal injection protocol originated in Oklahoma in 1977 and was quickly adopted by other states who were looking to replace the gruesome electric chair. The first drug in the sequence is thiopental, a potent and ultra fast-acting barbiturate. Thiopental's job is to render the inmate unconscious, unaware, and insensate to pain because the next two drugs in the sequence produce pain and suffering in the awake inmate. The second drug is pancuronium, a muscle paralytic drug, which stops breathing. The third drug of Oklahoma's triple-drug protocol is potassium chloride which stops the heart. The pain and suffering of the second and third drugs is not in dispute. After manufacturers stopped making thiopental, State executioners used another potent barbiturate called pentobarbital. Soon pentobarbital also became unavailable. At that point, State executioners selected a different type of first drug, a benzodiazepine drug called midazolam. Therein lies the rub. The use of the benzodiazepine midazolam and resulting "botched" executions triggered a string of lawsuits based on the pharmacology of lethal injection drugs and bringing pharmacological testimony for the first time before the Supreme Court of the United States.

Let Me Be Perfectly Clear

We live in a tremendously cruel society. Universal health care for all of our fellow human beings is actually a debated issue in this nation. We provide little treatment for the mentally ill among us and use prisons to cage the most severe of them. Individuals with the mental illness of drug dependence are considered morally defective and completely responsible for their own actions. We refuse to regulate guns and automatic weapons, resulting in the increasing use of innocent victims and children as target practice. Faced with the highest incarceration rate of any country in the world, we build more prisons and legislate more crimes. Young men and women are sent to foreign lands to kill the enemy. Foreign women and children die as a result of their collateral damage. We drive deeper the wedge between the rich and the poor, sending more people into poverty and desperation. We discriminate against each other based on gender, race, creed, and sexual preference. We wish harm to others not like us. We cast slurs so often the offense of the words are soon forgotten. We alone among Western civilizations carry out capital punishment despite the data that shows innocent men have been wrongly executed in our country. By these laws, we allow our leaders to carry out state-sanctioned homicide to a greater degree than the most savage countries of the world. We medicalize and sanitize the process of execution by using clinical medications, but rely on little medical and pharmacological knowledge in the selection and administration of lethal drugs. We allow the use of ineffective drugs administered by ineffective protocols which torture inmates before they die. We are not a nice people.

Capital Punishment by Lethal Drug Injection

The use of drugs for capital punishment goes back to ancient times. Socrates was put to death by drinking a brew made from hemlock, a poisonous plant that grows throughout the world and still causes a few cases of accidental poisoning in the United States.[1] Since Socrates, governments have carried out executions with quartering, gibbeting, decapitations (increased by the enthusiasm of Dr. Joseph-Ignace Guillotin), hanging, and firing squads. With the miraculous age of electricity came the invention of the electric chair for death by electrocution.[2] Next came cyanide gas executions in purpose-built prison gas chambers, perhaps reflecting the familiarity of mustard gas (a vesicant or "blister-forming" gas) used in WWI.

Lethal drug injections are the latest adaptation in the evolution of execution methods. Use of lethal drugs represents the medicalization of the death penalty, a method that appeared less painful and more humane.[3] Other reasons for the lethal injection method include the idea that juries were more likely to vote for the death penalty if it appeared more humane. In 1972 Oklahoma was facing a major repair bill for its electric chair and did not want to pay $200,000 or more for the construction of a new gas chamber. In contrast, executions using lethal drug protocols were said to cost only about $15 an inmate.[4]

Considering the plethora of potent and lethal chemicals in the world, to date, there are only about ten drugs used or proposed for use in lethal drug protocols for capital punishment. As outlined before in the Chapter narrative, the triple-drug lethal injection protocol first developed in Oklahoma was quickly duplicated and used in other states. We start there.

Oklahoma introduces a new method of execution using a three-drug lethal injection protocol

Thiopental. Thiopental was the first drug in Oklahoma's triple-drug lethal injection protocol. Thiopental is a barbiturate drug, and barbiturates cause sedation, general anesthesia, and at higher doses, produce coma and death. Thiopental was marketed by Hospira under the trade name Pentothal®. Thiopental is classified as an *ultra short-acting barbiturate*.[5]

Thiopental shares its mechanism of action with all barbiturate drugs and inhibits brain activity in three ways: working with the inhibitory neurotransmitter GABA to increase neuronal inhibition, working without GABA to increase neuronal inhibition, and further depressing the activity of brain neurons by blocking excitation.

Thiopental and other barbiturate drugs like amobarbital, pentobarbital, and secobarbital, are classified into the larger group of drugs known as central nervous system (CNS) depressants. Other types of CNS depressants include drugs like benzodiazepines (Valium®, Xanax®), opioid analgesics (morphine, OxyContin®), and over-the-counter drugs like the antihistamine diphenhydramine (Benadryl®). Alcohol, of course, is also a well-used and abused CNS depressant drug.

All CNS depressants are so named because their pharmacological effect is to inhibit the activity of cells in the brain, causing neuronal inhibition. However, brain neurons are not inhibited in an all-or-none fashion; some CNS depressants inhibit neurons to a greater degree than others. For example, barbiturates are among the most potent CNS depressant drugs, the benzodiazepines and opioids less so, and antihistamines the least. With too much depression of brain activity, the neurons that drive breathing cease to function and death occurs by respiratory depression and hypoxia.

The major toxicity due to administration of barbiturates is a dose-dependent depression of respiration.[6] This means that the greater the dose, the greater the depression of brain activity by barbiturates and the harder it is to breathe. Barbiturate drugs were initially marketed in the 1920s and 1930s and used before the time of FDA regulation. Before the development

---

[1] Hotti H, Rischer H (2017) The killer of Socrates: coniine and related alkaloids in the Plant Kingdom. Molecules 22(11). pii: E1962. doi: 10.3390/molecules22111962; Brtalik D et al. (2017). Intravenous poison hemlock injection resulting in prolonged respiratory failure and encephalopathy. J Med Toxicol. 13:180-182.

[2] *See* Denno D (2014) Lethal injection chaos post-*Baze*. Georgetown Law J 102:1331-1382 *and* Denno D (2007) The Lethal injection quandary: how medicine has dismantled the death penalty. Fordham Law Rev. 76:49-128, for extensive background and pertinent non-pharmacological legal issues.

[3] Curran WJ, Casscells W (1980) Sounding Board. The ethics of medical participation in capital punishment by intravenous drug injection. N Engl J Med. 302:226-230.

[4] Annas GJ (1985) Killing with kindness: why the FDA need not certify drugs used for execution safe and effective. Am J Public Health 75:1096-1099.

[5] This classification is important as some states incorporated this phrase in their Execution Statutes. For example. The State of Mississippi TITLE 99 – CRIMINAL PROCEDURE of the Mississippi Code, Chapter 19 – Judgment, Sentence, and Execution, § 99-19-51 Manner of execution of death sentence states: "The manner of inflicting the punishment of death shall be by continuous intravenous administration of a lethal quantity of **an ultra short-acting barbiturate or other similar drug** in combination with a chemical paralytic agent until death is pronounced by the county coroner where the execution takes place or by a licensed physician according to accepted standards of medical practice" [bold added]. When Mississippi ran out of thiopental, it substituted pentobarbital without legal challenge. When it ran out of pentobarbital and proposed the use of midazolam, a legal challenge was made with the drug expert providing pharmacological evidence that midazolam was NOT an "ultra-short-acting barbiturate or other similar drug."

[6] Rosenberg M, Weaver J (1991) General anesthesia. Anesth Prog. 38:172-186.

of the less toxic benzodiazepine drugs which largely replaced the use of barbiturates,[7] physicians were alarmed with the increase in barbiturate use and reported on the rise in barbiturate toxicity (poisonings).[8] Despite their greatly reduced use and availability, barbiturates are still ranked as the 15th most common type of drug to cause fatal drug toxicity due to poisoning.[9] For this reason, the few barbiturate drugs on the market today are all prescription-requiring drugs or drug combinations.

A review of the two studies that examined postmortem blood levels of thiopental after state execution concluded that the relatively low levels of thiopental could not guarantee that thiopental produced unconsciousness, unawareness, and an inmate that was insensate to pain.[10] Besides its use as the first drug in a triple-drug protocol, thiopental was used as the sole lethal injection drug in a single-drug protocol in 10 executions since the year 2010 (see Fig. 20.2 at end of this section).

Pancuronium. Pancuronium, like the newer analogs vecuronium, rocuronium, and cisatracurium, is classified as a neuro-muscular blocker or simply called a muscle paralytic drug. Pancuronium is the second drug used in Oklahoma's triple-drug protocol. Neuromuscular blockers work by blocking the action of acetylcholine, which is the neurotransmitter released from a nerve ending onto the muscle that causes the muscle to contract.[11] Clinical uses of neuromuscular blockers are to provide muscle relaxation for endotracheal intubation and to ensure patient immobility during surgery or mechanical ventilation.[12]

The clinical effects of pancuronium are shared by other neuromuscular blockers and include progressive loss of skeletal muscle contraction, first noted by drooping eyelids and muscle weakness.[13] Motor weakness progresses eventually to a total flaccid paralysis. The small, quick muscles of the eyes, jaw, and larynx relax before those of the arms, legs, and trunk of the body. Finally, the intercostal muscles that expand the ribs and the diaphragm are paralyzed, and breathing ceases. Without intubation and mechanical ventilation, death ensues from a lack of oxygen (hypoxia).

There are a few studies of the effect of neuromuscular blockers given in human volunteers without an anesthetic agent. In a classic 1947 paper, a complete description of the effects of one of the first muscle paralytic drugs, tubocurarine, was reported.[14] These researchers found that neuromuscular blockers had no effect on altering consciousness, or memory, and had no analgesic (pain-killing) effect. They concluded that these paralytic drugs should not be used alone for surgery as they may cause "serious psychic trauma." A later study, using trained anesthesiologists and the researchers themselves, found that in these awake subjects vecuronium had no effect on consciousness and, like the earlier study by Smith and colleagues, the most distress came from a feeling of shortness of breath and *air hunger*, even though they were artificially ventilated with supplemental oxygen at sufficient levels.[15] As early as 1950, clinicians realized that the use of paralytic drugs like vecuronium and pancuronium without adequate anesthesia leads to the possibility that a patient is awake but incapable of indicating distress or pain because of muscle paralysis.[16]

While these previous studies were done on the researchers themselves, who were trained in the procedures and knew what to expect, most research on the adverse effects of pancuronium and other neuromuscular blockers comes from clinical cases where conscious patients were completely paralyzed but unable to communicate with health care workers. In emergency care, patients who experienced paralysis without sedation or anesthesia reported dysphoria and severe pain.[17]

Patients in intensive care units who were paralyzed with pancuronium because they were intubated and on mechanical ventilators, but were not sedated and were conscious, reported that they felt "buried alive"; some thought they were already

[7] López-Muñoz F, Ucha-Udabe R, Alamo C (2005) The history of barbiturates a century after their clinical introduction. Neuropsychiatr Dis Treat. 1:329-343.

[8] Hargrove EA et al. (1952) Acute and chronic barbiturate intoxication recent advances in therapeutic management. Calif Med. 77:383-386; Miller RR, DeYoung DV, Paxinos J (1970) Hypnotic drugs. Postgrad Med J. 46:314-317; Wells F (1976) The moral choice in prescribing barbiturates. J Med Ethics 2:68-70.

[9] Roberts DM, Buckley NA (2011) Enhanced elimination in acute barbiturate poisoning – a systematic review. Clin Toxicol. 49:2-12.

[10] Zimmers, TA, Koniaris LG (2008) Peer-reviewed studies identifying problems in the design and implementation of lethal injection for execution. Fordham Urb. L.J. 35:919-929.

[11] Naguib M et al. (2015) Chapter 34: Pharmacology of Neuromuscular Blocking Drugs in *Miller's Anesthesia*, 5e. Ed. Murphy GS et al. Saunders, Elsevier, Philadelphia, PA, USA.

[12] Kovac AL (2009) Sugammadex: the first selective binding reversal agent for neuromuscular block. J Clin Anesth. 21:444-453; Vecuronium Bromide for Injection, Full Prescribing Information.

[13] Brenner GM, Stevens CW (2018) Chapter 7: Acetylcholine Receptor Antagonists, in *Brenner and Stevens' Pharmacology, 5e*. Elsevier, Philadelphia, PA, USA.

[14] Smith SM et al. (1947) The lack of cerebral effects of d-tubocurarine. Anesthesiol. 8:1-14.

[15] Topulos GP et al. (1993) The experience of complete neuromuscular blockade in awake humans. J Clin Anesth. 5:369-374.

[16] Brice DD et al. (1970) A simple study of awareness and dreaming during anaesthesia. Br J Anaesth. 42:535-542.

[17] Chong ID et al. (2014) Long-acting neuromuscular paralysis without concurrent sedation in emergency care. Am J Emerg Med. 32:452-456.

dead.[18] Most of these patients said they would rather die than go through 4 days of being paralyzed while conscious again. A study of patients who emerged from anesthesia but were still paralyzed from neuromuscular blockers gave reports of panic, suffocation, and a feeling of already being dead.[19] These experiences were horrific enough to trigger posttraumatic stress disorder (PTSD) in some unfortunate patients.

Pancuronium must not be given to an inmate unless the inmate is already in a state of General Anesthesia, otherwise there would be severe pain and suffering experienced by the inmate due to muscle paralysis while awake. Other muscle paralytic drugs that are proposed or were used in executions by various states include vecuronium, rocuronium, and cisatracurium.

Potassium chloride. The third and final drug in Oklahoma's triple-drug protocol is potassium chloride. Potassium is an element and potassium chloride is a salt.[20] Potassium chloride is a cardiac arresting drug and used to stop the heart. The heartbeat is regulated by electrolytes in the blood and surrounding tissue. Electrolytes can be thought of as the watery substance in blood and found in between the tissues and cells throughout the body. They are called electrolytes because they are fluids that contain ions (positively and negatively charged atoms) that the body uses for nerve activity and muscle contraction. Potassium chloride (KCl) contains positively charged potassium ions (K^+) and negatively charged chloride ions (Cl^-). IV injection of a high dose of potassium chloride changes the electrolytes bathing the heart and blocks heart muscle contraction. Stoppage of the heart, if not jump-started again very soon, leads to certain death.

Potassium chloride for injection is an electrolyte solution used for the treatment of hypokalemia, which means low blood-potassium levels.[21] Hypokalemia can be life threatening and can lead to dysfunction of excitable tissues such as cardiac, skeletal, and smooth muscle.[22] The low potassium in hypokalemia may result in muscular paralysis, respiratory failure, and cardiac abnormalities, which can be fatal.

Hyperkalemia, or above normal potassium in the blood, has been used for over 60 years as a way for cardiac surgeons to cause cardiac arrest so they can operate on a still heart.[23] Hyperkalemic solutions, also called cardioplegic solutions, contain high levels of potassium chloride and are intentionally administered in heart bypass surgeries to cause cardiac arrest. One clinical study that examined 30 heart surgery patients and found that cardiac arrest after high concentrations of potassium chloride occurred after an average of 44 s after administration.[24]

Potassium chloride for injection is also used in late-term abortions of a fetus with genetic or severe, nonviable abnormalities.[25] In these cases, potassium chloride is delivered directly into the fetal heart chamber or into the umbilical vein.

The earliest report of an accidental high dose of IV potassium chloride due to improper mixing was in a male patient who immediately complained of a severe pain moving up his arm (above the site of the IV) and a ringing in his ears.[26] The patient then lost consciousness, stopped breathing, and his heart stopped beating. Another case study in that same year reported that an IV infusion of potassium chloride produced severe pain at the site of the IV infusion.[27] In a forensic report of four IV potassium chloride-induced deaths at a hospital, one man who accidentally received a high-dose IV infusion of potassium chloride screamed out in pain.[28]

Potassium chloride at high IV concentrations injections is extremely painful because high concentrations of potassium ions depolarize (activate) pain nerve endings which are present in the veins.[29] Even potassium chloride at clinically used

[18] Perry SW (1985) Psychological reactions to pancuronium bromide. Am J Psychiatry 142:1390-1391.

[19] Thomsen JL et al. (2015) Awareness during emergence from anaesthesia: significance of neuromuscular monitoring in patients with butyrylcholinesterase deficiency. Br J Anaesth. 115 Suppl 1:i78-i88.

[20] Unlike sodium chloride (NaCl, which is table salt), potassium chloride injected IV at high concentrations causes extreme pain upon injection and stops the heart.

[21] *Potassium Chloride for Injection, Full Prescribing Information.*

[22] Kruse JA, Carlson RW (1990) Rapid correction of hypokalemia using concentrated intravenous potassium chloride infusions. Arch Intern Med. 150:613-617.

[23] Cardiac arrest means total stoppage of the heartbeat. Oliveira MA et al. (2014) Modes of induced cardiac arrest: hyperkalemia and hypocalcemia—literature review. Rev Bras Cir Cardiovasc. 29:432-436.

[24] Jakobsen Ø et al. (2013) Adenosine instead of supranormal potassium in cardioplegia: it is safe, efficient, and reduces the incidence of postoperative atrial fibrillation. A randomized clinical trial. J Thorac Cardiovasc Surg. 145:812-818.

[25] Isada NB et al. (1992) Fetal intracardiac potassium chloride injection to avoid the hopeless resuscitation of an abnormal abortus: I. Clinical issues. Obstet Gynecol. 80:296-299; Senat MV et al. (2002) Funipuncture for fetocide in late termination of pregnancy. Prenat Diagn. 22:354-356; Sfakianaki AK et al. (2014) Potassium chloride-induced fetal demise: a retrospective cohort study of efficacy and safety. J Ultrasound Med. 33:337-341.

[26] Lankton JW et al. (1973) Letter: Hyperkalemia after administration of potassium from nonrigid parenteral-fluid containers. Anesthesiology 39:660-661.

[27] Williams RH (1973) Potassium overdosage: a potential hazard of non-rigid parenteral fluid containers. Br Med J. 1:714-715.

[28] Wetherton AR et al. (2003) Fatal intravenous injection of potassium in hospitalized patients. Am J Forensic Med Pathol. 24:128-131.

[29] Parsons CL (2011) The role of a leaky epithelium and potassium in the generation of bladder symptoms in interstitial cystitis/overactive bladder, urethral syndrome, prostatitis and gynaecological chronic pelvic pain. BJU Int. 107:370-375; Ahluwalia A, Vallance P (1997) Evidence for functional responses to sensory nerve stimulation of rat small mesenteric veins. J Pharmacol Exp Ther. 281:9-14.

concentrations causes phlebitis and pain.[30] A similar solution of potassium ions kept soluble as the potassium acetate salt was accidentally injected in an inmate in Oklahoma.[31] Potassium acetate is substituted intentionally for potassium chloride as the third drug in Florida's current triple-drug protocol. Potassium acetate is essentially equivalent to potassium chloride.

Oklahoma replaces thiopental with pentobarbital as first drug in triple-drug protocol

In 2010 Oklahoma did not have any thiopental on hand to carry out further executions and thiopental was not available in the marketplace.[32] Oklahoma substituted another barbiturate for thiopental, called pentobarbital, as the first drug in the triple-drug protocol. Other states soon followed suit and some states switched from Oklahoma's triple drug lethal injection protocol to a single-drug protocol using only pentobarbital. Ohio was the first state to use pentobarbital as the sole agent in a lethal drug execution. Pentobarbital-only lethal injection is the method that was used the most since 2010, resulting in over 130 deaths (see Fig. 20.2).

Pentobarbital. Like thiopental, pentobarbital is a barbiturate drug and shares its general mechanism of action with thiopental (see earlier) and all barbiturates. Compared to thiopental, pentobarbital has a slightly slower onset of action and is classified as a short-acting barbiturate. There are no clinical studies determining the lethal dose of IV pentobarbital sodium in humans. However, the largest IV pentobarbital sodium dose ever administered to human volunteers is reported in an early pharmacokinetic study from the 1950s.[33] In two volunteers, 2.5 g pentobarbital were injected IV over 50 min. While blood concentrations were not determined in these volunteers, the authors note that following these large doses of IV pentobarbital, the volunteers were deeply anesthetized and stopped breathing. The subjects had to be put on a ventilator with oxygen "until spontaneous ventilation was deemed adequate." Such studies could not be performed today due to safety and ethical concerns, but it is clear that a 2.5 g dose given IV was a lethal dose in these two individuals as it caused them to stop breathing on their own. These volunteers would have died without the supportive measures of the artificial ventilator and oxygen supplementation.

Florida switches from pentobarbital to midazolam as first drug in triple-drug protocol

The decision to use midazolam (Versed®) as the first drug in a three-drug lethal injection protocol was made by Florida after its supply of pentobarbital ran out and it was no longer commercially available.[34] Unlike thiopental and pentobarbital, however, midazolam is not a barbiturate but rather a benzodiazepine. Other well-known benzodiazepines include alprazolam (Xanax®) and diazepam (Valium®). Benzodiazepine use by physicians largely replaced barbiturate use not because they were pharmacologically equivalent but because they were safer. For example, benzodiazepines have almost universally supplanted the older barbiturate drugs for the treatment of anxiety disorders.[35] Benzodiazepines are safer forms of drug treatment for these disorders because they do not present the risk of fatal overdose that the more powerful barbiturates do.

Midazolam, diazepam, and other benzodiazepines act at the same GABA receptor on brain neurons where GABA and barbiturates act.[36] Midazolam, diazepam, and all benzodiazepines do not increase the synthesis of GABA, but rather, enhance the effect of the existing GABA at the GABA receptor.[37] For drugs like midazolam to enhance GABA inhibition,

---

[30] Ervin SM (1987) The association of potassium chloride and particulate matter with the development of phlebitis. NITA 10:145-149.

[31] Someone at OKDOC erroneously ordered potassium acetate instead of potassium chloride and this error wasn't discovered until the time of the execution. The Warden decided to go ahead and use potassium acetate anyway.

[32] Hospira was the sole source of sodium thiopental in the United States. It was manufactured in Italy and after EU regulations regarding the restriction of drugs exported to the United States for use in lethal injections, it stopped production of this drug in its plant in Italy in 2011. *See* Kas K et al. (2016) Lethal drugs in capital punishment in USA: History, present, and future perspectives. Res Social Adm Pharm. 12:1026-1034.

[33] Brodie BB et al. (1953) The fate of pentobarbital in man and dog and a method for its estimation in biological material. J Pharmacol Exp Ther. 109:26-34.

[34] At the same time there is no domestic pharmaceutical market for prisons and correctional facilities to obtain any IV barbiturate drug formulations, international sources of IV barbiturates solutions are also unobtainable. *See* Gibson J, Lain CB (2015) Death penalty drugs and the international moral marketplace. Georgetown Law J. 103:1215-1274.

[35] Howie JG (1975) Psychological medicine. Psychotropic drugs in general practice. Br Med J. 2:177-179; Pieters T, Snelders S (2007) From King Kong pills to mother's little helpers—career cycles of two families of psychotropic drugs: the barbiturates and benzodiazepines. Can Bull Med Hist. 24:93-112.

[36] Chang L-R et al. (1981) Molecular sizes of benzodiazepine receptors and the interacting GABA receptors in the membrane are identical. FEBS Lett. 126:309-312; Sigel E, Barnard EA (1984) A gamma-aminobutyric acid/benzodiazepine receptor complex from bovine cerebral cortex. J. Biol. Chem. 259:7219-7223.

[37] Greenblatt DJ et al. (1983) Current status of benzodiazepines. N Engl J Med. 309:354-358.

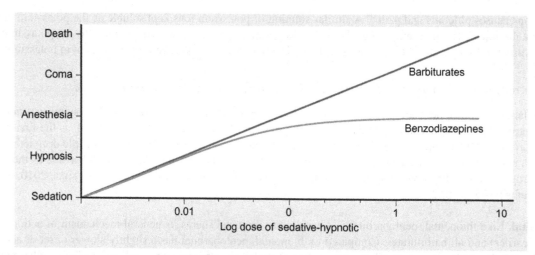

FIG. 20.1   Dose-response curves of barbiturates and benzodiazepines. The barbiturates exhibit a linear dose-response effect, which progresses from sedation to respiratory depression, coma, and death. Benzodiazepines exhibit a ceiling effect, which precludes severe CNS depression after oral administration of these drugs. Intravenous administration of benzodiazepines at clinical doses does not produce significant respiratory depression, except when other CNS depressants are coadministered. Benzodiazepines administered by either route do not produce anesthesia.[39]

GABA must be released naturally by the body's inhibitory neurons and be acting on the GABA receptors at the same time as the midazolam is present.[38] Midazolam helps GABA have a greater inhibitory effect. However without GABA present, midazolam does nothing to the GABA receptor and does not produce inhibition of the brain neurons. This is in contrast to barbiturates which activate GABA receptors without GABA present.

Importantly, GABA is a neurotransmitter produced in the brain in a limited amount. For that reason, midazolam effects are limited by the amount of GABA present in the brain and to the amount of GABA bound to GABA receptors. Midazolam therefore exhibits a ceiling effect and a limited ability to decrease brain activity (see Fig. 20.1). For this reason, midazolam is not approved as a sole general anesthetic agent, but only for the induction of anesthesia.

Because of this single mechanism of action, enhancing GABA inhibition only when GABA is present, midazolam is an extremely safe drug. It does not produce the potent CNS depressant activity of pentobarbital, thiopental, and other barbiturates. Although there are no intentional studies of large doses of benzodiazepines in the range of 500 mg IV like the midazolam dose used in lethal injection, there are studies of benzodiazepine overdose from unintentional or intentional suicide attempts that yield comparable blood levels. For example, clinical studies show that overdoses of benzodiazepines that lead to blood levels that are 10–20 times the therapeutic dose range produce no ill effect in benzodiazepine overdose patients.[40] In these studies, patients recover normally within a day, had no significant respiratory depression, and needed no assisted ventilation. Particularly important to the present case of lethal injection, patients overdosing on extremely high doses of benzodiazepine still responded to painful or noxious stimuli.

Midazolam's use in a triple-drug protocol is intended to produce a state of *general anesthesia* (unaware, unconscious, and insensate to pain) but cannot do so. Unlike pentobarbital, or another barbiturate in the single-drug protocol, midazolam is not intended to kill the condemned inmate. As the studies before suggest, midazolam is unable to kill an inmate even at a 500 mg dose used in lethal injection protocols. The second drug, vecuronium, a neuromuscular blocker, paralyzes the muscles throughout the body and therefore is lethal by respiratory depression. The third drug, potassium chloride, certainly is lethal by producing electrolyte disturbances that prevent the beating of the heart.

Soon other states began substituting midazolam as the first drug when pentobarbital was used up and unavailable. Media reports of botched executions in the last decade began with the use of midazolam and hydromorphone in Ohio's execution of 2014.[41] Due to the pain and suffering of suffocation produced by the second drug and the severe pain noted in individuals

---

[38]   D'Hulst C et al. (2009) The complexity of the GABA_A receptor shapes unique pharmacological profiles. Drug Disc. Today 14:866-875; Sieghart W et al. (2012) A novel GABA_A receptor pharmacology: drugs interacting with the $\alpha^+\beta^-$ interface. Brit. J. Pharmacol. 166:476-485. (D'Hulst et al. 2009, Sieghart et al. 2012).

[39]   Adapted from *Brenner and Stevens' Pharmacology*, 5th Edition. Elsevier, 2018.

[40]   Greenblatt DJ et al. (1977) Acute overdosage with benzodiazepine derivatives. Clin Pharmacol Ther. 21:497-514; Greenblatt DJ et al. (1978) Rapid recovery from massive diazepam overdose. JAMA 240:1872-1874; Allen MD et al. (1980) Pharmacokinetic study of lorazepam overdosage. Am J Psychiatry 137:1414-1415; Divoll M et al. (1981) Benzodiazepine overdosage: plasma concentrations and clinical outcome. Psychopharm. (Berl). 73:381-383.

[41]   The drug expert should not rely exclusively on media or witness reports of the inmate after lethal injection as support for certain pharmacological effects, although talking, grimacing, tearing, and gasping for breath are incompatible with the state of general anesthesia.

injected with potassium chloride while awake, it is clear that the first drug in a three-drug protocol must assuredly produce a state of general anesthesia in the condemned. The first drug in the triple-drug protocol, midazolam, cannot produce a state of general anesthesia and its use will surely or very likely cause severe pain and suffering from the subsequent injection of pancuronium and potassium chloride in the inmate.

Even though Florida executed more inmates with midazolam than Oklahoma, it was a case originating from Oklahoma (*Glossip v Gross*, see next section) that made it to the Supreme Court of the United States and sparked a number of lawsuits challenging the use of midazolam as the first drug in the three-drug lethal injection protocol. Unlike the previous first drugs in triple-drug protocols (thiopental and pentobarbital) no state has proposed a single-drug protocol using only midazolam. This is *prima facie* evidence that even the states don't think that midazolam is up to the task as a first drug and is a tacit admission that midazolam is not equivalent to the barbiturates.

Ohio uses midazolam and hydromorphone in new two-drug protocol

In January 2014, Ohio used an untested 2-drug lethal injection protocol after running out of pentobarbital. Following Florida's lead using the benzodiazepine midazolam as the first drug, Ohio injected the opioid analgesic hydromorphone (Dilaudid®) as the second drug. The theory behind the use of these two drugs to intentionally produce an overdose death was sound; it is known that the combination of benzodiazepines and opioids is a leading cause of drug overdose death in the United States. The use of the two-drug protocol, without pancuronium or another muscle paralytic, does not mask any symptoms of pain and suffering which led to the media reports of a botched execution.

Midazolam. The pharmacology of the IV benzodiazepine midazolam was elaborated above when Florida first replaced pentobarbital with midazolam as the first drug in a triple-drug protocol. Midazolam is a sedative-hypnotic drug and not a barbiturate or general anesthetic drug like pentobarbital or thiopental.

Hydromorphone. Hydromorphone is a moderate opioid analgesic drug, more potent than morphine but less potent than strong opioid analgesic fentanyl (coming up below). Hydromorphone is an opioid pain medication known better by its trade name Dilaudid®. Opioid pain medications, or opioid analgesics, are among the most powerful and dangerous drugs used in the clinic and prescribed to patients. Morphine is the gold standard of opioid analgesics and hydromorphone is about 10 times more potent than morphine. Other opioid analgesics in the same pharmacological class as hydromorphone include codeine and oxycodone (OxyContin®).

Hydromorphone is indicated for the management of pain in patients where an opioid analgesic is appropriate, that is, the treatment of moderate to severe pain.[42] Hydromorphone, like all opioids, works by binding to opioid receptors on pain neurons, which are brain and spinal cord cells that transmit pain information. Binding of hydromorphone with these opioid receptors on the pain neurons inhibits the activity of these pain neurons. The inhibition of pain neurons produces the analgesia, or relief of pain, that characterizes hydromorphone and other opioid analgesics.

The Ohio execution using midazolam and hydromorphone did not go well. The Ohio inmate gasped, snorted, and choked his way to death.[43] In spite of this well-publicized outcome, Arizona used midazolam and hydromorphone in their execution a few months later. It too did not go well, with the inmate gasping and struggling for nearly two hours before death was pronounced. By 2017, Ohio went back to a triple-drug protocol with midazolam as the first drug and Arizona went to a pentobarbital single-drug execution protocol.[44] To date, the double-drug protocol using midazolam and hydromorphone has not been repeated by any state.

Florida switches from midazolam to etomidate as first drug in a three-drug protocol

In 2017 Florida switched their first drug in a triple-drug lethal injection protocol from midazolam to etomidate, having previously used pentobarbital, and before that thiopental. To date, there have been five lethal executions completed using etomidate in Florida. No other state has used etomidate in a triple-drug or in a single-drug protocol.

Etomidate. In Florida's new triple-drug protocol, the first drug, etomidate, is used as a general anesthetic drug. Etomidate has a unique chemical structure, unlike barbiturates (pentobarbital) or benzodiazepines (midazolam).[45] Like pentobarbital,

---

[42] *Dilaudid*® (hydromorphone) Full Prescribing Information, Purdue Pharma LP, Stamford, CT, rev. 2013.

[43] See Berger E (2015) The Executioners' dilemmas. Univ Richmond Law Rev. 49:731-762 for an account of OH and AZ midazolam and hydromorphone double-drug executions.

[44] Malcom DR, Romanelli F (2017) The emergence of second-generation lethal injection protocols: a brief history and review. Pharmacother. 37:1249-1257.

[45] Forman SA (2011) Clinical and molecular pharmacology of etomidate. Anesthesiol. 114:695-707.

etomidate has multiple mechanisms of action. Like pentobarbital, but unlike midazolam, etomidate is classified as a general anesthetic agent. Studies of brain activity show that etomidate can produce a depression of brain activity like that produced by pentobarbital and other barbiturates.[46]

Firstly, etomidate enhances the ability of the natural inhibitory neurotransmitter, GABA, at the GABA receptor.[47] When GABA is present at its GABA receptor on a neuron, it changes the ion flow into the cell to make the neuron less active. Etomidate makes GABA work better when they are both at the GABA receptor and further decreases the activity of the neuron. Barbiturates (thiopental, pentobarbital) and benzodiazepines (midazolam, diazepam) share this GABA-enhancing mechanism of action with etomidate.

Secondly, etomidate, like barbiturates, acts on the GABA receptor by itself when GABA is not present.[48] By not relying on GABA being present to inhibit the brain neurons, etomidate can produce a greater inhibition and more widespread depression of the CNS. This GABA-independent action of etomidate is not shared by midazolam. Unlike barbiturates, there is no evidence that etomidate also blocks excitatory receptors on neurons, and like barbiturates and benzodiazepines, etomidate is not an analgesic drug.

While etomidate may be especially useful in patients with compromised cardiac function,[49] etomidate also has two adverse effects that are noted in clinical studies. Firstly, etomidate produces pain upon injection in about 20% of patients with IV administration.[50] Secondly, etomidate IV administration produces involuntary muscle movements or *myoclonus* in up to about 30% of patients.[51]

Because general anesthetics like etomidate do not exhibit a ceiling effect in their ability to inhibit neurons, large doses can cause overdose and death by respiratory and cardiac depression. The typical clinical dose is 0.3 mg/kg, or a dose of 30 mg etomidate in a 100 kg (220 lb.) inmate.[50] Reports of the lethal and toxic doses of etomidate are rare but a case of death following 80 mg of IV etomidate was reported as well as toxic effects after 250 mg of IV etomidate by continuous infusion.[52]

Nebraska goes with diazepam and fentanyl in new four-drug protocol

In 2017 Nebraska modified its lethal injection protocol to include four drugs: the benzodiazepine diazepam, the potent opioid analgesic fentanyl, the muscle paralytic cisatracurium, and potassium chloride, an agent that stops the heart.

Diazepam. Diazepam is a classic benzodiazepine sedative sold under the brand name of Valium® and now available from numerous generic pharmaceutical manufacturers. Other popular benzodiazepines include midazolam (Versed®) and alprazolam (Xanax®). Like midazolam (see earlier), diazepam is not a general anesthetic drug and is generally only a mild CNS depressant. Like midazolam, diazepam does not produce a state of unawareness, unconsciousness, and insensate to pain nor reduce the brain activity to the level of general anesthesia.

Diazepam for injection is available in vials containing 50 mg diazepam in 10 mL.[53] Clinical doses of diazepam range from 2 to 20 mg IV depending on the clinical indication and the severity of the patient's condition. The use of 200 mg of IV diazepam (from protocol amount above) will provide deep sedation and, in combination with the second drug fentanyl, would likely produce severe respiratory depression (see later).

Fentanyl. The 2nd drug in Nebraska's protocol is fentanyl, a potent opioid analgesic (painkiller) for the treatment of moderate to severe pain. Opioid pain medications, called *opioid analgesics*, are among the most powerful and dangerous drugs used in the clinic and prescribed to patients. Morphine is the gold standard of opioid analgesics, given for the treatment of moderate to severe pain.[49] Fentanyl is a synthetic opioid analgesic that is 100 times more potent than morphine.[54] Fentanyl

---

[46] Kim HM et al. (2012) Effects of etomidate on bispectral index scale and spectral entropy during induction of anesthesia by means of the raw electroencephalographic and electromyographic characteristics. Korean J Anesthesiol. 62:230-233; Lim TA, Lim KY (2006) BIS during etomidate-induced myoclonus. Anaesthesia 61:410-411.

[47] Herd MB et al. (2014) The general anaesthetic etomidate inhibits the excitability of mouse thalamocortical relay neurons by modulating multiple modes of GABAA receptor-mediated inhibition. Eur J Neurosci. 40:2487-2501.

[48] Forman SA (2011) *Op. cit.*

[49] *Etomidate (Amidate®) Full Prescribing Information*, Hospira, revised 2017.

[50] Aggarwal S et al. (2016) A comparative study between propofol and etomidate in patients under general anesthesia. Braz J Anesthesiol. 66:237-241.

[51] Chalmers P (1983) Etomidate-overdose by continuous infusion. Anaesthesia 38:506; Molina DK et al. (2008) Distribution of etomidate in a fatal intoxication. J Anal Toxicol. 32:715-718.

[52] *Diazepam for Injection*, Full Prescribing Information, Hospira, 2016.

[53] Brenner GM, Stevens CW (2018) *Brenner and Stevens' Pharmacology, 5th Ed.* Elsevier, Philadelphia PA.

[54] Grond S, Radbruch L, Lehmann KA (2000) Clinical pharmacokinetics of transdermal opioids: focus on transdermal fentanyl. Clin Pharmacokinet. 38:59-89.

is marketed by the brand name of Sublimaze® although many other formulations (e.g., transdermal patches and lozenges on a stick) and generic versions also exist. Morphine, fentanyl, and all opioid analgesics work to produce analgesia by binding to opioid receptors on pain neurons (brain cells) and in this way inhibit the activity of the pain neurons. The inhibition of pain neurons produces the analgesia, or relief of pain, that characterizes the therapeutic action of morphine, fentanyl, and other opioid analgesics.

While opioid analgesics are presently the best agents to treat pain and do so quite effectively, they are also a dangerous group of medicines that are responsible for many intentional and unintentional fatalities. Opioid analgesics work by inhibiting pain transmission in the CNS and do so by binding to opioid receptors on pain neurons. A more deadly problem is that morphine, fentanyl, and other opioids also bind to opioid receptors on brain neurons that control breathing and high doses of opioids produce respiratory depression.[55] Breathing ceases, and without oxygen in the blood, cardiac arrest and brain death from hypoxia ensues.

The use of fentanyl or other potent opioids also has the advantage of reversibility with the commonly available opioid antagonist, naloxone (Narcan®), should the lethal execution procedure need to be stopped.

Cisatracurium. Cisatracurium is a neuromuscular blocker or muscle paralytic drug in the same class as pancuronium (see earlier). Like pancuronium, cisatracurium works by blocking the action of acetylcholine which is the neurotransmitter released from a nerve ending onto the muscle that causes the muscle to contract. Should the doses and administration of diazepam and fentanyl not be sufficient to produce severe respiratory depression and death, the use of cisatracurium would mask any pain or suffering that may be experienced by the inmate.

Potassium chloride. Potassium chloride is a cardiac arresting drug and its actions were detailed before. IV injection of a high dose of potassium chloride changes the electrolytes bathing the heart and blocks heart muscle contraction. Potassium chloride at high concentration IV injections is extremely painful because high concentrations of potassium ions depolarize (activate) pain nerves present in the vasculature. Due to the severe pain noted in individuals injected with pancuronium and potassium chloride while awake, it is clear that the first two drugs in Nebraska' four-drug protocol must produce a state of general anesthesia in the inmate.

From 2010 to the end of 2018, there have been 8 different lethal drug protocols used for executions on 296 condemned inmates.[56] Over these 9 years, inmates were executed on average about once every week and a half, or more precisely, every 11.1 days. Fig. 20.2 shows that most executions (137) were done using a single-drug protocol, the barbiturate pentobarbital. Pentobarbital in a triple-drug protocol was about half as common at 69 deaths, and the oldest protocol of thiopental, pancuronium, and potassium chloride less than that. Before supplies ran out, 10 executions were carried out with thiopental in a single-drug protocol. Five executions were done using etomidate with a muscle paralytic and potassium chloride only in Florida. The two-drug protocol using midazolam and hydromorphone was only used twice with unsettlingly outcomes. The newest 4-drug protocol with diazepam and fentanyl was used just once in Nebraska.

The majority of inmates executed with only pentobarbital were killed by Texas officials. Texas rightly refused to switch to midazolam in a three-drug protocol when pentobarbital was no longer commercially available. Instead, Texas and a number of other states have turned to compounding pharmacies to obtain pentobarbital for lethal injection. This move is not without its own set of challenges. Compounding pharmacies as the source for lethal injection drugs is the topic of the next section.

Lethal Drugs From Compounding Pharmacies

The traditional role of a pharmacy was the compounding of medicines to fill a physician's prescription for the patient.[57] As pharmaceutical manufacturing companies developed in the late 19th century and medicines became cheaper and faster to manufacture on a large scale, pharmacies took on more of a retail characteristic in dispensing manufactured pills, tablets, and elixirs. However, the traditional role of compounding pharmacies was never completely lost and the compounding of drugs serves an essential role of modern health care.[58]

---

[55] White JM, Irvine RJ (1999) Mechanisms of fatal opioid overdose. Addiction 94:961-972.
[56] Data was gleaned from the Death Penalty Information website (www.deathpenalty.org), downloaded into Excel spreadsheets and analyzed to yield the figure data.
[57] Spark MJ (2014) Compounding of medicines by pharmacies: an update. Maturitas 78:239-240.
[58] Pergolizzi JV et al. (2013) Compounding pharmacies: who is in charge? Pain Pract. 13:253-257.

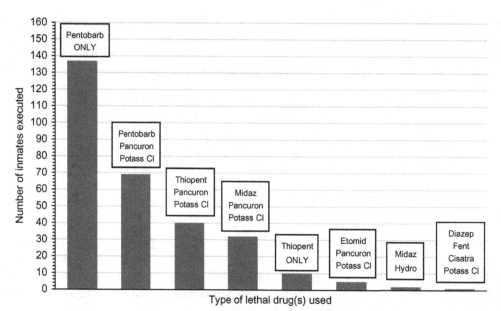

FIG. 20.2 Number of inmates executed from 2010 to 2018 and lethal injection drugs used. *Pentobarb*, pentobarbital; *Pancuron*, pancuronium; *Potass Cl*, potassium chloride; *Thiopent*, thiopental; *Midaz*, midazolam; *Etomid*, etomidate; *Hydro*, hydromorphone; *Diazep*, diazepam; *Fent*, fentanyl; *Cistra*, cisatracurium.

Much attention focused on the safety and reliability of compounded pharmacy products after the illnesses and deaths due to fungal meningitis from a contaminated batch of injection steroids used "off-label" to treat back pain that occurred in 2012.[59] Compounding pharmacies are regulated by State Boards of Pharmacy rather than the FDA. However, in the wake of this compounding pharmacy disaster, Congress passed the Drug Quality and Security Act, signed into Federal law in November 2013, which gives the FDA limited regulation over compounding pharmacies.[60] The Drug Quality and Security Act added a new source of drug manufacturers called "Out-Sourcing Facilities" for compounding pharmacies that voluntarily register (and pay fees) to be regulated. Now there are three types of drug suppliers: (1) FDA-approved pharmaceutical companies that market FDA-approved products and are strongly regulated by the FDA, (2) Out-Sourcing Facilities that are compounding pharmacy companies which voluntarily register with the FDA and are less strongly regulated by the FDA, and (3) traditional compounding pharmacies that are not registered with the FDA and not regulated by the FDA but are regulated by State Boards of Pharmacy.

Traditional compounding pharmacies are used when the commercially available manufactured product contains allergens that a person is allergic to, is not available in the dosage form needed, when two or more drugs need to be combined, or when a manufactured drug is not available.[61] Importantly, the use of a compounding pharmacy arises from a specific doctor-patient relationship, where an alternative to the commercially pharmaceutical manufacturer is justified based on specific patient characteristics recognized by the physician.

The FDA did a study of 36 samples of compounded drug products and found that 33% of them failed at least one quality test.[62] Quality tests done over 4 years (2006–2009) by the Missouri State Board of Pharmacy showed that drug product failure rates averaged 20%, with some drug potency tests showing results of 0%–450% of what the dose should be. The previous numbers are in contrast to the failure rate of FDA-approved prescription drugs, made by regulated pharmaceutical firms, which was less than 2%.[63] Since 2000, the FDA has issued warnings about quality tests and compounded drug products, including problems with potency, sterility, and the presence of contaminants or particulate matter not fully dissolved.

[59] Staes C et al. (2013) Description of outbreaks of health-care-associated infections related to compounding pharmacies, 2000-12. Am J Health Syst Pharm. 70:1301-1312.
[60] Qureshi N et al. (2014) Sterile compounding: clinical, legal, and regulatory implications for patient safety. J Manag Care Spec Pharm. 20:1183-1191.
[61] Spark et al. (2014) *Op.cit.*
[62] Sellers S, Utian WH (2012) Pharmacy compounding primer for physicians: prescriber beware. Drugs 72:2043-2050.
[63] Staes et al. (2013) *Op.cit.*

As detailed before, there is a greater risk of obtaining less quality drug formulations from compounding pharmacies than from FDA-approved manufacturers. For example, regulation and conformity to good manufacturing practices will be most stringent for FDA-approved pharmaceutical manufacturers, less so for outsourcing facilities, and nonexistent for traditional compounders. Of the approximately 7500 compounding pharmacies in the United States, including 3000 that make sterile solutions for injections, only about 2% participate in the industry's voluntary accreditation process.[63] Additionally, there is no statement of assurance in the proposed regulations that any testing of compounded lethal injection drugs will be done or that compounding pharmacies used will conform to standards or education and training for compounding of sterile solutions.[64]

Drug solutions formulated for injections can be contaminated by microorganisms and undergo chemical degradation (breakdown) and decreased stability of the drug. A study of the stability of sodium pentobarbital for injection compounded to mimic the same sodium pentobarbital for injection marketed as *Nembutal*® was investigated in a recent study.[65] In this study, compounded pentobarbital sodium solution was made to mimic the commercially available *Nembutal*® *Sodium Solution* (Pentobarbital for Injection) by dissolving the pentobarbital sodium into an aqueous solution of 40% propylene glycol and 10% ethanol. The pH was adjusted with small amounts of sodium hydroxide and hydrochloric acid.[66] The investigators found that there was no large-scale degradation of pentobarbital in their compounded pentobarbital sodium solution for as long as 6 years. The compounded pentobarbital solution showed about a 0.5% per year chemical degradation when stored in a locked drawer at room temperature. They report that the pentobarbital solution did show a yellow discoloration after about 2 years, noting that the commercial product, *Nembutal*® *Sodium Solution*, also showed this discoloration after about 2 years. They also reported that the potency of the compounded pentobarbital solution was equal to the commercially available solution by administration in a rodent model of anesthesia. Significantly, the researchers did not examine the pentobarbital solutions for microorganisms (bacteria, fungi) contamination. Typical tests carried out on compounded sterile preparations include the Bacterial Endotoxin test, which measures the amount of endotoxin in the sample. Endotoxins are bacterial cell wall components that signal the presence of gram-negative bacteria.[67] A second sterility test uses a membrane filtration procedure to filter out potential contaminants.

The American Pharmacists Association (APhA) adopted a policy on lethal injection drugs last year.[68] Their policy states:

*The American Pharmacists Association **discourages pharmacist participation in executions on the basis that such activities are fundamentally contrary to the role of pharmacists as providers of health care**.*

[bold added]

The International Academy of Compounding Pharmacists (IACP) also released a statement concerning the ethics of compounding lethal injection drugs, to wit[69]:

*While the pharmacy profession recognizes an individual practitioner's right to determine whether to dispense a medication based upon his or her personal, ethical and religious beliefs, **IACP discourages its members from participating in the preparation, dispensing, or distribution of compounded medications for use in legally authorized executions***.

[bold added]

The Supreme Court of the United States and Lethal Injection Drugs

Surprisingly, according to legal scholars, the existing body of law concerning the constitutionality of the execution methods used in capital punishment is extremely limited.[70] There was a SCOTUS decision in 1878 that upheld the constitutionality of execution by firing squad in Utah. A second SCOTUS opinion in 1889 upheld the use of the electric chair as constitutional under the Eighth Amendment.[71] But it was not until this century, almost 30 years after the first lethal drug execution,

---

[64] Thompsion RW, Belisle CB (2015) Respecting the risk of sterile compounding. Am J Health-System Pharmacology. 72:1269; Nemec EC et al. (2016) Design Considerations of a Compounded Sterile Preparations Course. Am J Pharm Educ. 80:12.

[65] Priest SM, Geisbuhler TP (2015) Injectable sodium pentobarbital: stability at room temperature. J Pharmacol Toxicol Methods 76:38-42.

[66] Exact same drug solution as described in the Full Prescribing Information for in *Nembutal*® *Sodium Solution. www.akorn.com/documents/catalog/ sell_sheets/76478-501-20.pdf.*

[67] Raetz CR, Whitfield C (2002) Lipopolysaccharide endotoxins. Annu Rev Biochem. 71:635-700.

[68] *www.pharmacist.com/apha-house-delegates-adopts-policy-discouraging-pharmacist-participation-execution.*

[69] IACP board updates position on compounding for lethal injections, at:*www.iacprx.org/?page=CC32315LethalIn.*

[70] Samburg MB (2009) Cruel and unusual? The bifurcation of eighth amendment inquiries after *Baze v. Rees.* Harv Civ Rights-Civ Lib Law Rev. 44:213-230.

[71] Like all of the Amendments in the beautifully terse Bill of Rights, the 8th Amendment simply states "Excessive bail shall not be required, nor excessive fines imposed, nor cruel and unusual punishments inflicted."

that SCOTUS considered for the first time the constitutionality of using drugs to carry out the death penalty. Two SCOTUS opinions set the context for current lethal drug injection protocols and are briefly reviewed next.

The first SCOTUS case, *Baze v. Rees*,[72] began in the Franklin Circuit Court for the Commonwealth of Kentucky in 2005. *Baze* and another death row inmate exhausted all their standard postconviction appeals and filed a civil suit against DOC Director *Rees*. The plaintiffs claimed that Kentucky's use of the triple-drug lethal injection protocol using thiopental, pancuronium, and potassium chloride was unconstitutional under the Eighth Amendment.[73] They alleged that the protocol might not be properly followed, resulting in significant pain and suffering. They also proposed an alternative protocol using a single-drug protocol with the barbiturate thiopental.[74]

The Supreme Court's decision to affirm the lower court rulings in *Baze* was rendered in seven different opinions, with little agreement by the Justices. Only five Justices clearly agreed that the Kentucky protocol was not unconstitutional.[73] The plurality opinion also laid out the two prongs that must be satisfied by a successful Eighth Amendment challenge of a lethal drug protocol. The first prong is that the execution protocol must show a "substantial risk of serious harm." The second prong is that an alternative method must be "feasible, readily implemented, and in fact significantly reduces a substantial risk of severe pain." *Baze* lost on the first prong partly because their arguments were based on the logistics of the execution procedure[75] and not the drugs themselves. The alternative method using thiopental in a single-drug protocol was rejected because in 2008 no state had yet used a single-drug protocol.[76]

Just 7 years later, SCOTUS would again take up the issue of lethal drugs used in state executions with the *Glossip v. Gross* case in 2015.[77] *Glossip* and other death row inmates at the Oklahoma State Penitentiary in McAlester, Oklahoma held that the use of midazolam as the first drug in a triple-drug protocol violated the 8th Amendment's "cruel and unusual punishments" clause. The inmates argued that midazolam, being a benzodiazepine, could not produce an inmate who was unconscious, unaware, and insensate to the pain of the second and third lethal injection drugs. SCOTUS in a 5-4 decision affirmed the lower courts ruling stating that "First, the prisoners failed to identify a known and available alternative method of execution that entails a lesser risk of pain, a requirement of all Eighth Amendment method-of-execution claims. See Baze v. Rees, 553 U.S. 35, 61, 128 S.Ct. 1520, 170 L.Ed.2d 420 (2008) (plurality opinion). Second, the District Court did not commit clear error when it found that the prisoners failed to establish that Oklahoma's use of a massive dose of midazolam in its execution protocol entails a substantial risk of severe pain."

Sixteen pharmacologists were organized and submitted an *amicus curiae* brief to SCOTUS as a neutral party in the *Glossip* case.[78] Clear and convincing evidence was provided that midazolam is a benzodiazepine and a sedative whereas thiopental and pentobarbital are barbiturates and general anesthetic drugs, that midazolam exhibits a ceiling effect which limits the depression of the brain unlike barbiturates, and that midazolam does not produce an unconscious and unaware state that makes an inmate insensate to painful stimuli. Instead, the majority Justices relied on the State's expert pharmacist who relied on no scientific references and famously cited drugs.com.

From the text of both the plurality and dissenting opinions, it appears that none of the justices paid much attention to the opinion of the sixteen pharmacology professors.[79] However, drug expert testimony on the misuse of midazolam as the first

---

[72] *Baze v. Rees*. 2008, 128 S. Ct. 1520. Supreme Court. Obviously you will want to go and read the opinions yourself. Yours truly, a pharmacologist, *will not do them justice*, so to speak.

[73] Samburg MB (2009) *Op. cit.*

[74] It is ironic that SCOTUS rejected the inmate's alternative method of a single-drug barbiturate protocol. This is now the most common method of execution and accounts for more than half of all lethal drug executions since 2010. *Baze* bringing up the issue of an alternative method of lethal injection also forced SCOTUS to rule on alternative methods, setting a standard which haunted *Glossip* and other decisions.

[75] For example, they successfully argued against an IV catheter placed in the neck for drug administration; the defendants already switched the protocol to IV placement in the arm before the case was heard by SCOTUS.

[76] The State of Ohio pioneered the use of a single-drug protocol with thiopental in 2009.

[77] *Glossip v. Gross*. 2015, 136 S. Ct. 20. Supreme Court.

[78] Available at: *www.americanbar.org/content/dam/aba/publications/supreme_court_preview/BriefsV5/14-7955_amicus_neither_pharm.authcheckdam.pdf*.

[79] The 16 pharmacologists were as follows: Edward Bilsky, Ph.D. at the University of New England in Biddeford ME, Charles Chavkin, Ph.D. at the University of Washington in Seattle WA, Kathryn A. Cunningham, Ph.D. at the University of Texas Medical Branch in Galveston TX, Kenneth E. McCarson, Ph.D. at the University of Kansas Medical Center in Kansas City KS, Christopher R. McCurdy, Ph.D. at the University of Florida in Gainesville FL, Jay McLaughlin, Ph.D. at the Torrey Pines Institute for Molecular Studies in Port St. Lucie FL, S. Stevens Negus, Ph.D. at Virginia Commonwealth University in Richmond VA, Dennis J. Paul, Ph.D. at the Louisiana State University School of Medicine in New Orleans LA, Frank Porreca, Ph.D. at the University of Arizona College of Medicine in Tucson AZ, Paul L. Prather, Ph.D. at the University of Arkansas for Medical Sciences in Little Rock AR, Sandra C. Roerig, Ph.D. at Louisiana State University Health Sciences Center in Shreveport LA, Kelly M. Standifer, Ph.D. at the University of Oklahoma College of Pharmacy in Oklahoma City OK, John R. Traynor, Ph.D. at the University of Michigan Medical School in Ann Arbor MI, Ellen Unterwald, Ph.D. at Temple University School of Medicine in Philadelphia PA, David R. Wallace, Ph.D. at the Oklahoma State University Center for Health Sciences in Tulsa OK, and Linda Werling, Ph.D. at the George Washington University School of Medicine and Health Sciences in Washington DC. Any of these 16 pharmacologists might be worth contacting when a drug expert is needed. Tell them I sent you.

drug in a triple-drug protocol was finally effective for the first time in a case heard in the United States District Court for the Southern District of Ohio Eastern Division (Columbus). Judge Merz granted a preliminary injunction and stay of execution to death row inmates based on the pharmacology of midazolam.[80] On initial appeal, the federal district court ruling was upheld; however, that same appeals court *en banc* reversed the federal district court ruling. Similar drug expert testimony on the inadequacy of midazolam in lethal injections is ongoing in a number of states that use the triple-drug protocol with midazolam as the first drug. It appears that a tipping point with midazolam was been reached with judges in the latest cases amenable to science and agreeing with well-established pharmacological testimony of midazolam.

Alternative Methods of Execution

The definition of an alternative method as promulgated by the *Glossip* decision is a "known and available alternative method of execution that entails a lesser risk of pain." In response to current or expected legal challenges, the legislatures of some states have proposed or enacted alternative methods of execution. The following execution methods were enacted but not implemented at the time of this writing.

Missouri's proposed use of propofol in a new triple-drug protocol

Propofol. In 2013 the state of Missouri proposed the use of propofol, an intravenously administered general anesthetic drug, as the first drug in a triple-drug protocol.[81] Propofol and its brand name of Diprivan® became well known after the death of Michael Jackson following administration of propofol to him by his personal physician. Propofol has wide use in various clinical settings and five FDA-approved indications including induction and maintenance of general anesthesia.[82]

When the maker of propofol found out it was supplied to the Missouri Department of Corrections (MDOC), it demanded return of the drug. As the propofol is made in Austria, the European Union threatened to impose strict export restrictions on propofol if Missouri used it for a lethal execution. Other medical groups and the FDA pressured Missouri as any export restrictions to the United States would threaten availability of a much-used and important therapeutic agent. Finally, in late 2013, Missouri officials abandoned the use of propofol as the first drug in a triple-drug protocol and the Governor ordered the MDOC to develop a new lethal injection execution protocol.

Nevada goes with a new three-drug protocol

The Nevada Execution Protocol, revised in June, 2018, describes a new triple-drug lethal injection procedure including a benzodiazepine sedative (midazolam), a potent opioid analgesic (fentanyl), and the muscle paralytic, cisatracurium. They dropped the heart-stopping potassium chloride as the third and final drug used in most triple-drug protocols.

Midazolam. The benzodiazepine midazolam is the first drug in Nevada's new lethal injection protocol. While midazolam cannot produce general anesthesia, but only deep sedation, the use of midazolam with the second drug, the strong opioid fentanyl, produces severe respiratory depression (see later).

Fentanyl. Fentanyl is a potent opioid analgesic, about 100 times more potent than morphine. A full description of fentanyl used in Nebraska's lethal injection protocol is given before.

Cisatracurium. The third and final drug in Nevada's protocol is cisatracurium. Cisatracurium is a neuromuscular blocker or muscle paralytic drug in the same class as pancuronium, vecuronium, and cisatracurium.[83] Like pancuronium, vecuronium, and rocuronium, cisatracurium works by blocking the action of acetylcholine which is the neurotransmitter released from a nerve ending onto the muscle that causes the muscle to contract.[11] Clinical uses of neuromuscular blockers are to provide muscle relaxation for endotracheal intubation, and to ensure patient immobility during surgery or mechanical ventilation.[84]

---

[80] Magistrate Judge Merz decision was made on Jan 16, 2017 and is available at: *assets.documentcloud.org/documents/3421284/Death-penalty-opinion.pdf.*
[81] Dresser R (2014) Drugs and the death penalty. Hastings Center Report, Jan-Feb issue:9-10.
[82] *Diprivan (propofol) injectable emulsion, USP* (2017) Full prescribing information, Fresenius-Kabi, Lake Zurich, IL.
[83] *Cisatracurium Besylate (Nimbex®) Injection*, Full Prescribing Information, Abbot Labs.
[84] Kovac AL (2009) Sugammadex: the first selective binding reversal agent for neuromuscular block. J Clin Anesth. 21:444-453.

The use of a muscle paralytic after midazolam and fentanyl is unnecessary and may mask any problems in the administration of the first two drugs. Note that Nevada dropped the use of the traditional third drug, namely, potassium chloride, which is painful and unneeded if the first two drugs produce their deadly effect.

California's proposes a single-drug protocol using a barbiturate

California, usually so forward-thinking and *avant-garde*, sought an alternative lethal injection protocol went back to the future by proposing a single-drug protocol in 2015. California DOC released a protocol for public comments stating that one out of a possible of four barbiturate drugs (amobarbital, pentobarbital, secobarbital, or thiopental) would be used for lethal drug executions. There was no mention of the use of a compounding pharmacy to obtain the barbiturate drugs, so an analysis of available IV barbiturates was done to assess the feasibility of California's protocol.

Currently, only one formulation of sodium pentobarbital for injection is commercially available and approved by the FDA. This is *Nembutal® Sodium Solution* (Pentobarbital Sodium for Injection, USP) manufactured by Akorn, Inc. a subsidiary of Oak Pharmaceuticals, Inc. There are two additional barbiturate drugs marketed as injection solutions listed by the FDA; *Brevital® Sodium* and *Phenobarbital Sodium Injection, USP*. The first one, *Brevital® Sodium,* is the trade name of methohexital sodium for injection, USP and is manufactured by Par Pharmaceutical Companies in Chestnut Ridge, NY. The second barbiturate injection solution, *Phenobarbital Sodium Injection, USP* is manufactured by West-Ward Pharmaceuticals in Eatontown, NJ.

The manufacturer of *Nembutal® Sodium Solution* (Pentobarbital Sodium for Injection, USP), Akorn Pharmaceuticals (part of Oak Pharmaceuticals), recently announced that it would not sell any of its products to correctional institutions[85] stating in a letter to Office of State Comptroller, State of New York that "Akorn strongly objects to the use of its products to conduct or support capital punishment through lethal injection or other means. To prevent the use of our products in capital punishment, Akorn will not sell any product directly to any prison or other correctional institution."[86] As the sole supplier of FDA-approved and marketed pentobarbital sodium for IV injection, Akorn has made pentobarbital sodium IV solutions from commercial pharmaceuticals unobtainable by correctional institutions to use in lethal injections.

The first of the two additional barbiturate IV solutions on the market is *Brevital® Sodium,* methohexital sodium for injection, USP and is manufactured by Par Pharmaceutical Companies. In response to the possible use of *Brevital® Sodium* as part of a three-drug lethal injection protocol by the State of Indiana, Department of Corrections, Par Pharmaceuticals issued a news release that stated "As a pharmaceutical company, Par's mission is to help improve the quality of life. The state of Indiana's proposed use is contrary to our mission. Par is working with its distribution partners to establish distribution controls on Brevital® to preclude wholesalers from accepting orders from departments of correction."[87] As Par Pharmaceuticals is sole supplier of FDA-approved methohexital sodium for injection, the use of this barbiturate IV solution as an alternative to the use of pentobarbital is a moot point.

The only other barbiturate IV solution on the commercial market is *Phenobarbital Sodium Injection, USP* manufactured by West-Ward Pharmaceuticals, a subsidiary of the London based Hikma Pharmaceuticals. This IV barbiturate formulation is also no longer available for purchase by correctional institutions. The company issued a statement when it imposed its restrictions on shipments to correctional facilities stating, "Hikma strongly objects to the use of any of its products in capital punishment."[88] At the same time there is no domestic pharmaceutical market for prisons and correctional facilities to obtain any IV barbiturate drug formulations, international sources of IV barbiturates solutions are also unobtainable.[89]

After public responses, including those of the author, California DOC altered the proposed protocol in July 2017 to using one of two barbiturates, pentobarbital or thiopental. To date, there have been no inmates executed using California's single-drug protocol.[90]

[85] Silverman, E (2015) Akorn takes steps to prohibit its drugs from being used for executions. Wall Street Journal, March 4, 2015. *blogs.wsj.com/pharmalot/2015/03/04/akorn-takes-steps-to-prohibit-its-drugs-from-being-used-for-executions/.*

[86] Joseph Bonaccorsi, General Counsel of Akorn to Mr. Patrick Doherty, Director of Corporate Governance, State of New York, Office of the State Comptroller. *www.osc.state.ny.us/press/releases/mar15/akorn_letter.pdf.*

[87] Stephen Mock, Par Pharmaceutical Statement on Brevital® Sodium, Par Pharmaceutical Companies Inc, Woodcliff Lake, NJ, May 28, 2014 news release. *pr.parpharm.com/phoenix.zhtml?c=81806&p=irol-newsArticle&ID=1935104.*

[88] Hikma Is Latest Firm to Stop Drugs Being Sold for Lethal Injections, in-pharmatechnologist.com, May 20, 2013. *www.in-pharmatechnologist.com/Processing/Hikma-is-Latest-Firm-to-Stop-Drugs-Being-Sold-for-ethalInjections.*

[89] Gibson J, Lain CB (2015) Death Penalty Drugs and the International Moral Marketplace. Georgetown Law J. 103:1215-1274.

[90] And likely to remain that way for quite a while. In March, 2019, California governor Gavin Newsom signed an executive order issuing a reprieve to all 730 death row inmates, joining Ohio's new governor in enacting a moratorium on the death penalty.

Oklahoma legislates a nitrogen gas alternative

Oklahoma is a real pioneer state when it comes to lethal execution protocols. It was the first state to propose a lethal drug injection protocol, the first state to switch from thiopental to pentobarbital, and now the first state to legislate the use of nitrogen gas as an alternative method to lethal drug injection.

Nitrogen gas as a major component in air was isolated and discovered in the 18th century.[91] Nitrogen gas is an inert gas, meaning it is nontoxic and nonreactive with the chemicals of the body. Indeed, every breath we take contains three times more nitrogen than oxygen; air is made up of about 78% nitrogen, 21% oxygen, about 1% carbon dioxide (and growing), and minute amounts of other rare gases.[92] While oxygen is used in all cells of the body to create energy from glucose, nitrogen passes in and out of the blood unused. Nitrogen is not metabolized like other drugs after entering the blood stream and eliminated from the body almost entirely by the lungs.[93]

Nitrogen hypoxia. The main effect of high concentrations of nitrogen gas inhalation in humans is nitrogen hypoxia. Nitrogen gas at high concentrations decreases the amount of oxygen in the air, producing hypoxia. Hypoxia is a condition of lowered oxygen in the blood and, if it lasts long enough, severely affects the brain causing irreversible damage.[94]

A clinical study of brief nitrogen hypoxia was done in three healthy volunteers to study the effects of reduced blood oxygen to various organs.[95] In this study, the subjects were fitted with masks connected to room air and pure (100%) nitrogen gas. The subjects were told to exhale as deeply as possible on room air, then the valve switched to pure nitrogen gas and they were instructed to overventilate and breathe as deeply as possible at the rate of 20 breaths per minute. Measurements of breathing and blood oxygen and other parameters were obtained in real time during the nitrogen gas inhalation, for up to 20 s. The authors noted that when the breathing of nitrogen gas went on for 8–10 s, the subjects reported visual disturbances. After 15–16 s, the subjects experienced some "clouding of consciousness" and impairment of vision. Those subjects that breathed nitrogen gas for 17–20 s became unconscious, which was observed to occur with a generalized muscular reaction (*convulsion*). There were no fatalities in the study as the researchers switched from nitrogen gas to room air as soon as the subjects became unconscious.

Fatalities have occurred by persons unknowingly entering a chamber or room filled with high concentrations of nitrogen gas in industrial settings, but they are rare.[96] It is estimated that nitrogen hypoxia deaths occurs at a rate of eight fatalities per year in the United States. However, suicide by inert gas inhalation, including the use of nitrogen gas, is an increasingly common method of suicide.[97]

Nitrogen and helium gas use in suicide. There are numerous case reports of suicides linked to the use of helium[98] or nitrogen gas[99] inhalation. Helium is an inert gas that is colorless, tasteless, and odorless. When placed in a plastic bag secured around the victims head, the helium inside the bag will quickly replace the oxygen and unconsciousness will occur within seconds and death in a few minutes. Helium use in suicide was promulgated in the literature of several *right to die* organizations and individuals, both in the United States[100] and abroad,[101] and including *how-to* manuals with detailed instructions.

Unlike the carbon dioxide (CO_2) gas that is typically used in animal euthanasia, helium or nitrogen allows the animal's CO_2 to be exhaled and levels of CO_2 to maintain normality.[102] It is the buildup of CO_2 in the blood (hypercapnia) that triggers a struggle to breathe and produces gasping and "breathlessness."

---

[91] Straka L et al. (2013) Suicidal nitrogen inhalation by use of scuba full-face diving mask. J Forensic Sci. 58:1384-1387.

[92] Liu W et al. (2011) Application of medical gases in the field of neurobiology. Med Gas Res. Jun 27;1(1):13. doi: 10.1186/2045-9912-1-13.

[93] Doolette DJ, Mitchell SJ (2001) The physiological kinetics of nitrogen and the prevention of decompression sickness. Clin Pharmacokinet. 40:1-14.

[94] Brierley JB (1977) Experimental hypoxic brain damage. J Clin Pathol Suppl 11:181-187; Graham DI (1977) Pathology of hypoxic brain damage in man. J Clin Pathol Suppl 11:170-180.

[95] Ernsting J (1963) The effect of brief profound hypoxia upon the arterial and venous oxygen tensions in man. J Physiol. 169:292-311.

[96] Straka L et al. (2013) Op. cit.

[97] Byard RW (2018) Changing trends in suicides using helium or nitrogen - A 15-year study. J Forensic Leg Med. 58:6-8.

[98] See the following references and references therein: Ogden RD, Wooten RH (2002) Asphyxial suicide with helium and a plastic bag. Am J Forensic Med Pathol. 23:234-237; Auwaerter V et al. (2007) Toxicological analysis after asphyxial suicide with helium and a plastic bag. Forensic Sci Int. 170:139-141; Schön CA, Ketterer T (2007) Asphyxial suicide by inhalation of helium inside a plastic bag. Am J Forensic Med Pathol. 28:364-367.

[99] See the following references and references therein: Straka L et al. (2013) Op. cit.; Harding BE, Wolf BC (2008) Case report of suicide by inhalation of nitrogen gas. Am J Forensic Med Pathol. 29:235-237; Madentzoglou MS et al. (2013) Nitrogen-plastic bag suicide: a case report. Am J Forensic Med Pathol. 34:311-314.

[100] Ogden RD, Wooten RH (2002) Op. cit.

[101] Ogden RD et al. (2010) Assisted suicide by oxygen deprivation with helium at a Swiss right-to-die organisation. J Med Ethics 36:174-179.

[102] Llonch P et al. (2013) Assessment of unconsciousness in pigs during exposure to nitrogen and carbon dioxide mixtures. Animal 7:492-498.

Nitrogen gas that has reduced the air to an oxygen content to less than 25% of normal concentrations can produce loss of consciousness in seconds and death within minutes.[103] In general, there are no significant pathological findings during a nitrogen hypoxia suicide. Nitrogen is a normal component of the blood so toxicological analysis of an autopsy blood sample cannot be used to determine the cause of death.

A number of states have laws allowing for alternative execution methods if lethal injection drugs are unavailable or proven constitutionally unacceptable. States with alternative methods of execution include Oklahoma using nitrogen gas (above), and Mississippi and Alabama who also enacted laws for the alternative use of nitrogen gas in executions. The electric chair can still be used to carry out the death penalty in Tennessee and Utah enacted legislation to use a firing squad.[104] Even hanging is allowed in New Hampshire "if for any reason the commissioner [of corrections] finds it to be impractical to carry out the punishment of death by administration of the required lethal substance or substances."[105]

Epilogue and Conclusions

The Supreme Court noted in *Glossip* that:

> *Because it is settled that capital punishment is constitutional, it necessarily follows that there must by a constitutional means of carrying it out. And because some risk of pain is inherent in any method of execution, we have held that the Constitution does not require the avoidance of all risk of pain. After all, while most humans wish to die a painless death, many do not have that good fortune. Holding that the Eighth Amendment demands the elimination of essentially all risk of pain would effectively outlaw the death penalty altogether.*[106]

It is anachronistic to think that death by lethal drugs cannot be made painless. As stated by a noted legal scholar, seventeen million patients a year are rendered unconscious and insensate to pain using drugs during surgeries, with slicing through the skin and cutting of tissues, with greater than 99.9% reliability.[107] SCOTUS wrongly thinks that if they demand painless executions, the death penalty would not be possible. This is an opinion biased by the unscientific choice of drugs, inadequate monitoring of inmate consciousness, and the mistake-ridden performance of prison execution teams. The typical three-drug lethal drug protocol used a second and third drug that can produce pain themselves, as the second drug can produce pain and suffering from paralysis of breathing muscles and the third drug intense burning pain. In spite of this, the U.S. Supreme Court has never once invalidated any state's chosen procedure under the Eighth Amendment's cruel and unusual punishment standard.

Many so-called *botched* executions resulted from the improper placement of IV catheters and inexperience of performing IV drug administration yet not one state considered delivering drugs by intramuscular (IM) administration. Barbiturates and other lipid soluble drugs will deliver peak drug concentrations to the bloodstream from an IM injection nearly as fast as from an IV delivery. IM administration involves sticking a needle into the muscle mass of the thigh, arm, or buttocks; a skill that most of us could do after a few simple practice sessions. Another route unconsidered by the states is transdermal administration of lethal drugs by a patch formulation, presented next.

Lethal drugs delivered to the condemned inmate's bloodstream by a skin patch (transdermal administration) is a route universally applicable for all inmates. Every condemned inmate has skin, but not every inmate has accessible veins for IV administration. There is no skill or training in the placement of a patch on the upper arm or thigh, unlike the much needed skill and training needed for the proper placement of an intravenous catheter.

Fentanyl, a powerful opioid analgesic already used in lethal injection, is available in a transdermal formulation.[108] There are analogs of fentanyl that are super-potent, including carfentanil which is a veterinary drug used to tranquilize rhinos and elephants. Carfentanil is sold under the brand name of Wildnil® and is the most potent opioid commercially available. Powerful highly lipophilic opioids in high doses and in combination with high doses of lipophilic barbiturates formulated in lethal drug patches may produce uneventful executions.

No matter what one professes to think or believe about capital punishment, if it is to occur,[109] death must be the *sole punishment* and not enhanced by pain or torture. Putting someone to death should be a professional and a solemn act of

---

[103] Harding BE, Wolf BC (2008) *Op. cit.*

[104] Professor Denno makes a good case for the use of the firing squad. See Denno D (2016) The firing squad as "a known and available alternative method of execution" post-*Glossip*. Univ Michigan J Law Reform 49:749-793.

[105] Drug Penalty Information Center at *deathpenaltyinfo.org/lethal-injection*.

[106] *Glossip*, 135 S. Ct. at 2732-33 (internal alterations and citations omitted).

[107] Berger E (2016) Gross error. Washington Law Rev. 91:929-1004.

[108] See Chapter 4 *The Power of the Poppy*.

[109] Only a small percentage of animal species kill its own kind.ᵃ Humans can rise a little above the brute animals by making the procedure as humane as possible. ᵃExamples include sharks, snakes, alligators and crocs, hyenas, wolves, lions, and some primates such as monkeys and humans.

state-sanctioned homicide. It is also wrong-headed to think that a condemned inmate should suffer a tortuous and painful death to somehow equate with the pain and suffering wrought upon the victims. The goal of capital punishment is the termination of living, the ultimate loss of human life to the condemned inmate, which is *sufficient punishment in itself*. Any additional tortuous pain and suffering that occurs in carrying out a death sentence is inherently unconstitutional or at least unconscionable.[110]

At the heart of the drug expert's concern is not the matter of capital punishment but of the method and choice of lethal drugs. It was illogical, unscientific, and nonpharmacological to substitute a strong barbiturate general anesthetic like pentobarbital for a mere sedative benzodiazepine like midazolam. However, scientific and pharmacological advice was sought by very few state DOCs with regard to the choice of lethal drugs when revising lethal injection protocols.[111] Trial judges did not do their job as gatekeeper and testimony from the State's expert was heard without adequate *Daubert* challenge.

The call for pharmacologist drug experts to serve the community, the state, or even the nation is one of passion not for the morality of lawmakers supporting capital punishment but for the pharmacology of the drugs being used. It is a passion for the pharmacological truth, or as damn close as present-day science can get us, not the fight for or against capital punishment. As much as a climate scientist might feel in the presence of a staunch global warming denier, the sentient pharmacologist may become equally frustrated when learning of the lethal injection *switcheroo* from a barbiturate to a benzodiazepine. As the best cure for frustration is action, it is a goal of this book that pharmacologists throughout the land answer the call to participate in lethal injection cases as expert witnesses. Additionally, it is hoped that the attorneys of the condemned inmates, both Federal Public Defenders and *pro bono* bigshots, consult with pharmacologists for their knowledge and testimony needed to defend drug truth in the courtroom.

A broader "call to pharms" concerns the impact of pharmacological truths in the justice system. Because of the overwhelming role drug use plays in our society, a drug expert is needed to assure that legal decisions are based on solid scientific data. As one of the few remaining truths in today's contentious and surreal social environment, scientific knowledge and expertise are crucial to the equitable operation of our justice system. It is the drug experts, the professors of pharmacology, which can provide this knowledge to judges and juries to maintain a solid foundation in all matters, large and small, of drug use in legal proceedings.

[Narrative continued]
The condemned inmate enters the execution chamber and is strapped onto the gurney. He is in shorts and a scrub top with buttons down the front. Medical personnel in white gowns, gloves, and masks attach EKG and EEG leads to the inmate. The prison execution team enters and places one lethal drug patch on the upper arm of the inmate. Medical personnel monitor the heart rate and brain waves and when the inmate is thought to be dead, send in the state's coroner to physically examine the inmate and pronounce death. If this does not occur in 15 min, a second lethal injection patch is placed on the inmate's other arm. Additional lethal drug patches are placed on the inmate's thighs if needed. If the inmate survives 1 h after the fourth and last patch, supportive measures will be started with emergency transfer to appropriate medical facilities.

Lay and media witnesses to the execution reported that the inmate closed his eyes 44 s after the first patch placement and remained quiet throughout the procedure. At 1 min and 14 s after the patch placement some witnesses noted a few quick gasps, which persisted for about 20 s. Breathing slowed to imperceptible levels and ceased after 3 min. The EKG and EEG flatlined at 3 min and 30 s. The state's coroner examined the inmate and pronounced him dead at 4 min and 44 s after the procedure began.

---

[110] SCOTUS in their *Glossip* and *Bayes* opinions think it is okay to experience some pain during execution but not "sure or very likely severe pain."

[111] When a rare commission or committee is set up to gather expert advice, as in Tennessee, the DOC may not heed their advice anyway. Trial testimony from the Deputy Commissioner of the TN DOC at the Nashville, Tennessee lethal injection case heard by Chancellor Lyle at the Davidson County Chancery Court, July 18, 2018.

Appendix A: List of medical schools by city and state, including phone number

State/other	City	Medical school	Phone
Alabama	Birmingham	University of Alabama School of Medicine	(205) 934-1997
	Mobile	University of South Alabama College of Medicine	(251) 460-7189
Arkansas	Little Rock	University of Arkansas for Medical Sciences	(501) 686-5350
Arizona	Glendale	Arizona College of Osteopathic Medicine	(888) 247-9277
	Mesa	School of Osteopathic Medicine in Arizona	(866) 626-2878
	Phoenix	University of Arizona College of Medicine—Phoenix	(602) 827-2001
	Tucson	University of Arizona College of Medicine—Tucson	(520) 626-4555
California	Irvine	University of California, Irvine, School of Medicine	(949) 824-5926
	La Jolla	University of California, San Diego School of Medicine	(858) 534-1501
	Loma Linda	Loma Linda University School of Medicine	(909) 558-8633
	Los Angeles	University of California, LA David Geffen School of Medicine	(310) 825-6373
	Los Angeles	University of Southern California, Keck School of Medicine	(323) 442-1100
	Pomona	College of Osteopathic Medicine of the Pacific	(909) 469-5335
	Sacramento	University of California, Davis, School of Medicine	(916) 734-4800
	San Francisco	University of California, San Francisco, School of Medicine	(415) 476-2342
	Stanford	Stanford University School of Medicine	(650) 725-3900
	Vallejo	Touro University College of Osteopathic Medicine	(888) 880-7336
Connecticut	Farmington	University of Connecticut School of Medicine	(860) 679-2413
	New Haven	Yale School of Medicine	(203) 785-4672
Colorado	Aurora	University of Colorado School of Medicine	(303) 724-5375
	Parker	Rocky Vista University College of Osteopathic Medicine	(720) 875-2800
District of Columbia	Washington, DC	Georgetown University School of Medicine	(202) 687-3922
	Washington, DC	George Washington University School of Medicine	(202) 994-2987
	Washington, DC	Howard University College of Medicine	(202) 806-5677

Continued

State/other	City	Medical school	Phone
Florida	Boca Raton	Florida Atlantic University, Charles E. Schmidt College of Medicine	(561) 297-3000
	Bradenton	Lake Erie College of Osteopathic Medicine Bradenton Campus	(941) 756-0690
	Fort Lauderdale	Nova Southeastern University College of Osteopathic Medicine	(866) 817-4068
	Gainesville	University of Florida College of Medicine	(352) 846-2473
	Miami	University of Miami Leonard M. Miller School of Medicine	(305) 243-6545
	Miami	Florida International University Herbert Wertheim College of Medicine	(305) 348-0570
	Orlando	University of Central Florida College of Medicine	(407) 266-1000
	Tallahassee	Florida State University College of Medicine	(850) 644-1855
	Tampa	University of South Florida College of Medicine	(813) 974-2229
Georgia	Atlanta	Emory University School of Medicine	(404) 727-5640
	Atlanta	Morehouse School of Medicine	(404) 752-1720
	Augusta	Medical College of Georgia at Augusta University	(706) 721-2231
	Macon	Mercer University School of Medicine	(478) 301-4022
	Suwanee	Georgia College of Osteopathic Medicine	(866) 282-4544
Hawaii	Honolulu	University of Hawaii, John A. Burns School of Medicine	(808) 692-1000
Illinois	Chicago	Northwestern University The Feinberg School of Medicine	(312) 503-0340
	Chicago	Rush Medical College of Rush University Medical Center	(312) 942-3237
	Chicago	University of Chicago, The Pritzker School of Medicine	(773) 702-3004
	Chicago	University of Illinois College of Medicine	(312) 996-3500
	Downers Grove	Chicago College of Osteopathic Medicine	(800) 458-6253
	Maywood	Loyola University Chicago Stritch School of Medicine	(708) 216-3223
	North Chicago	Chicago Medical School, Franklin University of Medicine	(847) 578-3000
	Springfield	Southern Illinois University School of Medicine	(217) 545-3318
Indiana	Indianapolis	Indiana University School of Medicine	(317) 278-3048
Iowa	Des Moines	Des Moines University College of Osteopathic Medicine	(800) 240-2767
	Iowa City	University of Iowa Carver College of Medicine	(319) 335-8064
Kansas	Kansas City	University of Kansas School of Medicine	(913) 588-5200
Kentucky	Lexington	University of Kentucky College of Medicine	(859) 323-5079
	Louisville	University of Louisville School of Medicine	(502) 852-5184
	Pikeville	Kentucky College of Osteopathic Medicine	(606) 218-5406
Louisiana	New Orleans	Louisiana State University School of Medicine in NOLA	(504) 568-4808
Maine	Biddeford	University of New England College of Osteopathic Medicine	(207) 602-2329
Maryland	Baltimore	Johns Hopkins University School of Medicine	(410) 955-3180
	Baltimore	University of Maryland School of Medicine	(410) 706-7410
	Bethesda	Uniformed Services University, F. Edward Hebert School of Medicine	(301) 295-3016
Massachusetts	Boston	Boston University School of Medicine	(617) 638-4147
	Boston	Harvard Medical School	(617) 432-1501
	Boston	Tufts University School of Medicine	(617) 636-6565
	Worcester	University of Massachusetts Medical School	(508) 856-8100

Continued

State/other	City	Medical school	Phone
Michigan	Ann Arbor	University of Michigan Medical School	(734) 764-8175
	Detroit	Wayne State University School of Medicine	(313) 577-1335
	East Lansing	Michigan State University College of Human Medicine	(517) 353-1730
	Rochester	Oakland University William Beaumont School of Medicine	(248) 370-3634
	East Lansing	Michigan State University College of Osteopathic Medicine	(517) 353-7740
Minnesota	Rochester	Mayo Clinic School of Medicine	(507) 284-3268
	Minneapolis	University of Minnesota Medical School	(612) 624-1188
Mississippi	Jackson	University of Mississippi School of Medicine	(601) 984-1010
	Hattiesburg	William Carey University College of Osteopathic Medicine	(601) 318-6235
Missouri	Columbia	University of Missouri—Columbia School of Medicine	(573) 882-1566
	Kansas City	University of Missouri—Kansas City School of Medicine	(816) 235-1808
	Kansas City	Kansas City University, College of Osteopathic Medicine	(877) 425-0247
	Kirksville	A.T. Still University—Kirksville College of Osteopathic Medicine	(866) 626-2878
	St. Louis	Saint Louis University School of Medicine	(314) 977-9801
Nebraska	Omaha	Creighton University School of Medicine	(402) 280-2600
	Omaha	University of Nebraska College of Medicine	(402) 559-4204
Nevada	Henderson	Touro University Nevada College of Osteopathic Medicine	(702) 777-1750
	Las Vegas	University of Nevada Las Vegas, School of Medicine	(702) 895-3011
New Hampshire	Hanover	Geisel School of Medicine at Dartmouth	(603) 650-1200
New Jersey	Camden	Cooper Medical School of Rowan University	(856) 361-2800
	Newark	Rutgers New Jersey Medical School	(973) 972-4300
	Piscataway	Rutgers, Robert Wood Johnson Medical School	(732) 235-6300
	Stratford	Rowan University School of Osteopathic Medicine	(856) 566-7050
New Mexico	Albuquerque	University of New Mexico School of Medicine	(505) 272-2321
New York	Albany	Albany Medical College	(518) 262-6008
	Bronx	Albert Einstein College of Medicine	(718) 430-2000
	Brooklyn	State University of New York Downstate Medical Center College of Medicine	(718) 270-3776
	Buffalo	Jacobs School of Medicine at the University at Buffalo	(716) 829-2775
	Hempstead	Hofstra Northwell School of Medicine at Hofstra University	(516) 463-7516
	New York	Columbia University College of Physicians and Surgeons	(212) 305-3592
	New York	CUNY School of Medicine	(212) 650-7718
	New York	Icahn School of Medicine at Mount Sinai	(212) 659-9001
	New York	Mount Sinai School of Medicine of New York University	(212) 263-5372
	New York	Weill Cornell Medicine	(212) 746-6005
	New York	Touro College of Osteopathic Medicine—New York	(212) 851-1199
	Old Westbury	New York Institute of Technology College of Osteopathic Medicine	(516) 686-3747
	Rochester	University of Rochester School of Medicine and Dentistry	(585) 275-0017
	Stony Brook	Stony Brook University School of Medicine	(631) 444-1785
	Syracuse	State University of New York Upstate Medical University	(315) 464-4513
	Valhalla	New York Medical College	(914) 594-4900

Continued

State/other	City	Medical school	Phone
North Carolina	Durham	Duke University School of Medicine	(919) 684-2455
	Chapel Hill	University of North Carolina at Chapel Hill School of Medicine	(919) 966-4161
	Winston-Salem	Wake Forest School of Medicine of Wake Forest Baptist Medical Center	(336) 716-5026
Ohio	Athens	Ohio University Heritage College of Osteopathic Medicine	(800) 345-1560
	Cincinnati	University of Cincinnati College of Medicine	(513) 558-7391
	Cleveland	Case Western Reserve University School of Medicine	(216) 368-2825
	Columbus	Ohio State University College of Medicine	(614) 292-1200
	Dayton	Wright State University Boonshoft School of Medicine	(937) 775-2933
	Rootstown	Northeast Ohio Medical University	(330) 325-2511
	Toledo	The University of Toledo College of Medicine	(419) 383-4243
Oklahoma	Oklahoma City	University of Oklahoma College of Medicine	(405) 271-2265
	Tulsa	OSU College of Osteopathic Medicine	(918) 561-8234
Oregon	Portland	Oregon Health & Science University School of Medicine	(503)494-8220
Pennsylvania	Erie	Lake Erie College of Osteopathic Medicine	(814) 866-6641
	Hershey	Pennsylvania State University College of Medicine	(717) 531-8521
	Philadelphia	Drexel University College of Medicine	(215) 991-8561
	Philadelphia	Lewis Katz School of Medicine at Temple University	(215) 707-7000
	Philadelphia	Perelman School of Medicine at the University of Pennsylvania	(215) 898-6796
	Philadelphia	Sidney Kimmel Medical College at Thomas Jefferson University	(215) 955-6980
	Philadelphia	Philadelphia College of Osteopathic Medicine	(800) 999-6998
	Pittsburgh	University of Pittsburgh School of Medicine	(412) 648-8975
	Scranton	Geisinger Commonwealth School of Medicine	(570) 504-7000
Rhode Island	Providence	The Warren Alpert Medical School of Brown University	(401) 863-3330
South Carolina	Columbia	University of South Carolina School of Medicine	(803) 216-3301
	Greenville	University of South Carolina School of Medicine Greenville	(803) 733-3200
	Spartanburg	Edward Via College of Osteopathic Medicine—Carolinas Campus	(864) 327-9800
South Dakota	Sioux Falls	University of South Dakota, Sanford School of Medicine	(605) 357-1300
Tennessee	Harrogate	Lincoln Memorial University—DeBusk College of Osteopathic Medicine	(800) 325-0900
	Johnson City	East Tennessee State University James H. Quillen College of Medicine	(423) 439-6315
	Memphis	University of Tennessee Health Science Center College of Medicine	(901) 448-5529
	Nashville	Meharry Medical College	(615) 327-6204
	Nashville	Vanderbilt University School of Medicine	(615) 322-5191

Continued

State/other	City	Medical school	Phone
Texas	Austin	University of Texas at Austin Dell Medical School	(512) 495-5555
	Bryan	Texas A&M Health Science Center College of Medicine	(979) 436-0200
	Dallas	University of Texas Southwestern Medical School	(214) 648-2509
	Edinburg	University of Texas Rio Grande Valley School of Medicine	(888) 882-4026
	El Paso	Texas Tech University Health Sciences Paul L. Foster School of Medicine	(915) 215-4300
	Ft. Worth	University of North Texas, Texas College of Osteopathic Medicine	(800) 535-8266
	Galveston	University of Texas Medical Branch School of Medicine	(409) 772-2671
	Houston	Baylor College of Medicine	(713) 798-4951
	Houston	McGovern Medical School at the University of Texas Health Science Center	(713) 500-5010
	Lubbock	Texas Tech University Health Sciences Center School of Medicine	(806) 743-3000
	San Antonio	University of Texas School of Medicine at San Antonio	(210) 567-4432
	San Antonio	University of Incarnate Word School of Osteopathic Medicine	(210) 283-6994
Utah	Salt Lake City	University of Utah School of Medicine	(801) 581-6436
Vermont	Burlington	University of Vermont College of Medicine	(802) 656-2156
Virginia	Blacksburg	Edward Via College of Osteopathic Medicine—Virginia Campus	(540) 231-6138
	Charlottesville	University of Virginia School of Medicine	(434) 924-5118
	Lynchburg	Liberty University College of Osteopathic Medicine	(434) 592-7444
	Norfolk	Eastern Virginia Medical School	(757) 446-5800
	Richmond	Virginia Commonwealth University School of Medicine	(804) 828-9788
	Roanoke	Virginia Tech Carilion School of Medicine	(540) 526-2559
Washington	Seattle	University of Washington School of Medicine	(206) 543-1060
	Spokane	Washington State University Elson S. Floyd College of Medicine	(509) 358-7944
	Yakima	Pacific Northwest University, College of Osteopathic Medicine	(866) 329-0521
West Virginia	Huntington	Marshall University Joan C. Edwards School of Medicine	(304) 691-1700
	Lewisburg	West Virginia School of Osteopathic Medicine	(800) 356-7836
	Morgantown	West Virginia University School of Medicine	(304) 293-6607
West Virginia	Huntington	Marshall University Joan C. Edwards School of Medicine	(304) 691-1700
	Lewisburg	West Virginia School of Osteopathic Medicine	(800) 356-7836
	Morgantown	West Virginia University School of Medicine	(304) 293-6607
Wisconsin	Madison	University of Wisconsin School of Medicine and Public Health	(608) 263-8668
	Milwaukee	Medical College of Wisconsin	(414) 456-8213
US territories			
Puerto Rico	Bayamon	Universidad Central del Caribe School of Medicine	(787) 798-6904
	Caguas	San Juan Bautista School of Medicine	(787) 743-3038
	Ponce	Ponce Health Sciences University School of Medicine	(787) 840-2575
	San Juan	University of Puerto Rico School of Medicine	(787) 765-2363
Northern Mariana Islands	Saipan	The University of Loyola at CNMI (Commonwealth of the Northern Mariana Islands)	(670) 234-8008

Note: At present, there are no medical schools in Alaska, Delaware, Idaho, Montana, and Wyoming, nor the US Territories of American Samoa, Guam, or the U.S. Virgin Islands.

Appendix B: Sample letter of engagement for the drug expert

Craig W. Stevens, Ph.D.
Professor of Pharmacology
Department of Pharmacology and Physiology
OSU-Center for Health Sciences
1111 W. 17th Street
Tulsa, Oklahoma 74107-1898

Ph: 918.561.8234 FAX: 918.561.8276 email: cw.stevens@okstate.edu

October 20, 2016

██████████████
████████████
████████

Oklahoma City, Oklahoma 73102   tel. (405) ████████   email: ████████████

RE:_____ [insert case info]

Dear ████████:

The purpose of this letter is to confirm my engagement as a Pharmacology expert witness/litigation consultant ('drug expert') for you and the firm. I will act in the capacity of a consultant in performing the services that you request of me on matters relevant to the above-mentioned case, including phone consultations and office meetings, research, analysis, litigation reports, and other consulting services as you deem necessary. In addition, I will also be available, at your request and in accordance to our joint arrangement and schedules, to testify as an expert witness at a deposition, hearing and/or trial in a civil or criminal action or in any arbitration should such services be needed.

The fees and expenses for services shall be based upon the following fee schedule:
Rate for conference calls, meetings, records review, research/analysis, reports: $250/hour
Rate for deposition and/or trial testimony*: $400/hour

*rate begins/ends with departure from/arrival back to my office in Tulsa, OK. Rate for cases involving out of state and/or overnight travel is capped at $2,500/day excluding travel, meal, and lodging expenses. **For all expenses and services rendered, the contracting law firm is responsible for payment.**

Please confirm this letter of engagement by signing below and scan and attach in an email sent to **cw.stevens@okstate.edu**.

Thank you for this opportunity to serve you and the firm.

Sincerely,

_____   Date:___Oct. 20, 2016_____
Craig W. Stevens, Ph.D. – LITIGATION CONSULTANT
Professor of Pharmacology

Accepted and agreed on by (*signed*):

_____   Date:_____

Printed Name:_____

Appendix C: Sample invoice for the drug expert

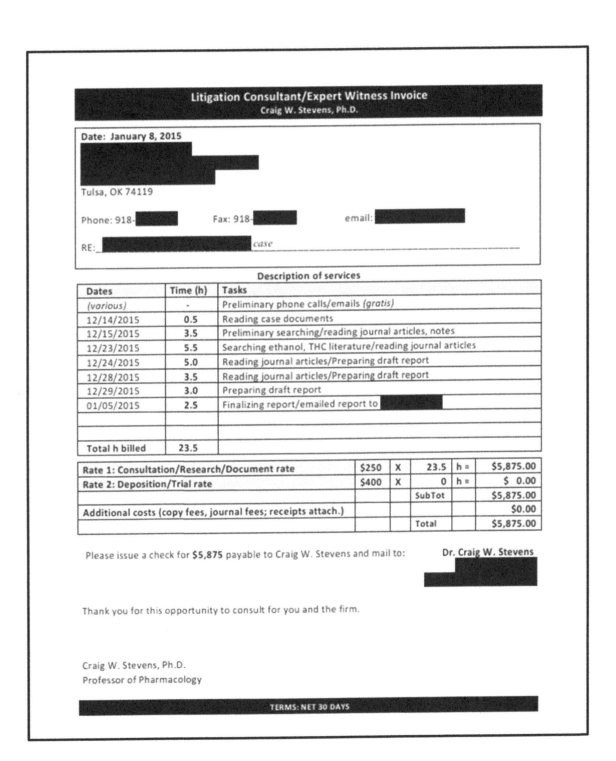

Litigation Consultant/Expert Witness Invoice
Craig W. Stevens, Ph.D.

Date: January 8, 2015

Tulsa, OK 74119

Phone: 918-██████   Fax: 918-██████   email: ██████████

RE: ████████████████ *case*

Description of services

Dates	Time (h)	Tasks
(various)	-	Preliminary phone calls/emails *(gratis)*
12/14/2015	0.5	Reading case documents
12/15/2015	3.5	Preliminary searching/reading journal articles, notes
12/23/2015	5.5	Searching ethanol, THC literature/reading journal articles
12/24/2015	5.0	Reading journal articles/Preparing draft report
12/28/2015	3.5	Reading journal articles/Preparing draft report
12/29/2015	3.0	Preparing draft report
01/05/2015	2.5	Finalizing report/emailed report to ████████
Total h billed	**23.5**	

Rate 1: Consultation/Research/Document rate	$250	X	23.5	h =	$5,875.00
Rate 2: Deposition/Trial rate	$400	X	0	h =	$ 0.00
				SubTot	$5,875.00
Additional costs (copy fees, journal fees; receipts attach.)					$0.00
				Total	$5,875.00

Please issue a check for **$5,875** payable to Craig W. Stevens and mail to: **Dr. Craig W. Stevens**
████████

Thank you for this opportunity to consult for you and the firm.

Craig W. Stevens, Ph.D.
Professor of Pharmacology

TERMS: NET 30 DAYS

Appendix D: Excerpt of litigation report

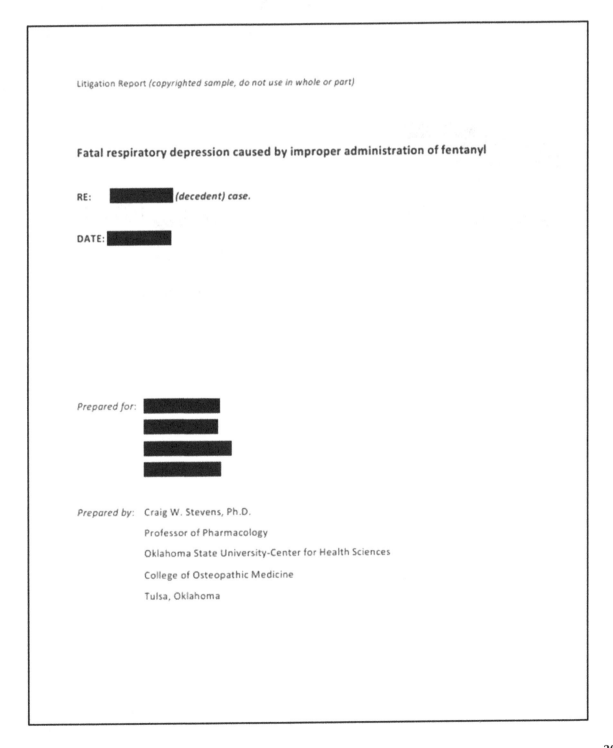

Litigation Report *(copyrighted sample, do not use in whole or part)*

Fatal respiratory depression caused by improper administration of fentanyl

RE: ███████ *(decedent) case.*

DATE: ████████

Prepared for: ██████████
██████████
██████████
██████████

Prepared by: Craig W. Stevens, Ph.D.

Professor of Pharmacology

Oklahoma State University-Center for Health Sciences

College of Osteopathic Medicine

Tulsa, Oklahoma

Resources

The following case documents and information were examined in the preparation of this report ████████, pharmacy records, ambulance and police reports ████████ Toxicology Report, and Food and Drug Administration (FDA) Prescribing Labels and documents. Additionally, a thorough search and reading of the medical and pharmacological journal literature concerning fentanyl and its side effects was done. This above information, along with over 30 years experience as a Pharmacologist, formed the basis for my expert opinion given below.

Narrative

The decedent, ████████, was diagnosed with stage 1 pancreatic cancer in the summer of ████████ had a history of asthma and chronic obstructive pulmonary disease (COPD). In ████, she began to experience escalating pain and sought treatment ████ ██ aggressively treated her with strong opioid analgesics, including IV morphine (DURAMORPH®), IV hydromorphone (DILAUDID®), fentanyl transmucosal lozenges (ACTIQ®) and fentanyl transdermal skin patches (DURAGESIC®). ████████ obtained treatment for pain from ████ from ████████ ████████. She died during the night or early morning of ████████.

A brief introduction to the opioid analgesics administered to ████████ is presented next.

A. Background on Opioid Analgesic Medications administered to ████████

Opioid pain medications, called *opioid analgesics*, are among the most powerful and dangerous drugs used in the clinic and prescribed to patients. Morphine is the gold standard of opioid analgesics, given for the treatment of moderate to severe pain. Besides morphine, opioid analgesics include other well-known pain medications such as codeine, oxycodone (OXYCONTIN), meperidine (DEMEROL®), and hydromorphone (DILAUDID). There are also a number of combination opioid products as well, such as hydrocodone/acetaminophen (NORCO, LORTAB, VICODIN) and many others. They are among the most prescribed medicines in the USA. Morphine, and all opioids, work by binding to opioid receptors on pain neurons (brain cells) and in this way inhibit the activity of the pain neurons. The inhibition of pain neurons produces the analgesia, or relief of pain, that characterizes morphine and other opioid analgesics (Brenner and Stevens, 2013).

While opioid analgesics are presently the best agents to treat pain and do so quite effectively, they are also a dangerous group of medicines that are responsible for many intentional and unintentional fatalities. The major adverse effect of all opioid drugs is respiratory depression. Opioids produce respiratory depression by direct inhibitory effect on brainstem respiratory neurons. The mechanism of respiratory depression also involves a reduction in the responsiveness of the brainstem neurons to increases in carbon dioxide in the blood. Patients and abusers who receive a high dose of opioids and who are not promptly treated with an opioid antagonist (antidote) and ventilation support can die from opioid overdose due to fatal respiratory depression. Breathing ceases and cardiac arrest and brain death ensues.

The Food and Drug Administration (FDA) approves the indications and use of all prescribed medicines marketed in the USA. In reaction to the increasing opioid overdose fatalities, the FDA increased awareness by sending out warning notices and announcements. For example in the case of fentanyl patches, in July 2005 the FDA sent out letters to health care providers and the public stressing that the directions on the product label and package insert should be followed exactly in order to avoid overdose. However the FDA continued to receive reports of deaths and life-threatening side effects after doctors inappropriately prescribed the fentanyl patch or patients incorrectly using it. A second warning letter was issued in 2007 entitled "Second safety warning on fentanyl skin patch: Deaths and serious injuries from improper use." It was stated that "it is crucial doctors prescribe these products appropriately and that patients use them correctly" (FDA News Release 12-21-2007).

In spite of these repeated warnings and many others to health care providers, there did not appear to be any drop in opioid-related fatalities across the nation. More recently the FDA used its authority to regulate drugs to employ Risk Evaluation and Mitigation Strategy (REMS) programs for opioids which mandates education and registration requirements for health care providers who prescribe transmucosal fentanyl products and fentanyl transdermal skin patches. The REMS programs for these opioid analgesics went into effect in 2011 and 2012.

1. MORPHINE (generic oral, IV formulation as DURAMORPH)

Morphine is the oldest of opioid analgesic drugs and was originally isolated from the unripe seed pod of poppy plants (Brenner and Stevens, 2013). It is available in different formulations (drug preparations) for oral, intravenous (IV), intrathecal, and epidural administration. One of the trade names of injectable morphine is DURAMORPH. It is also available in a generic oral tablet formulation as Morphine sulfate-immediate release (MSIR) in dosage strengths of 15 or 30 mg per tablet (FDA Prescribing Label)

Morphine remains in the body for a long time; only half of the morphine is metabolized by 1.5–2 hours (elimination half-life), although more sensitive studies extend this half-life to 4-6 hours. The major pathway of morphine sulfate metabolism is conjugation with D-glucuronic acid to produce the 3- and 6-glucuronide metabolites (M3G and M6G; about 50% and 15%, respectively). M6G has been shown to have analgesic activity but crosses the blood-brain barrier poorly, while M3G has no significant analgesic activity.

2. Hydromorphone (DILAUDID)

Hydromorphone is a strong opioid analgesic structurally similar to morphine and about 10 times more potent. Hydromorphone injection is indicated for the relief of moderate to severe pain such as that due to surgery, cancer, or trauma. Hydromorphone is extensively metabolized via glucuronidation in the liver, with greater than 95% of the dose metabolized to hydromorphone-3-glucuronide along with minor amounts of 6-hydroxy reduction metabolites. Both metabolites are inactive (FDA Label).

3. Hydrocodone/acetaminophen (NORCO, LORTAB, VICODIN)

NORCO, LORTAB, and VICODIN are some brand names of the combination formulation of hydrocodone and acetaminophen supplied in a tablet form for oral administration. Hydrocodone is a semisynthetic opioid analgesic with actions qualitatively similar to those of codeine and morphine. Like all opioids, hydrocodone binds to opioid receptors on pain neurons as described above. In addition to analgesia, hydrocodone like other opioids may be habit-forming and lead to drug dependence and addiction. Use of hydrocodone-containing products also carries the risk of respiratory depression. Acetaminophen is a member of the NSAID (Non-Steroidal Anti-Inflammatory Drug) drug class that includes common over-the-counter agents such as ibuprofen and aspirin. Acetaminophen by itself is available in a number of formulations including the brand name product TYLENOL.

Hydrocodone/acetaminophen is available in 4 different dosage strengths of hydrocodone (2.5, 5.0, 7.5 and 10 mg hydrocodone) in combination with a constant amount of acetaminophen (325 mg). LORTAB tablets are indicated for the relief of moderate to moderately severe pain (FDA Prescribing Label).

4. Fentanyl Transmucosal Oral Lozenges (ACTIQ)

Fentanyl is a strong opioid analgesic drug estimated to be 50-100 times more potent than morphine (Kuhlman et al. 2003). It is used for the treatment of moderate to severe pain. Fentanyl is available in different forms including an IV injection formulation and a transdermal skin patch formulation for around-the-clock pain treatment (DURAGESIC, see below). It is not available for normal oral administration in pill or tablet form, but is available as a transmucosal oral lozenge formulation which consists of what is essentially a fentanyl lollipop (ACTIQ). ACTIQ comes in 200 mcg, 400 mcg, 600 mcg, 800 mcg, 1200 mcg and 1600 mcg dosage strengths. Peak plasma concentrations of fentanyl occur about 25 minutes after use of ACTIQ (Striesand et al. 1991).

ACTIQ is available only through a restricted program called the Transmucosal Immediate Release Fentanyl (TIRF) Risk Evaluation and Mitigation Strategy (REMS) program. This program was put in place by the FDA to reduce the fatalities associated with overdose, misuse and abuse of fentanyl transmucosal drugs. Outpatients, healthcare professionals who prescribe to outpatients, pharmacies, and distributors are required to enroll in the program. For inpatient administration (e.g., hospitals, hospices, and long-term care facilities that prescribe for inpatient use) patient and prescriber enrollment is not required.

Litigation report - ████ *case*

C. Integration of Medical Literature on Fatal Respiratory Depression caused by Fentanyl with the Specifics of Fentanyl administered to ████████████

There is no doubt that opioid analgesic overdose is at epidemic levels among patients in the USA (see §A above). A review of medical malpractice suits filed by parties representing patients who died from fatal respiratory depression while administered opioid analgesic yielded the finding that one of the most common risk factors was medication administration errors when starting, converting, or changing opioid analgesic doses (Rich et al. 2011). An additional report examining the root causes for opioid-related overdose deaths in the USA confirmed that a common factor was physician knowledge deficit, and cited in particular, overestimating the tolerance to respiratory depression conferred by prior use of opioids in patients (Webster et al. 2011).

In the case of ████████, physicians at ████ demonstrated a knowledge deficit in the use *per se* and in the initial dosing of fentanyl in both transmucosal and transdermal formulations (see medical error list below).

.

.

.

.

E. Conclusion

Given that ████████████ was administered powerful and dangerous opioid analgesics including fentanyl by ████████; given that ████████ suffered from moderate to severe COPD which is a known risk factor for opioid-induced fatal respiratory depression; given that greater initial doses than approved by the FDA for the transmucosal fentanyl (Actiq) and for the transdermal fentanyl (Duragesic) were administered to ████████████; given that both transmucosal fentanyl (Actiq) and transdermal fentanyl (Duragesic) are to be used only in opioid-tolerant patients and that ████ ████ did not meet the criteria for opioid tolerance; and given that fentanyl patches in particular were used in violation of FDA-approved labeling, it is my expert opinion that the death of ████ ████████ was due to medical errors and negligence on the part of ████ and its staff causing fatal respiratory depression due to improper use of fentanyl opioid analgesics.

I reserve the right to amend this report should further information become available.

I declare under penalty of perjury that I have examined the report and all the statements contained herein, and to the best of my knowledge, they are true, correct and complete. My opinions stated herein are based on reasonable degree of scientific and medical certainty.

_____   Date: _____

Craig W. Stevens, Ph.D.
Professor of Pharmacology

REFERENCES CITED

Anderson DT, Muto JJ. (2000) Duragesic transdermal patch: postmortem tissue distribution of fentanyl in 25 cases. J Anal Toxicol. 24:627-634.

Bohnert AS, Valenstein M, Bair MJ, Ganoczy D, McCarthy JF, Ilgen MA, Blow FC. (2011) Association between opioid prescribing patterns and opioid overdose-related deaths. J. American Med Assoc 305:1315-1321.

Brenner, GM and Stevens, CW. (2013) *Pharmacology*, 4th edition. Pharmacology textbook for medical and health professional students, Saunders/Elsevier, Philadelphia/London.

Dahan A, Yassen A, Bijl H, Romberg R, Sarton E, Teppema L, Olofsen E, Danhof M. (2005) Comparison of the respiratory effects of intravenous buprenorphine and fentanyl in humans and rats. Br J Anaesth. 94:825-834.

Dahan A, Yassen A, Romberg R, Sarton E, Teppema L, Olofsen E, Danhof M. (2006) Buprenorphine induces ceiling in respiratory depression but not in analgesia. Br J Anaesth. 96:627-632.

Grond S, Radbruch L, Lehmann KA (2000) Clinical pharmacokinetics of transdermal opioids: focus on transdermal fentanyl. Clin Pharmacokinet. 38:59-89.

Kuhlman JJ Jr, McCaulley R, Valouch TJ, Behonick GS. (2003) Fentanyl use, misuse, and abuse: a summary of 23 postmortem cases. J Anal Toxicol. 27:499-504.

Appendix E: Excerpt of drug expert deposition

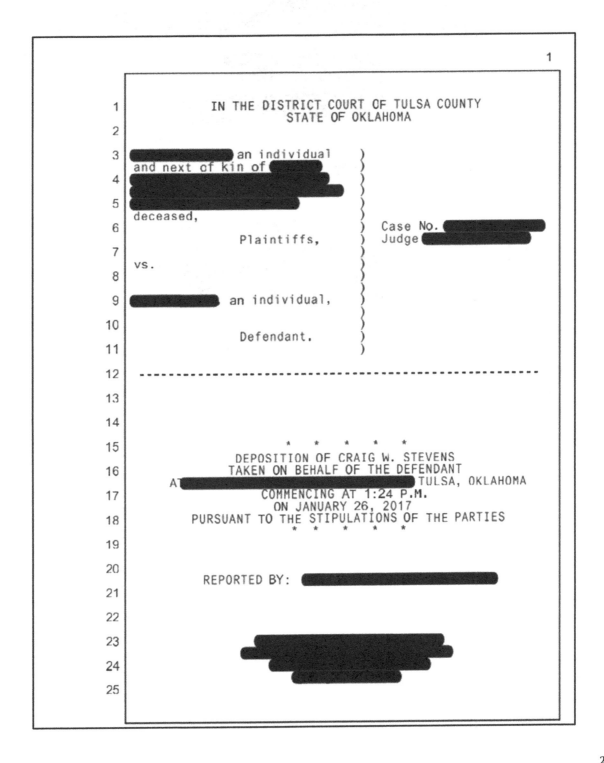

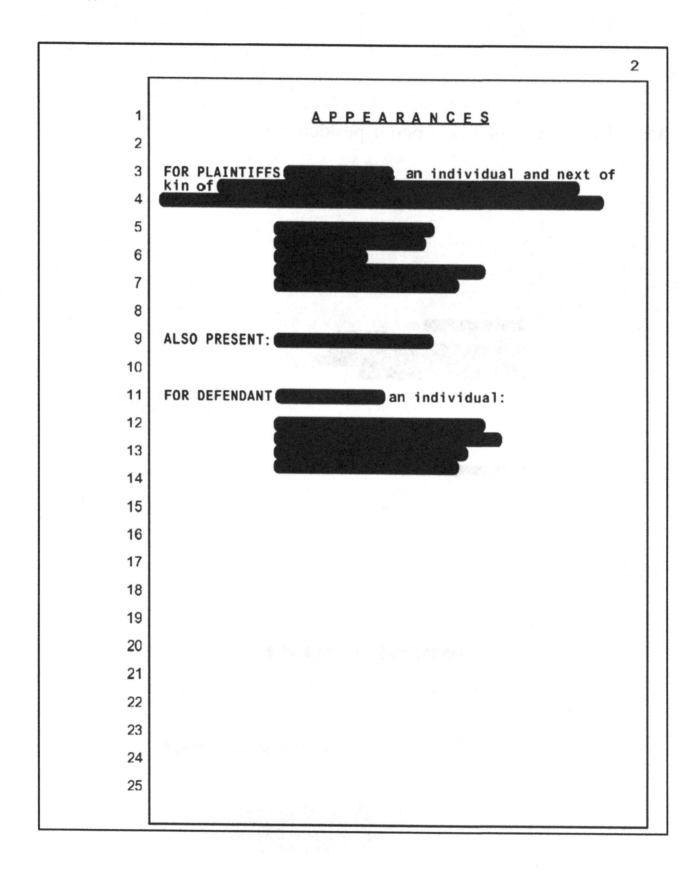

3

1   S T I P U L A T I O N S

2

3   IT IS HEREBY STIPULATED AND AGREED by and between
    the parties hereto that the notice for the taking of the
    deposition is waived and that the same may be taken at

4   this time and place.
        IT FURTHER STIPULATED AND AGREED that all

5   objections, except as to the form of the questions, are
    reserved to the time of trial, with the same force and

6   effect as if made at the taking of the deposition.

7

8

9   C O N T E N T S

    WITNESS   **PAGE**

10 CRAIG W. STEVENS
            EXAMINATION BY ████████████   4

11   REQUESTED INFORMATION...................   37
            REQUESTED INFORMATION...................   42

12   REQUESTED INFORMATION...................   43
            REQUESTED INFORMATION...................   44

13   EXAMINATION BY ████████   73
            EXAMINATION BY ██████████████   80

14   EXAMINATION BY ████████   92
            SIGNATURE PAGE........................   94

15   REPORTER'S CERTIFICATE.................   95

16

17

18

19

20

21

22

23

24

25

1   <u>**CRAIG W. STEVENS**</u>

2 being first duly sworn to testify the truth, the whole

3 truth, and nothing but the truth, testified as follows:

4   *   *   *   *   *   *   *   *

01:09PM 5   EXAMINATION

6 BY MR. ███████████

7   Q.   Would you state your name for the record,

8 please.

9   A.   Craig W. Stevens, S-T-E-V-E-N-S.

01:24PM 10   Q.   And I understand you have a Ph.D.?

11   A.   I have a Ph.D. in pharmacology.

12   Q.   If I refer to you as Doctor for short, would

13 that be fine?

14   A.   That's fine, thank you.

01:24PM 15   Q.   Tell us what pharmacology is.

16   A.   Pharmacology is the study of drugs in all its

17 various aspects, including beneficial effects, adverse

18 effects, toxicology and any other pertinent issues

19 having to do with drug administration.

01:25PM 20   Q.   Are you a toxicologist?

21   A.   I am not formally degreed in toxicology.

22 Toxicology is a subdiscipline of the broader degree of

23 pharmacology.

24   Q.   If you connect forensic to pharmacology, what

01:25PM 25 does that entail?

Craig W. Stevens, January 26, 2017   5

1   A.   Forensic, my understanding of it is someone
2 that may be involved with usually legal or medical-legal
3 proceedings.
4   Q.   You're involved in legal-medical proceedings,
01:25PM 5 are you not?
6   A.   I am.
7   Q.   Are you a forensic pharmacologist?
8   A.   I'm a pharmacologist who does, I guess you
9 could say, forensic work.
01:25PM10   Q.   Are you a licensed forensic pharmacologist?
11   A.   No, I am not licensed in that regard.
12   Q.   Are you board certified as a forensic
13 pharmacologist?
14   A.   No, I am not.
01:26PM15   Q.   Are you board certified in any area that a
16 doctor can be board certified by the American Board of
17 Medical Specialties?
18   A.   No. I'm a Ph.D. and not a physician, per se,
19 so those board eligibilities are not applicable to my
01:26PM20 training.
21   Q.   Do you know Dr. ███████████████████
22   A.   I don't believe I do.
23   Q.   Well, he's the chief forensic toxicologist at
24 the office of the chief medical examiner. Does that
01:26PM25 help you?

1   A.   No, I don't know him.

2   Q.   His CV shows that he's certified as a fellow of

3   the American Board of Forensic Toxicology. He has a

4   license number of ███████. Do you have anything similar to

01:27PM 5   that?

6   A.   No, I do not.

7   Q.   We talked about my son before we started here.

8   And apparently if you don't get a tenured professor

9   track when you get your Ph.D., you do, I guess, a

01:27PM 10   postdoctorate research fellowship?

11   A.   That's a little bit of a mischaracterization.

12   It's not a matter of if you don't get the tenure track

13   job. It's a matter that most of your tenure track jobs

14   require you to do postdoctorate training first. So I

01:28PM 15   went directly from my Ph.D. to a post-doc without

16   attempting to get a tenure track job.

17   Q.   You didn't attempt to get a tenured

18   professorship once you got your Ph.D.?

19   A.   Not until I finished my post-doc, because in my

01:28PM 20   field in many medical fields at a medical school you

21   have to have a post-doc. It's a requirement before you

22   can apply for a professorship.

23   Q.   Did you apply for a professorship at the

24   University of Minnesota, where you did your

01:28PM 25   postdoctorate research fellowship?

Appendix F: Excerpt of a court transcript cross-examination

```
 1   strike someone?
 2        A.  It's possible for sure.
 3           MR. ████████  That's all I have, Judge.
 4        THE COURT:  Yes, sir.  Cross-examination on --
 5           MR. ████████  Yes.
 6        THE COURT:  -- Mr. ████████s questions or the
 7   Court's.
 8           MS. ████  Thank you, Your Honor.
 9                    CROSS-EXAMINATION
10   BY MS. ████:
11        Q.  I'm going to see if I understand this correctly.
12   You are actually testifying that with certainty -- someone
13   with that level that ████████ had, are you trying to
14   say with certainty you can say how he was acting?
15        A.  Yes, I am.
16        Q.  All right.  Do you believe that there are other
17   experts, articles that will say that you have the ability
18   to predict someone's actions even when you were not
19   present?
20        A.  I guess I'm not sure what articles you're
21   referring to or --
22        Q.  Are there any?
23        A.  I did not research that in this particular
24   report.
25        Q.  Okay.  So at this time you're not aware of any
```

1   articles that would support your testimony that you, not

2   having been present when this incident occurred, can say

3   how ███████████████ was acting?

4   A. I'm aware of all of the articles here which

5   support my testimony, I believe, that show without a doubt

6   this level of methamphetamine can cause aggression,

7   violence, psychotic behavior.

8   Q. And that's what I'm getting out, because now when

9   I'm talking to you, you say "can cause," okay? Now, you

10   would agree with me that there is a lot of evidence out

11   there to support that methamphetamine is bad, correct?

12   A. Yes, that's correct.

13   Q. Methamphetamine can cause people to act in ways

14   that they might normally not act?

15   A. For sure.

16   Q. Methamphetamine can cause people to be

17   aggressive?

18   A. And it does, yes.

19   Q. And are you suggesting then that every single

20   person that uses methamphetamine is aggressive to another

21   person?

22   A. That could be an interesting experiment. I don't

23   know.

24   Q. I'm not asking you about an interesting

25   experiment. I said are you testifying that every single

1   person that uses methamphetamine is going to be aggressive?

2   A.   I am testifying that methamphetamine at that

3   level in the blood --

4   Q.   Again, I'm going to --

5   A.   -- will cause aggression.

6   MR. █████████:   Judge, I would ask that --

7   MS. █████:   Judge, I would ask that this --

8   MR. █████████:   -- the witness be allowed to

9   answer the question.

10   MS. █████:   -- be instructed to answer my

11   question.

12   THE COURT: One moment. One moment. My court

13   reporter can only get one person talking at one time.

14   There was an objection; he answered it.

15   You had said something to me, Ms. █████, and I'm

16   sorry, I did not hear it. There were multiple people

17   talking. What did you ask?

18   MS. █████:   Because I'm asking the question, I

19   have asked it twice so far, and it's not been answered. I

20   would ask if you would instruct the witness to answer the

21   question that I'm asking.

22   THE COURT: The question I thought was answered

23   when he said that a person with that level of

24   methamphetamine in the blood would have demonstrated levels

25   of aggressiveness.

DISTRICT COURT OF OKLAHOMA - OFFICIAL TRANSCRIPT

1	MS. ████: But that was not --
2	THE COURT: Was that your answer?
3	THE WITNESS: That's correct, Your Honor.
4	THE COURT: And then --
5	MS. ████: And, again, that was not my question.
6	THE COURT: -- what was the question?
7	MS. ████: My question, Your Honor, was are you
8	testifying that anyone who uses methamphetamine would
9	necessarily then be aggressive?
10	THE COURT: No. But with that level of
11	intoxication they would be. Is that a fair summary of your
12	testimony?
13	THE WITNESS: That's very good, Your Honor.
14	Q. (By Ms. ████) Now, you said that you reviewed the
15	defendant's statements. which statements of the defendant
16	did you review?
17	A. I listened to the 911 call.
18	Q. Uh-huh.
19	A. And then I read police transcripts that were
20	provided to me I believe as a word document of an interview
21	with the defendant.
22	Q. Was that an interview that the defendant had with
23	detectives?
24	A. I believe so.
25	Q. Was it like numerous pages, a fairly thick

Appendix G: Sample toxicology reports

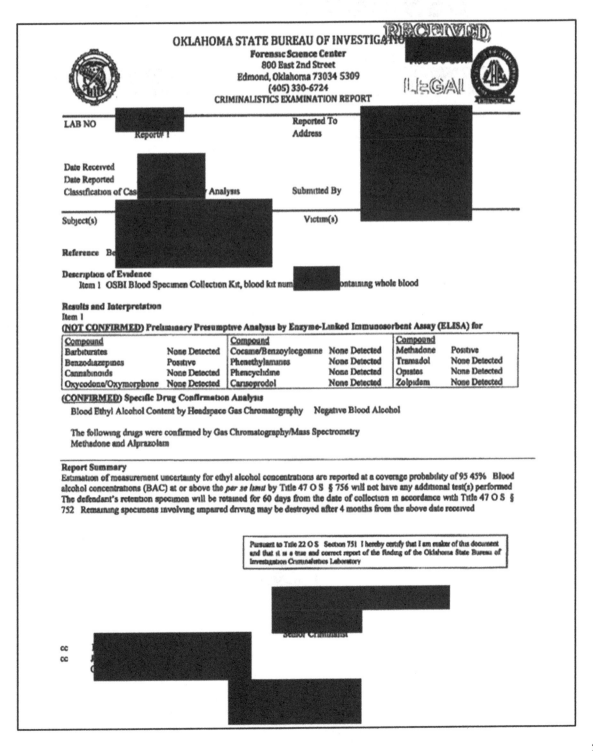

OKLAHOMA STATE BUREAU OF INVESTIGATION
Forensic Science Center
800 East 2nd Street
Edmond, Oklahoma 73034 5309
(405) 330-6724
CRIMINALISTICS EXAMINATION REPORT

RECEIVED

LEGAL

LAB NO

Reported To
Address

Date Received
Date Reported
Classification of Case   Analysis   Submitted By

Subject(s)   Victim(s)

Reference

Description of Evidence
Item 1 OSBI Blood Specimen Collection Kit, blood kit num   ntaining whole blood

Results and Interpretation
Item 1
(NOT CONFIRMED) Preliminary Presumptive Analysis by Enzyme-Linked Immunosorbent Assay (ELISA) for

Compound		Compound		Compound	
Barbiturates	None Detected	Cocaine/Benzoylecgonine	None Detected	Methadone	Positive
Benzodiazepines	Positive	Phenethylamines	None Detected	Tramadol	None Detected
Cannabinoids	None Detected	Phencyclidine	None Detected	Opiates	None Detected
Oxycodone/Oxymorphone	None Detected	Carisoprodol	None Detected	Zolpidem	None Detected

(CONFIRMED) Specific Drug Confirmation Analysis

Blood Ethyl Alcohol Content by Headspace Gas Chromatography   Negative Blood Alcohol

The following drugs were confirmed by Gas Chromatography/Mass Spectrometry
Methadone and Alprazolam

Report Summary
Estimation of measurement uncertainty for ethyl alcohol concentrations are reported at a coverage probability of 95 45% Blood alcohol concentrations (BAC) at or above the *per se limit* by Title 47 O S § 756 will not have any additional test(s) performed The defendant's retention specimen will be retained for 60 days from the date of collection in accordance with Title 47 O S § 752 Remaining specimens involving impaired driving may be destroyed after 4 months from the above date received

Pursuant to Title 22 O S Section 751 I hereby certify that I am maker of this document and that it is a true and correct report of the finding of the Oklahoma State Bureau of Investigation Criminalistics Laboratory

Senior Criminalist

cc
cc

BOARD OF MEDICOLEGAL INVESTIGATIONS
OFFICE OF THE CHIEF MEDICAL EXAMINER

901 N.Stonewall
Oklahoma City, Oklahoma   73117

REPORT OF LABORATORY ANALYSIS

ME CASE NUMBER: 14█████████

DECEDENT'S NAME: █████████

MATERIAL SUBMITTED: BLOOD, VITREOUS, URINE, LIVER, BRAIN,
                     GASTRIC

LABORATORY NUMBER: █████

DATE RECEIVED: █████

HOLD STATUS: 5 YEARS

SUBMITTED BY: █████████

MEDICAL EXAMINER █████████

NOTES: Addendum to the report dated 03█████

ETHYL ALCOHOL:

Blood:

Vitreous:

Other:

CARBON MONOXIDE

Blood:

TESTS PERFORMED:

EIA - (Heart Blood) - Amphetamine, Methamphetamine, Fentanyl, Cocaine, Opiates, PCP, Barbiturates, Benzodiazepines
(The EIA panel does not detect Oxycodone, Methadone, Lorazepam or Clonazepam)

RESULTS:

AMPHETAMINE
POSITIVE - (Less than 0.06 mcg/mL) - (Heart Blood)

METHAMPHETAMINE
0.13 mcg/mL - (Heart Blood)

█████████
02/11/2015
DATE

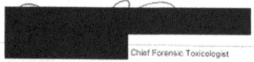

Chief Forensic Toxicologist

Jan 21 2010 10:40 APT DUTT CONSTRUCTION 4058444004   3/4

BOARD OF MEDICOLEGAL INVESTIGATIONS
OFFICE OF THE CHIEF MEDICAL EXAMINER
901 N.Stonewall
Oklahoma City, Oklahoma 73117

REPORT OF LABORATORY ANALYSIS

OFFICE USE ONLY

Rh _____ Co _____

I hereby certify that this is a true
and correct copy of the original
document. Valid only when copy
bears imprint by the office seal.

By _____

Date _____

ME CASE NUMBER: 09█   LABORATORY NUMBER:

DECEDENT'S NAME: DATE RECEIVED:

MATERIAL SUBMITTED: HOLD STATUS: 30 DAYS

SUBMITTED BY: MEDICAL EXAMIN

NOTES:

ETHYL ALCOHOL:

Blood: NEGATIVE (HEART)

Vitreous:

Other:

CARBON MONOXIDE

Blood:

TESTS PERFORMED:
BLOOD BASES
BLOOD EIA - Amphetamine, Methamphetamine, Cocaine, Opiates*, PCP, Barbiturates, Benzodiazepines, Fentanyl*
* This test does not detect Oxycodone, Methadone, Lorazepam, Nitrobenzodiazepines.

RESULTS:
BLOOD (FEMORAL)
COCAINE - POSITIVE LESS THAN 0.03 mcg/mL
BENZOYLECGONINE - 0.19 mcg/mL

DATE   ....
                                    .... M.D., Deputy Chief Forensic Toxicologist

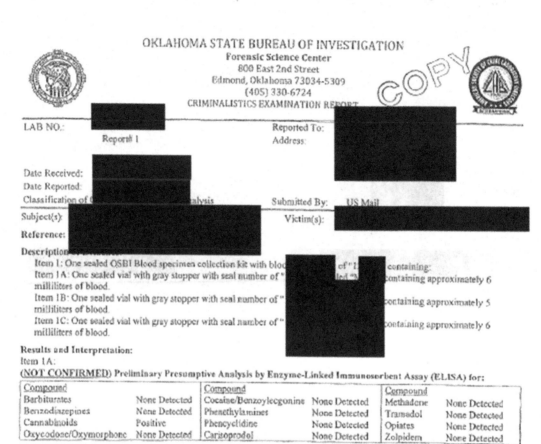

OKLAHOMA STATE BUREAU OF INVESTIGATION
Forensic Science Center
800 East 2nd Street
Edmond, Oklahoma 73034-5309
(405) 330-6724
CRIMINALISTICS EXAMINATION REPORT

LAB NO.:   Reported To:
       Report# 1   Address:

Date Received:
Date Reported:
Classification of ☐   analysis   Submitted By: US Mail
Subject(s):   Victim(s):
Reference:

Description ☐
   Item 1: One sealed OSBI Blood specimen collection kit with bloc☐ of "1☐ containing:
   Item 1A: One sealed vial with gray stopper with seal number of "☐led "☐ containing approximately 6
   milliliters of blood.
   Item 1B: One sealed vial with gray stopper with seal number of "☐ containing approximately 5
   milliliters of blood.
   Item 1C: One sealed vial with gray stopper with seal number of "☐ containing approximately 6
   milliliters of blood.

Results and Interpretation:
Item 1A:
(NOT CONFIRMED) Preliminary Presumptive Analysis by Enzyme-Linked Immunosorbent Assay (ELISA) for:

Compound		Compound		Compound	
Barbiturates	None Detected	Cocaine/Benzoylecgonine	None Detected	Methadone	None Detected
Benzodiazepines	None Detected	Phenethylamines	None Detected	Tramadol	None Detected
Cannabinoids	Positive	Phencyclidine	None Detected	Opiates	None Detected
Oxycodone/Oxymorphone	None Detected	Carisoprodol	None Detected	Zolpidem	None Detected

(CONFIRMED) Specific Drug Confirmation Analysis:
   Blood Ethyl Alcohol Content by Headspace Gas Chromatography: Negative Blood Alcohol
   No drugs detected by Alkaline drug screen.
   The following compounds were confirmed by Gas Chromatography/Mass Spectrometry:
   Delta-9-Tetrahydrocannabinol: 8.32± 0.65 ng/mL
   11-Nor-Delta-9-Tetrahydrocannabinol-9-Carboxylic Acid: 105± 8 ng/mL
Items 1B and 1C not analyzed.

Report Summary:
Estimations of measurement uncertainty are reported at a coverage probability of 95.45%. The defendant's retention specimen
will be retained for 60 days from the date of collection in accordance with Title 47 O.S. § 752. Remaining specimens involving
impaired driving may be destroyed after 4 months from the above date received.

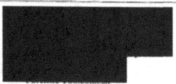

Pursuant to Title 22 O.S., Section 751, I hereby certify that I am maker of this document,
and that it is a true and correct report of the finding of the Oklahoma State Bureau of
Investigation Criminalistics Laboratory.

14-03-040

cc: Department of Public Safety

Appendix H: Sample medical records

Patient Name: ▇▇▇▇▇		MRN: ▇▇▇▇	Admission#: ▇▇▇▇

Medication Administration Record

Medications

Medication Name: morphine (Morphine IV) (Morphine 10 mg/1 mL inj)

Admin Date/Time: ▇▇ 19:34 CST	Charted Date/Time: ▇▇ 19:34 CST

Ingredients: MORP10I 5 mg 0.5 mL

Admin Details: (Auth) IV Push, Left Upper Arm

Pain Intensity 4

Action Details: Order ▇▇▇▇ 18:57 CST; Perform ▇▇▇▇ 19:34 CST; VERIFY: ▇▇▇▇ 1/5/2016 19:34 CST

Reason for Medication: ▇▇▇▇ 19:34 CST

Pain

Medication Name: LORazepam (Lorazepam IVP) (Lorazepam 2mg/1ml inj)

Admin Date/Time: ▇▇ 19:18 CST	Charted Date/Time: ▇▇ 19:43 CST

Admin Details: Electronically Reviewed and Signed

PRN medication effectiveness: Non pain medication, Yes

Action Details: Order ▇▇▇▇ 18:57 CST; Perform ▇▇▇▇ 19:42 CST; VERIFY: ▇▇▇▇ 19:42 CST

Medication Name: atropine ophthalmic (Atropine ophth 1%) (Atropine 1% ophth soln 5 mL)

Admin Date/Time: ▇▇ 19:15 CST	Charted Date/Time: ▇▇ 19:16 CST

Ingredients: Atropine ophth 1% 4 drop(s)

Admin Details: (Auth) PO

Action Details: Order ▇▇▇▇ 18:57 CST; Perform ▇▇▇▇ 19:16 CST; VERIFY: ▇▇▇▇ 19:16 CST

Reason for Medication: ▇▇▇▇ 19:16 CST

Congestion

Medication Name: morphine (Morphine IV) (Morphine 10 mg/1 mL inj)

Admin Date/Time: ▇▇ 19:15 CST	Charted Date/Time ▇▇ 19:43 CST

Admin Details: Electronically Reviewed and Signed

Pain Intensity: 4; Pain Scale Type: FLACC Pain scale; PRN medication effectiveness: Pain medication; Purpose of PRN medication: Pain reduction

Action Details: Order ▇▇▇▇ 18:57 CST; Perform ▇▇▇▇ 19:43 CST; VERIFY: ▇▇▇▇ 19:43 CST

Medication Name: LORazepam (Lorazepam IVP) (Lorazepam 2mg/1ml inj)

Admin Date/Time: ▇▇ 18:48 CST	Charted Date/Time ▇▇ 19:42 CST

Ingredients: LORA2I 2 mg 1 mL

Admin Details: (Auth) IV Push, Left Arm

Action Details: Order ▇▇▇▇ 18:57 CST; Perform ▇▇▇▇ 19:42 CST; VERIFY: ▇▇▇▇ 19:42 CST

Reason for Medication: ▇▇▇▇ 19:42 CST

Agitation

Patient Name: ▇▇▇▇	Patient Type: Inpatient Hospice (HOS)
Admit / Discharge: ▇▇▇▇	Report Request ID: ▇▇▇▇
Print Date / Time: 1/26/2016 10:01 CST Page 55 of 61	OPI: ▇▇▇▇

Patient Name: ▓▓▓▓▓▓▓▓▓▓ MRN: ▓▓▓▓▓▓ Admission#: ▓▓▓▓▓▓▓

Emergency Documentation

SKIN: Skin exam normal, Skin exam included findings of skin warm, dry, and normal in color, no rash.
EKG INTERPRETATION (15:39 LS)
12 LEAD EKG INTERPRETATION: 12 lead EKG interpreted by Emergency Department Physician, 12 lead EKG shows, sinus tachycardia, Interpretation:, Conduction normal, ST segments normal, T waves, Axis normal, Clinical impression:, with sinus arrythmia.
O2SAT INTERPRETATION (15:38 LS)
O2SAT: Continuous pulse oximetry, Oxygen saturation 95%, on 3L, via nasal cannula, Oxygen saturation interpretation: Low normal, Intervention required: patient observed, Intervention required: Oxygen administration.
LAB INTERPRETATION (15:39 LS)
INTERPRETATION: I reviewed the lab results.
RADIOLOGY INTERPRETATION
INTERPRETER: Preliminary review of x-rays by, ED Physician. (15:39 LS)
  Preliminary review of CT scans by, Radiologist. (17:12 LS)
CHEST: Films of the chest show, copd. (15:39 LS)
  Chest CT, severe motion - RML ? acute pe vs chronic pe vs motion. (17:12 LS)
DIAGNOSIS (19:33 LS)
FINAL: PRIMARY: Hypoglycemia, ADDITIONAL: Chest pain, unspecified, copd with exacerbation, hyperlipidemia, hypertension.
DOCTOR NOTES
RE-EVALUATION: Routine re-evaluation, after administration of IV fluids, Routine re-evaluation, after observation, Routine re-evaluation, after administration of oxygen therapy, The patient's condition has improved. (19:32 LS)
CRITICAL CARE: Time spent providing critical care to patient was 30-74 minutes, spent time with pt, reviewing old records, talking to consultant, stabilizing, talking to vrad, etc. (19:33 LS)
D/W: Discussed this case with Dr. hosp, to admit. (19:32 LS)
EVENTS
ATTENDING: ▓▓▓▓▓▓▓▓▓▓ saw the patient at ▓▓▓▓▓▓▓▓ 14:30. (14:30 LS)
TRANSFER: Triage to Emergency Bay 3 34. ▓▓▓▓▓▓ CYE)
  Removed from Emergency Bay 3 34. (19:52 CYE)
DISPOSITION
PATIENT: Disposition: Admit to floor from ER. (17:47 LS)
  EVD: No travel to EVD infected area in 21 day, Discharge Vitals: Vital signs rechecked, Suspected abuse: No abuse/neglect suspected, Disposition Transport: Cart, Condition: Fair, Patient left the department. (19:52 CYE)
PRESCRIPTION
  No recorded prescriptions

Patient Name: ▓▓▓▓▓▓▓▓	Patient Type: Inpatient (IPW)
Admit / Discharge: ▓▓▓▓▓▓▓▓	Report Request ID: ▓▓▓▓▓▓
Print Date / Time: 1/26/2016 10:10 CST	OPI: ▓▓▓▓

Page 8 of 1,019

Patient Name: ▓▓▓▓▓▓▓▓▓▓ MRN: ▓▓▓▓▓▓ Admission#: ▓▓▓▓▓▓

Discharge Summary

DATE OF ADMISSION: ▓▓▓▓▓▓ WORK TYPE #: 08
DATE OF DISCHARGE: ▓▓▓▓▓▓
PHYSICIAN: ▓▓▓▓▓▓▓▓▓▓ PHYS #: ▓▓▓▓▓▓

DISCHARGE SUMMARY

DISCHARGE DIAGNOSES:
1. Chronic hypoxemic respiratory failure from chronic obstructive pulmonary disease.
2. Hypoglycemia.

CONSULTATIONS:
1. Pulmonary/Critical Care.
2. Palliative care.
3. Hospice.

HOSPITAL COURSE:
This patient is a 74-year-old woman that presents with weakness She had recently been hospitalized here with low glucose and weakness. Please see ▓▓▓▓▓▓▓▓'s dictated history and physical for full details. The patient was admitted for hypoglycemia and chest pain, and COPD. Dr. ▓▓▓▓▓ took over her care the following day. She was evaluated for hypoglycemia. During her course, she had worsening exacerbation of her COPD. She started requiring BiPAP. Eventually, it was discovered that an outside pharmacy had given her glipizide instead of Levaquin and that was most likely responsible for her profound hypoglycemia. Eventually, the hypoglycemia resolved and her main problem continued to be respiratory failure. She did not show any improvement in her respiratory failure and eventually hospice was consulted. She was transferred to the hospice service under the care of Dr Bradley.

DISCHARGE MEDICATIONS
Per Hospice Service.

▓▓▓▓▓▓▓▓▓▓▓▓

DD: ▓▓▓▓ 49:21
DT: ▓▓▓▓ 58:14
Original Job #: ▓▓▓▓▓▓
Job #: ▓▓▓▓▓▓

cc: ▓▓▓▓▓▓▓▓
▓▓▓▓▓▓▓▓

Patient Name ▓▓▓▓▓▓▓ Patient Type: Inpatient (IPW)
Admit / Discharge: ▓▓▓▓▓▓▓ Report Request ID: ▓▓▓▓▓▓
Print Date / Time 1/26/2016 10:10 CST Page 16 of 1,019 OPI: ▓▓▓▓▓▓

Appendix I: Sample pharmacy records

INTEGRIS Clinics
Practice Management

Name: ▮▮▮▮   D.O.B. ▮▮▮▮

Allergies: PCN Sulfa ELS	Cresta eyes only PCN							
Date:	1/20/11	10/5/11	1/5/12	4/4/12	11/13/12	2/26/13	3/7/13	4/24/13
Vitals								
Weight	173	178 61"	182	179.4	177	183.3	182.7	188.3
Height								
Temperature			97.1			98.2	97.6	97.6
Pulse	94	83	78	95	83	80	75	85
Respirations	18	18	20	20	18	20	20	20
Blood Pressure	134/66	124/70	123/100	116/63	131/75	132/75	134/74	133/58
Pain scale	7	5-6	4	6-7	7	4	5	4 4A
Medication/Dose/Frequency								
Cymbalta 60m 1/day	✓	✓	✓	✓	✓	✓	✓	✓
Flonase 2/1 sprays each nostril day	✓	✓	✓	✓	✓	✓	✓	✓
Lyrica 100m 1/BID	✓	✓	✓	✓	✓	✓	✓	✓
Singulair 10, 1/day	✓	✓	✓	✓	✓	✓	✓	✓
Symbicort 160/4.5 prn	✓	✓	✓		✓	✓	✓	✓
Xanax 0.5m 1 q 6° prn DC	✓		✓		✓	✓		
Albuterol MDI prn	✓	✓	✓	✓	✓	✓	✓	✓
Pepcid OTC prn	✓	✓	✓	✓	✓	PRN	✓	✓
Klonopin 0.5m 1, q 8° prn	✓	✓	✓	✓	✓	✓	✓	✓
Tramadol 50m 2/1 BID					✓	✓	✓	1-2 q 8 prn

227

Your Prescription Record | Pharmacy | Walgreens

Prescription Records

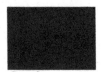

Female

Confidential Patient Information

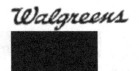

Walgreens

Fill Date ⇵	Prescription ⇵	NDC #	Qty	Pharmacist	Prescriber ⇵	Insur/Claim Ref# ⇵	Price ⇵
	MONTELUKAST 10MG TABLETS RX #: 0639835-07869	00378520103	30	ADP		AETNA/ 131548345128807999	$20.00
	CYMBALTA 60MG CAPSULES (NEW) RX #: 0667455-07869	00002327030	30	MMR		AETNA/ 131548345561805999	$35.00
	FLUTICASONE 50MCG NASAL SP (120INH) RX #: 0674079-07869	50383070018	16	ADP		AETNA/ 131553708508803000	$20.00
	MONTELUKAST 10MG TABLETS RX #: 0639835-07869	00378520103	30	ADP		AETNA/ 131792475560829999	$20.00
	CYMBALTA 60MG CAPSULES (NEW) RX #: 0667455-07869	00002327030	30	ADP		AETNA/ 131792475138805999	$35.00
	LYRICA 100MG CAPSULES RX #: 0971304-07869	00071101568	60	ADP		AETNA/ 131792475331815999	$35.00
	FLUTICASONE 50MCG NASAL SP (120INH) RX #: 0674079-07869	50383070018	16	ADP		AETNA/ 131792475536819999	$20.00

Appendix J: Alcohol charts for males and females

APPENDIX I
ALCOHOL CHART FOR MALES

Prepared by the Wisconsin Department of Transportation

Body Weight	Number of Drinks											
	1	2	3	4	5	6	7	8	9	10	11	12
100 lb.	.038	.075	.113	.150	.188	.225	.263	.300	.338	.375	.413	.450
110 lb.	.034	.066	.103	.137	.172	.207	.241	.275	.309	.344	.379	.412
120 lb.	.031	.063	.094	.125	.156	.188	.219	.250	.281	.313	.344	.375
130 lb.	.029	.058	.087	.116	.145	.174	.203	.232	.261	.290	.320	.348
140 lb.	.027	.054	.080	.107	.134	.161	.188	.214	.241	.268	.295	.321
150 lb.	.025	.050	.075	.100	.125	.151	.176	.201	.226	.251	.276	.301
160 lb.	.023	.047	.070	.094	.117	.141	.164	.188	.211	.234	.258	.281
170 lb.	.022	.045	.066	.088	.110	.132	.155	.178	.200	.221	.244	.265
180 lb.	.021	.042	.063	.083	.104	.125	.146	.167	.188	.208	.229	.250
190 lb.	.020	.040	.059	.079	.099	.119	.138	.158	.179	.198	.217	.237
200 lb.	.019	.038	.056	.075	.094	.113	.131	.150	.169	.188	.206	.225
210 lb.	.018	.036	.053	.071	.090	.107	.125	.143	.161	.179	.197	.215
220 lb.	.017	.034	.051	.068	.085	.102	.119	.136	.153	.170	.188	.206
230 lb.	.016	.032	.049	.065	.081	.098	.115	.130	.147	.163	.180	.196
240 lb.	.016	.031	.047	.063	.078	.094	.109	.125	.141	.156	.172	.188

APPENDIX 2
ALCOHOL CHART FOR FEMALES

Prepared by the Wisconsin Department of Transportation

Body Weight	Number of Drinks											
	1	2	3	4	5	6	7	8	9	10	11	12
90 lb.	.053	.106	.159	.212	.265	.318	.371	.424	.477	.530	.583	.636
100 lb.	.047	.094	.141	.188	.235	.282	.329	.376	.423	.470	.517	.564
110 lb.	.042	.084	.126	.168	.210	.252	.294	.336	.378	.420	.482	.504
120 lb.	.038	.076	.114	.152	.190	.228	.266	.304	.342	.380	.418	.456
130 lb.	.036	.072	.108	.144	.180	.216	.252	.228	.324	.360	.396	.432
140 lb.	.033	.066	.099	.132	.165	.198	.231	.264	.297	.330	.363	.396
150 lb.	.031	.062	.093	.124	.155	.186	.217	.248	.279	.310	.341	.372
160 lb.	.028	.056	.084	.112	.140	.168	.196	.224	.252	.280	.308	.336
170 lb.	.027	.054	.081	.108	.135	.162	.189	.216	.243	.270	.297	.324
180 lb.	.026	.052	.078	.104	.130	.156	.182	.208	.234	.260	.286	.312
190 lb.	.025	.050	.075	.100	.125	.150	.175	.200	.225	.250	.275	.300
200 lb.	.023	.046	.069	.092	.115	.138	.161	.184	.207	.230	.253	.276
210 lb.	.022	.044	.066	.088	.110	.132	.154	.176	.198	.220	.242	.264

Appendix K: Excerpt of *Daubert* motion against the drug expert

IN THE DISTRICT COURT OF ████████
STATE OF OKLAHOMA

████████ and ████████   )
)
                   Plaintiffs,)
)
)   Case No: CJ-████████
vs.   )
)   )
████████████   )
)
An Oklahoma limited liability company,)
)
                   Defendant.   )

PLAINTIFF'S DAUBERT MOTION TO EXCLUDE DEFENDANT'S EXPERT WITNESS TESTIMONY BY CRAIG STEVENS, Ph.D.

COMES NOW, Plaintiff, ████████ by and through her attorney of record, ████████, and hereby presents Plaintiff's Daubert Motion to Exclude Defendant's Expert Witness Testimony by Craig Stevens, Ph.D. at trial under Okla. Stat. Tit. 12 § 2702.

Defendant plans to present evidence through its witness, Craig Stevens, Ph.D., that it is his "expert opinion that the plaintiff, ████████████████████████ ████████████████████████████ ████████ *See Exhibit 1, p.15* – report of Craig Stevens, Ph.D.

Said opinions of Dr. Stevens do not fall under the standards of *Daubert*, as codified by the State of Oklahoma in 12 O.S. § 2702, and therefore must be excluded. Furthermore, the prejudicial nature of a prescription drug interaction in the minds of the jury is the basis for Defendant desiring to present such evidence. However, it is clear that the probative value of such evidence under our evidentiary rules must outweigh the undoubted prejudicial effect and thus must be excluded.

I.

DR. STEVENS' REPORT AND OPINONS DO NOT MEET THE STANDARDS OF ADMISSIBILIYY UNDER DAUBERT AND 12 O.S. §2702 AND MUST BE EXCLUDED

Defendant, as the party seeking to present expert opinion testimony, has the burden of establishing admissibility by a preponderance of the evidence. *See Bourjaily v. United States,* 483 U.S. 171, 175(1987). This Court is well aware of its gate keeping function when expert testimony pursuant to Oklahoma Statute Title 12 §§ 2702 and 2703 is offered. *See Christian v. Gray,* 2003 OK 10, 65 P.3d 591 and *Twyman v. The GHK Corp.,* 2004 OK CIV APP 53, 93 P.3d 51 (adopting the procedures set forth in *Daubert v. Merrell Dowell Pharmaceuticals, Inc.,* 509 U.S. 579 (1993) replacing the prior *Frye* test). In *Daubert,* the Supreme Court established guidelines for district courts to use in determining the admissibility of expert testimony pursuant to Rules 702 and 104 of the Federal Rules of Evidence. In *Daubert,* the Court emphasized the trial judge's "gatekeeping" role with respect to expert proof on scientific issues. *Daubert* at 597-598. Although there is no single criterion for determining whether a specific scientific methodology is reliable, the *Daubert* Court identified the following four factors that a district court should consider when evaluating the scientific validity of expert testimony: (1) the testability of the expert's hypotheses; (2) whether the expert's methodology has been subjected to peer review; (3) the rate of error associated with the methodology; and (4) whether the methodology is generally accepted within the scientific community. *Daubert* at 593-594.

The State of Oklahoma has adopted the standard of admissibility with regard to expert testimony as set forth in the *Daubert* case in *Christian.* The Oklahoma Supreme Court has held that a Court must consider whether the expert is proposing to testify as to (1) scientific knowledge that (2) will assist the trier of fact to understand or determine a fact in issue. *Christian* at 598, citing *Daubert* at 592-593.

Appendix L: Drug tests available at commercial laboratories

Test Summary Sheet for:

NMS LABS

Test Code 1874B

Test Name Drug Screen (10 Panel), Blood

Purpose
Drug of Abuse Monitoring; Forensic Analysis; Screening for a Class of Drugs and Quantitation of Positive Findings

Method(s)
Enzyme-Linked Immunosorbent Assay (ELISA)

Suggested CPT Code(s)
80307

New York State Approval Status
Approved

Turnaround Time
4 days (If Positive: 8 days)

Test Includes

Analyte(s)	Synonym(s)
Amphetamines	
Barbiturates	
Benzodiazepines	
Cannabinoids	
Cocaine / Metabolites	
Methadone / Metabolite	
Methamphetamine / MDMA	

https://www.nmslabs.com/tests/1874B

Analyte(s)	Synonym(s)
Opiates	
Oxycodone / Oxymorphone	
Phencyclidine	Angel Dust; PCP; Sherm

Test Also Known As

Adderall; Amfetamine; Cannabis; Coke; Crack; Desoxyn®; Dextroamphetamine; Ecstasy; Heroin; Levoamphetamine; Marijuana; Meth; Molly; THC; Tranquilizer

Reflex Tests

Test Code	Test Name
50010B	Amphetamines Confirmation, Blood
50011B	Barbiturates Confirmation, Blood
50012B	Benzodiazepines Confirmation, Blood
50013B	Cannabinoids Confirmation, Blood
50014B	Cocaine and Metabolites Confirmation, Blood
50015B	Methadone and Metabolite Confirmation, Blood
50016B	Opiates - Free (Unconjugated) Confirmation, Blood
50017B	Phencyclidine Confirmation, Blood

The CPT Codes provided in this document are based on AMA Guidelines and are for informational purposes only. NMS Labs Does not assume responsibility for billing errors due to Reliance on the CPT Codes listed in this document.

Appendix M: Retrograde calculation of blood alcohol concentration (BAC)

The formula for calculating back in time to the time of the motor vehicle accident from a known blood sample obtained later is as follows:

$$BAC_{\text{at time of accident}} = BAC_{\text{of blood sample}} + (T_{\text{time elapsed (h)}} \times E_{\text{elimination rate per hour, \% BAC}})$$

In the Chapter 17 case, the patron's BAC from the blood draw was 0.072% and the time elapsed from obtaining the blood sample and the MVA was 1.5 hours, which are plugged into the equation. The following table shows the formula, calculations made, and the BAC that results from using the low range estimate of 0.010 for the elimination rate of alcohol per hour (left side of the following table) or 0.025 for the high range of elimination rate (right side of the following table).

Low elimination rate range (0.010/h)	High elimination rate range (0.025/h)
$BAC_{\text{at time of accident}} = 0.072 + (1.5 \times 0.010)$	$BAC_{\text{at time of accident}} = 0.072 + (1.5\ h \times 0.025)$
$BAC_{\text{at time of accident}} = 0.072 + 0.015$	$BAC_{\text{at time of accident}} = 0.072 + 0.0375$
$BAC_{\text{at time of accident}} = 0.087 = 0.08\ \%\ BAC$	$BAC_{\text{at time of accident}} = 0.1095 = 0.10\ \%\ BAC$

Index

Note: Page numbers followed by *f* indicate figures, *t* indicate tables, *b* indicate boxes, and *np* indicate footnotes.

Printed in the United States
By Bookmasters